Postoperative Joint MR Imaging

Editor

LUIS S. BELTRAN

MAGNETIC RESONANCE IMAGING CLINICS OF NORTH AMERICA

www.mri.theclinics.com

Consulting Editors
SURESH K. MUKHERJI
LYNNE S. STEINBACH

November 2022 • Volume 30 • Number 4

ELSEVIER

1600 John F. Kennedy Boulevard ● Suite 1800 ● Philadelphia, Pennsylvania, 19103-2899

http://www.mri.theclinics.com

MAGNETIC RESONANCE IMAGING CLINICS OF NORTH AMERICA Volume 30, Number 4
November 2022 ISSN 1064-9689, ISBN 13: 978-0-323-81387-7

Editor: John Vassallo (j.vassallo@elsevier.com)
Developmental Editor: Arlene Campos

Magnetic Resonance Imaging Clinics of North America (ISSN 1064-9689) is published quarterly by Elsevier Inc., 360 Park Avenue South, New York, NY 10010-1710. Months of issue are February, May, August, and November. Business and Editorial Offices: 1600 John F. Kennedy Blvd., Ste. 1800, Philadelphia, PA 19103-2899. Customer Service Office: 3251 Riverport Lane, Maryland Heights, MO 63043. Periodicals postage paid at New York, NY and additional mailing offices. Subscription prices are $408.00 per year (domestic individuals), $1053.00 per year (domestic institutions), $100.00 per year (domestic students/residents), $455.00 per year (Canadian individuals), $1069.00 per year (Canadian institutions), $573.00 per year (international individuals), $1069.00 per year (international institutions), $100.00 per year (Canadian students/residents), and $275.00 per year (international students/residents). International air speed delivery is included in all *Clinics* subscription prices. All prices are subject to change without notice. **POSTMASTER:** Send address changes to *Magnetic Resonance Imaging Clinics*, Elsevier Health Sciences Division, Subscription Customer Service, 3251 Riverport Lane, Maryland Heights, MO 63043. Customer Service (orders, claims, online, change of address): Elsevier Health Sciences Division, Subscription **Customer Service, 3251 Riverport Lane, Maryland Heights, MO 63043. Tel:1-800-654-2452 (U.S. and Canada); 314-447-8871 (outside U.S. and Canada). Fax: 314-447-8029. E-mail: journalscustomerservice-usa@elsevier.com (for print support); journalsonlinesupport-usa@elsevier.com (for online support).**

Reprints. For copies of 100 or more of articles in this publication, please contact the Commercial Reprints Department, Elsevier Inc., 360 Park Avenue South, New York, NY 10010-1710. Tel.: 212-633-3874; Fax: 212-633-3820; E-mail: reprints@elsevier.com.

Magnetic Resonance Imaging Clinics of North America is covered in the *RSNA Index of Imaging Literature, MEDLINE/PubMed (Index Medicus),* and *EMBASE/Excerpta Medica.*

Contributors

CONSULTING EDITORS

SURESH K. MUKHERJI, MD, MBA, FACR
Clinical Professor of Radiology and Radiation
Oncology, University of Illinois, Peoria, Illinois;
Robert Wood Johnson Medical School,
Rutgers University, New Brunswick, New
Jersey; Faculty, Otolaryngology–Head Neck
Surgery, Michigan State University,
Farmington Hills, Michigan; National Director of
Head and Neck Radiology, ProScan Imaging,
Carmel, Indiana, USA

LYNNE S. STEINBACH, MD, FACR
Emeritus Professor of Radiology on Full Recall,
Department of Radiology and Biomedical
Imaging, University of California, San
Francisco, San Francisco, California, USA

EDITOR

LUIS S. BELTRAN, MD
Director of Musculoskeletal Ultrasound,
Division of Musculoskeletal Imaging and
Intervention, Department of Radiology,
Assistant Professor, Harvard Medical School,
Brigham and Women's Hospital, Boston,
Massachusetts, USA

AUTHORS

LUIS AGUILELLA, PhD
Department of Orthopedics, Hospital de la
Ribera, Valencia, Spain

MOHAMMAD A. ALFAQIH, MD, DABR
Assistant Professor of Radiology, King Saudi
University, College of Medicine, King Saud
Univeristy Medical City, Riyadh, Saudi Arabia

TOLUWALASE ASHIMOLOWO, MD
Summit Radiology, Atlanta, Georgia, USA

ROCIO AUBAN, MD
Department of Radiology, Hospital de
Manises, Valencia, Spain

JONATHAN C. BAKER, MD
Associate Professor of Radiology,
Musculoskeletal Section, Mallinckrodt
Institute of Radiology, St Louis, Missouri,
USA

LUIS S. BELTRAN, MD
Director of Musculoskeletal Ultrasound,
Division of Musculoskeletal Imaging and
Intervention, Department of Radiology,
Assistant Professor, Harvard Medical School,
Brigham and Women's Hospital, Boston,
Massachusetts, USA

JENNY T. BENCARDINO, MD
Division of Musculoskeletal Radiology,
Department of Radiology, Penn Medicine,
University of Pennsylvania, Philadelphia,
Pennsylvania, USA

CHRISTOPHER J. BURKE, MBChB
Department of Radiology, NYU Langone
Medical Center, NYU Langone Orthopedic
Hospital, New York, New York,
USA

LUIS CEREZAL, MD, PhD
Department of Radiology, Diagnóstico Médico Cantabria, Santander, Spain

SAEED DIANAT, MD
Division of Musculoskeletal Radiology, Department of Radiology, Penn Medicine, University of Pennsylvania, Philadelphia, Pennsylvania, USA

JAN FRITZ, MD, PD, RMSK
Department of Radiology, Division of Musculoskeletal Radiology, NYU Grossman School of Medicine, NYU Langone Medical Center, NYU Langone Orthopedic Hospital, New York, New York, USA

SOTERIOS GYFTOPOULOS, MD, MBA, MSc
Department of Radiology, NYU Langone Medical Center, Department of Orthopedic Surgery, NYU Langone Orthopedic Hospital, New York, New York, USA

JAIME ISERN-KEBSCHULL, MD, PhD
Musculoskeletal Unit Specialist, Department of Radiology, Hospital Clinic, University of Barcelona, Barcelona, Spain

RITI M. KANESA-THASAN, MD
Assistant Professor of Clinical Radiology, Department of Radiology, Division of Musculoskeletal Imaging, University of Pennsylvania, Philadelphia, Pennsylvania, USA

ARA KASSARJIAN, MD, FRCPC
Founder and Consultant Radiologist, Elite Sports Imaging, SL, Tournament Staff Physician, Madrid Open Tennis, Madrid, Spain

IMAN KHODARAHMI, MD, PhD
Department of Radiology, NYU Langone Medical Center, NYU Langone Orthopedic Hospital, New York, New York, USA

JAMES LINKLATER, OAM, MBBS (Hons), B Med Sc (Hons), FRANZCR
Radiologist and Chief Executive Officer, Castlereagh Imaging & Illawarra Radiology Group, Sydney, New South Wales, Australia

EVA LLOPIS, MD
Department of Radiology, Hospital de la Ribera, IMSKE, Valencia, Spain

LAWRENCE LO, MD
Assistant Professor of Clinical Radiology, Hospital of the University of Pennsylvania, Penn Medicine University City, Philadelphia, Pennsylvania, USA

MARIAM A. MALIK, MD
Instructor of Radiology, Musculoskeletal Section, Mallinckrodt Institute of Radiology, St Louis, Missouri, USA

WILLIAM C. MEYERS, MD, MBA
President and Chairman, Vincera Institute, Professor of Surgery, Sidney Kimmel Medical College at Jefferson, Philadelphia, Pennsylvania, USA

WILLIAM B. MORRISON, MD, FACR
Professor of Radiology, Thomas Jefferson University Hospital, Philadelphia, Pennsylvania, USA

FRANCISCO DEL PIÑAL, PhD
Instituto de cirugía plástica y de la mano, Hospital de la Lux, Madrid y Hospital Mutua Montañesa, Santander, Spain

JOHANNES B. ROEDL, MD, PhD
Associate Professor of Clinical Radiology, Department of Radiology, Thomas Jefferson University Hospital, Philadelphia, Pennsylvania, USA

MOHAMMAD SAMIM, MD, MRCS
Department of Radiology, NYU Langone Orthopedic Hospital, New York, New York, USA

XAVIER TOMAS, MD, PhD
Head of Musculoskeletal Unit, Department of Radiology, Hospital Clinic, University of Barcelona, Barcelona, Spain

HILARY UMANS, MD
Lenox Hill Radiology & Imaging Associates, New York, New York, USA; Department of Radiology, Albert Einstein College of Medicine, Bronx, New York, USA

ADAM C. ZOGA, MD, MBA
Professor of Diagnostic Radiology, Vice Chair of Clinical Practice, Director of Musculoskeletal MRI, Department of Radiology, Thomas Jefferson University Hospital, Philadelphia, Pennsylvania, USA

Contents

Postoperative MR imaging of joints is now commonly requested, yet artifacts caused by metallic orthopedic implants remain a significant challenge during image interpretation. Effective artifact reduction is essential to identify postsurgical complications, such as prosthesis loosening, infection, adverse local tissue reaction, and periarticular soft tissue injuries. This article reviews basic and advanced metal artifact reduction MR imaging techniques applied to various clinical protocols for successful postoperative MR imaging of small and large joints.

Following anterior shoulder instability surgery, patients may present with new or recurrent symptoms. Postoperative imaging, including MR imaging, may be obtained for these patients to assess the integrity of the repaired tissues and orthopedic fixation hardware or grafts. Familiarity with different operative techniques and their expected normal appearances and complications helps in the appropriate interpretation of these imaging studies. This article provides an overview of the current treatment guidelines and surgery options for patients with anterior shoulder instability and reviews the normal and abnormal postoperative imaging appearances of the shoulder joint after treatment with the most common surgical stabilization techniques.

MR imaging is crucial in the evaluation of symptomatic patients who have undergone rotator cuff surgery. Familiarity with anatomic rotator cuff repair and the other surgical options for irreparable cuff tears, expected normal postoperative findings, and potential complications is essential for better MR imaging interpretation.

Elbow injuries are a growing problem particularly among overhead athletes, because more children and adolescents are participating in sporting activities. The goal of surgical management of elbow injuries is to restore the capsuloligamentous and osseous contributions to stability. However, postoperative MR imaging evaluation is difficult because of the variety of surgical techniques available, and the lack of postoperative MR imaging for suspected complications because many are diagnosed clinically and a revision may be performed without imaging. This article reviews some of the commonly performed surgical techniques for select elbow injuries, with their postoperative MR imaging findings and complications.

In this article we will do an overview of the general and specific complications that occur after the most common wrist and hand surgeries. Knowledge of the different surgical techniques is essential for postoperative imaging evaluation. General complications include infection, complex regional pain syndrome, problems related with the surgical approach (open or arthroscopic) and bone healing problems. The most frequent fractures of the wrist with specific complications are distal radius fractures and scaphoid fractures as associated with tendon ruptures secondary to friction, nonunion or secondary malignment. We will briefly review the different approaches for triangular fibrocartilage injuries, including acute and degenerative lesions. Scapholunate instability is the most common instability and an important indication for surgery with pin fixation in the acute setting and arthroplasty or arthrodesis in the chronic irreparable injuries. One of the most common surgeries of the wrist is carpal tunnel release, although complications are uncommon, radiologists should be familiar with the normal appearance and pathological changes after surgery. Trapeziometacarpal joint osteoarthritis is frequent especially in postmenopausal women and has several treatment options depending on the stage.

Postoperative imaging of the hip used to be dominated by radiographs, computed tomography, and occasionally nuclear medicine studies, given that most surgeries were arthroplasties or, less commonly, core decompressions. The indications and procedures performed have expanded well beyond arthroplasties and now include labral procedures (resections, repairs, and reconstructions), osteochondroplasties, acetabuloplasties, and removal of loose bodies, among others. As a result, postoperative evaluation of the hip now often includes MR imaging and MR arthrography. This article discusses normal postoperative appearances and some of the more common complications associated with hip arthroscopy and hip arthroplasty with a focus on MR imaging.

MR imaging evaluation can be valuable in patients with prior surgery for athletic pubalgia presenting with new, recurrent, or persistent groin pain. The clinical and interventional history as well as comparison with preoperative imaging is essential for imaging interpretation. Imagers should be aware of expected and unexpected postoperative findings. MR imaging findings concerning for infection, new injury, contralateral injury, or concomitant sources of symptoms (such as hip pathology) should be reported when present.

In this article, we describe the postoperative appearances of the reconstructed ligaments of the knee focusing on the anterior cruciate ligament (ACL). The expected evolving signal alterations of the graft over time are also reviewed. The postoperative appearance of the ligamentous reconstruction in patients with multiligamentous knee injuries (MLKI) and isolated PCL tears are also discussed.

Surgery to treat a torn meniscus is a common orthopedic procedure, and radiologists are frequently asked to image patients with new or recurrent knee pain after meniscus surgery. However, surgery alters the MR imaging appearance of the meniscus, making the diagnosis of recurrent tear a diagnostic challenge. This article reviews relevant anatomy of the meniscus, surgical techniques used to treat meniscus tear, the roles of conventional MR imaging and MR arthrography to assess the postoperative meniscus, and the key MR imaging findings to distinguish the intact postoperative meniscus from recurrent tear.

Many surgical procedures and operations are used to treat ankle and foot disorders. Radiography is the first-line imaging for postoperative surveillance and evaluation of pain and dysfunction. Computed tomography scans and MR imaging are used for further evaluation. MR imaging is the most accurate test for soft tissues assessments. MR imaging protocol adjustments include basic and advanced metal artifact reduction. We chose a surgical approach to select the common types of procedures and discuss the normal and abnormal postoperative MR imaging appearances, highlighting potential complications. This article reviews commonly used surgical techniques and their normal and abnormal MR imaging appearances.

MAGNETIC RESONANCE IMAGING CLINICS OF NORTH AMERICA

SERIES OF RELATED INTEREST

Advances in Clinical Radiology
Neurologic Clinics
PET Clinics
Radiologic Clinics

VISIT THE CLINICS ONLINE!
Access your subscription at:
www.theclinics.com

PROGRAM OBJECTIVE
The goal of Magnetic *Resonance Imaging Clinics of North America* is to keep practicing physicians up to date with current clinical practice by providing timely articles reviewing the state of the art in patient care.

TARGET AUDIENCE
All practicing physicians and healthcare professionals who provide patient care utilizing findings from Magnetic Resonance Imaging.

LEARNING OBJECTIVES
Upon completion of this activity, participants will be able to:
1. Review various surgical techniques, both traditional and novel, for accurately diagnosing and evaluating postoperative musculoskeletal repair findings.
2. Discuss common challenges in diagnosing and interpreting postoperative imaging studies of musculoskeletal repair.
3. Recognize MRI imaging as the preferred diagnostic, evaluation, and interpretation tool for postoperative musculoskeletal repair findings.

ACCREDITATION
The Elsevier Office of Continuing Medical Education (EOCME) is accredited by the Accreditation Council for Continuing Medical Education (ACCME) to provide continuing medical education for physicians.

The EOCME designates this journal-based CME activity enduring material for a maximum of 10 *AMA PRA Category 1 Credit*(s)™. Physicians should claim only the credit commensurate with the extent of their participation in the activity.

All other healthcare professionals requesting continuing education credit for this enduring material will be issued a certificate of participation.

DISCLOSURE OF CONFLICTS OF INTEREST
The EOCME assesses conflict of interest with its instructors, faculty, planners, and other individuals who are in a position to control the content of CME activities. All relevant conflicts of interest that are identified are thoroughly vetted by EOCME for fair balance, scientific objectivity, and patient care recommendations. EOCME is committed to providing its learners with CME activities that promote improvements or quality in healthcare and not a specific proprietary business or a commercial interest.

The planning committee, staff, authors and editors listed below have identified no financial relationships or relationships to products or devices they or their spouse/life partner have with commercial interest related to the content of this CME activity:
Luis Aguilella; Mohammad A. Alfaqih, MD, DABR®; Toluwalase Ashimolowo, MD; Rocio Auban; Jonathan C. Baker, MD; Luis Beltran, MD; Jenny T. Bencardino, MD; Christopher J. Burke, MBChB; Luis Cerezal, MD, PhD; Francisco del Piñal; Saeed Dianat, MD; Soterios Gyftopoulos, MD, MBA, MSc; Jaime Isern-Kebschull, MD, PhD; Riti M. Kanesa-thasan, MD; Ara Kassarjian, MD, FRCPC; Iman Khodarahmi, MD, PhD; Pradeep Kuttysankaran; James Linklater, OAM, MBBS (Hons), B Med Sc (Hons), FRANZCR; Eva Llopis, MD; Lawrence Lo, MD; Mariam A. Malik, MD; William B. Morrison, MD, FACR; Johannes B. Roedl, MD, PhD; Mohammad Samim, MD, MRCS; Doreen Thomas-Payne, MSN, BSN, RN, PMHNP-BC; Xavier Tomas, MD, PhD; Hilary Umans, MD; Adam Zoga, MD, MBA

The planning committee, staff, authors and editors listed below have identified financial relationships or relationships to products or devices they or their spouse/life partner have with commercial interest related to the content of this CME activity:
Jan Fritz, MD: *Researcher*: Siemens AG, BTG International, Zimmer Biomed, DePuy Synthes, QED, SyntheticMR; *Advisor*: Siemens AG, SyntheticMR, GE Healthcare, QED, BTG, ImageBiopsy Lab, Boston Scientific, Mirata Pharma; *Patent Beneficiary*: Siemens Healthcare

UNAPPROVED/OFF-LABEL USE DISCLOSURE
The EOCME requires CME faculty to disclose to the participants:
1. When products or procedures being discussed are off-label, unlabelled, experimental, and/or investigational (not US Food and Drug Administration [FDA] approved); and
2. Any limitations on the information presented, such as data that are preliminary or that represent ongoing research, interim analyses, and/or unsupported opinions. Faculty may discuss information about pharmaceutical agents that is outside of FDA-approved labelling. This information is intended solely for CME and is not intended to promote off-label use of these medications. If you have any questions, contact the medical affairs department of the manufacturer for the most recent prescribing information.

TO ENROLL
To enroll in the *Magnetic Resonance Imaging Clinics of North America* Continuing Medical Education program, call customer service at 1-800-654-2452 or sign up online at http://www.theclinics.com/home/cme. The CME program is available to subscribers for an additional annual fee of USD 281.00.

METHOD OF PARTICIPATION

In order to claim credit, participants must complete the following:

1. Complete enrolment as indicated above.
2. Read the activity.
3. Complete the CME Test and Evaluation. Participants must achieve a score of 70% on the test. All CME Tests and Evaluations must be completed online.

CME INQUIRIES/SPECIAL NEEDS

For all CME inquiries or special needs, please contact elsevierCME@elsevier.com.

Foreword
Postoperative Joint MR Imaging

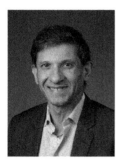 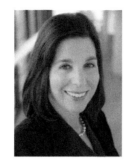

Suresh K. Mukherji, MD, MBA, FACR   Lynne S. Steinbach, MD, FACR
Consulting Editors

Radiologists are increasingly asked to evaluate joints for complications following surgery. This can be daunting for many reasons. There are many different types of surgery that we need to understand. Has a tendon been removed or redirected? What is normal baseline appearance following surgery, and can it mimic preoperative criteria for abnormality? Does the expected appearance change over time? What are the technical aspects that we should employ to best see the joint and surrounding structures against a background of metallic and micrometallic artifact as well as scar tissue?

Thanks to Luis Beltran, editor of this issue of *Magnetic Resonance Imaging Clinics of North America*, these challenges have been outlined, elucidated, and discussed with diagrams and examples in different articles written by a select group of esteemed musculoskeletal MR imagers with world-class expertise in their subject. These authors guide the reader through crucial aspects of postoperative joint MR imaging.

What sequences and parameters are best to use for MR postoperative imaging? This is discussed in the first article on technical considerations. Items such as evaluation of bone loss in glenohumeral instability, the variable appearance of the rotator cuff tendon over the first year following surgery, new rotator cuff repair techniques, elbow ligament reconstruction and ulnar nerve translocation, and total wrist arthrodesis are examples of what is discussed in articles on the postoperative upper-extremity joints. The last half of the issue reviews postoperative imaging of the lower-extremity joints. Subjects include evaluation of adverse local tissue reactions to total hip arthroplasty, the normal appearance of postoperative surgery for athletic pubalgia that can sometimes be confused for pathology based on preoperative criteria, cruciate ligament surgical complications, evaluation for recurrent meniscal tear, and tricky nonanatomic reconstruction of ankle ligaments.

We hope that you will find this reference a comprehensive and up-to-date synopsis on postoperative joint MR imaging and will refer to it when you get those challenging cases. Thanks to those who participated in this project for your hard work and great accomplishment.

Suresh K. Mukherji, MD, MBA, FACR
University of Illinois & ProScan Imaging
Carmel, IN 46074, USA

Lynne S. Steinbach, MD, FACR
Department of Radiology and Biomedical Imaging
University of California
San Francisco 505 Parnassus
San Francisco, CA 9413-0628, USA

E-mail addresses:
sureshmukherji@hotmail.com (S.K. Mukherji)
lynne.steinbach@ucsf.edu (L.S. Steinbach)

1064-9689/22/© 2022 Published by Elsevier Inc.

Preface
Postoperative Joint MR Imaging

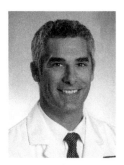

Luis S. Beltran, MD
Editor

It has been my pleasure to serve as guest editor for the current issue of *Magnetic Resonance Imaging Clinics of North America* entitled, "Postoperative Joint MR Imaging." Postoperative MR imaging of the joints can be a very challenging endeavor due to artifacts and the altered anatomy that can occur from the various operative procedures that are performed throughout the numerous joints in the body. It is essential to be able to know why these artifacts occur and how they can be minimized using conventional and advanced artifact reduction techniques. The image interpreter should also understand the anatomic changes that occur in joints following surgery. Having a thorough knowledge of the technical considerations, the anatomy, and normal and abnormal imaging appearances throughout the main joints in the body is critical in the management of patients with postoperative joint pain symptoms. In this issue, we present a collection of 10 unique review articles, starting with a comprehensive up-to-date primer on the technical considerations of postoperative MR imaging of joints, followed by a shoulder-to-toe approach toward discussing

postoperative MR imaging in the most frequently operated and imaged joints of the body. The authors of these articles are well-respected, national, and international leaders in the field of Musculoskeletal Radiology. I am very grateful and proud of the work that the authors have presented in this issue, and I would like to take this opportunity to thank them for their tremendous effort to make this issue a success. I hope that the readers will find the inciteful discussions and image-rich material provided in these articles to be informative and relevant to daily clinical practice.

Luis S. Beltran, MD
Division of Musculoskeletal Imaging
and Intervention
Department of Radiology
Harvard Medical School
Brigham and Women's Hospital
75 Francis Street
Boston, MA 02115, USA

E-mail address:
lbeltran@bwh.harvard.edu

Magn Reson Imaging Clin N Am 30 (2022) xiii
https://doi.org/10.1016/j.mric.2022.07.004
1064-9689/22/© 2022 Published by Elsevier Inc.

Postoperative MR Imaging of Joints
Technical Considerations

Christopher J. Burke, MBChB*, Iman Khodarahmi, MD, PhD,
Jan Fritz, MD, PD, RMSK

KEYWORDS

• MRI • Postoperative • Arthroplasty • Metal reduction • Implants • Artifacts • Prosthesis • SEMAC

KEY POINTS

- As more patients require MR imaging in the postoperative setting, particularly after orthopedic osteosynthesis and joint replacements, optimizing MRI protocols with effective metal artifact reduction is essential.
- Common metallic orthopedic implant-induced artifacts on MR imaging scans include signal dephasing, signal loss, signal pile-up, failed fat suppression, and geometric distortions.
- Basic methods to reduce metallic artifacts include using fast and turbo spin-echo sequences, high transmit and receiver bandwidths, and thin slice thickness.
- Bandwidth-adjusted short tau inversion recovery (STIR) provides robust fat suppression around metallic implants. Dixon-based fat suppression may suffice for orthopedic implants producing only small metal artifacts.
- Advanced methods to reduce metal artifacts include slice encoding for metal artifact correction (SEMAC) and multiacquisition with variable-resonance image combination (MAVRIC).

INTRODUCTION

Postoperative joint MR imaging in the presence of metallic orthopedic implants is safe and now commonplace. Demand is expected to steadily increase based on the high numbers of osteosyntheses, reconstructive surgeries, and joint arthroplasty procedures in the United States annually, the latter of which is expected to increase to nearly 4 million by 2030.[1] Common indications include the evaluation of implant integrity and periprosthetic tissues, such as bone, synovium, ligaments, and muscle-tendon units. Despite postoperative joint MR imaging being safe, metallic implant-induced artifacts continue to represent a challenge to the radiologist. Common artifacts include signal loss, signal pile-up, failed fat suppression, and geometric distortions. Advances in MR imaging hardware and sequence software now allow artifact mitigation with various techniques, resulting in substantially fewer artifacts, less obscuration of periprosthetic tissues, and overall unprecedented image quality.

MR imaging of metallic implants requires prospective pulse sequence modifications and optimizations to counteract implant-induced alteration of the magnetic fields mainly caused by magnetic susceptibility differences between the metallic components and surrounding human tissue and fluid. The effects of implant-induced alterations on MR images depend mainly on the strength of the external magnetic field, sequence type, and metallic alloys of the orthopedic implants, but also depend on size, shape, and spatial orientation.

Although formerly introduced to refer to a set of modifications applied to fast spin-echo pulse sequences,[2] nowadays, the term MARS MR imaging, defined as metal artifact reduction sequence MR imaging, is primarily used as an umbrella

Department of Radiology, NYU Langone Medical Center & Langone Orthopedic Hospital, 301 East 17th Street, 6th Floor, Radiology, New York, NY 10003, USA
* Corresponding author.
E-mail address: Christopher.Burke@nyulangone.org

Magn Reson Imaging Clin N Am 30 (2022) 583–600
https://doi.org/10.1016/j.mric.2022.03.002
1064-9689/22/© 2022 Elsevier Inc. All rights reserved.

term to refer to the group of basic and advanced concepts, modifications, techniques, and dedicated pulse sequences used to optimize metal artifact reduction and image quality around metallic implants.[3] As an alternative, the acronym MAR, defined as metal artifact reduction, may be used, which comes with the additional advantage of being universally applicable to describe MR imaging and computed tomography (CT) metal artifact reduction techniques. Nowadays, all major vendors offer a variety of MAR/MARS techniques.

This article addresses strategies for modifying pulse sequences and creating protocols for optimal MR imaging of postoperative joints and arthroplasty implants.

GENERAL CONSIDERATIONS

Metallic implants introduce magnetic field inhomogeneities due to the susceptibility differences between tissues and metal, with the resultant spin precession frequency offsets causing a variety of artifacts.[4] Metallic implant-induced inhomogeneities in the B_0 magnetic field affect the in-plane frequency encoding direction and through-plane slice-selection direction when using 2-dimensional (2D) pulse sequences.

On MR images, metal-induced artifacts include signal voids resulting from intravoxel T2* dephasing, and erroneous shift of signal intensities along the in-plane readout direction and through-plane slice direction, leading to a 3-dimensional (3D) composite of areas with artifactual signal loss and signal hyperintense areas caused by signal pile-up.

Standard methods to reduce metallic artifacts include fast/turbo spin-echo pulse sequences with high transmit and receiver bandwidths (BWs), thin slice thickness, and short tau inversion recovery (STIR) fat suppression. Optionally, the image matrix size may be increased to optimize spatial resolution; however, this will not influence signal displacement and artifact size. Optimizing these parameters comes at the cost of reduced signal-to-noise ratio (SNR), which in turn may require increasing the number of acquisitions and often longer acquisition times.

For postoperative MR imaging with metallic orthopedic implants, using longer than usual echo train length has been recommended as a means to reduce the size of implant-induced metallic artifacts. However, dedicated quantitative and qualitative evaluations showed that high receiver BW and minimized inter-echo spacing are the effective parameters for metal artifact reduction, whereas long echo trains fail to reduce implant-related metal artifacts but cause degradation of image quality around the implant with resultant larger-appearing total metal artifacts.[5]

Other techniques, such as view-angle tilting (VAT), and advanced multispectral and multispatial advanced metal artifact reduction, including multiacquisition variable-resonance image combination (MAVRIC) and slice encoding for metal artifact correction (SEMAC), are clinically available products offered by multiple vendors. Many of those techniques can be used in combination.

MAVRIC and SEMAC are advanced metal artifact reduction techniques embedded into specialized test introvert spin-echo pulse sequences, which are specifically aimed to address metal artifacts by applying multiple excitations during pulse sequence acquisition, resulting in MR imaging scans with minimized overall implant-induced metallic artifacts.[6]

SAFETY ASPECTS

There are important safety considerations associated with MR imaging of metallic orthopedic implants. Very few metallic orthopedic implants and joint replacement prostheses bear the Food and Drug Administration (FDA) label "MR safe." Most are "MR conditional," and, therefore, most implants are scanned "off-label."[7] Certain categories of hazards, particularly heating and displacement, should be considered.[8]

MR imaging of commonly used implants is associated with variable degrees of periprosthetic tissue heating. The principles of heat induction by radiofrequency transmission have been extensively studied.[9] The trend of musculoskeletal MR imaging toward 3.0 T may raise patient safety concerns due to the higher imparted radiofrequency energy at 3.0 T than 1.5 T.[10]

Interestingly, an in vitro model evaluating the spatial temperature rises of 4 different total hip arthroplasty implant constructs using the spectrum of clinically available metal artifact reduction techniques found higher temperature rises at 1.5 T than 3.0 T, which may be related to wavelength differences of the radiofrequency pulses.[11] Furthermore, compressed sensing-accelerated SEMAC MR imaging was not associated with higher degrees of heating than the high-bandwidth turbo spin-echo techniques.

In addition, investigators have pointed out that MR imaging–related heat deposition is low compared with the heat deposition of cemented prostheses.[7,12] The exothermic reaction of methyl methacrylate cement polymerization generates 50° to 70°C in vitro and up to 48°C in vivo. This degree of heat deposition is several-fold higher than heat deposition from MR imaging at 1.5 T and

> **Box 1**
> **Clinical best practice considerations for postoperative MR imaging of joints in patients with metallic orthopedic implants**
>
> Execute pulse sequences in the normal mode
>
> Use lower than normal radiofrequency flip and refocusing angles
>
> Limit the number of echoes per echo train
>
> Use low-energy radiofrequency pulse modes
>
> Use low-gradient performance modes
>
> Execute pulse sequences within permitted specific absorption rates
>
> Observe specific energy dose limits
>
> Exercise patient communication after every pulse sequence
>
> Perform MR imaging examinations under direct observation.

3.0 T. Thus, the risk of MR imaging–related implant heating is considered low.

MR imaging–related displacement with fixated orthopedic implants outside the central nervous system is typically less of a concern in postoperative MR imaging of joints.

As part of best clinical practice, several considerations may be applied to postoperative MR imaging of joints in patients with metallic orthopedic implants to limit the imparted energy and gradient effects (**Box 1**). All examinations should be performed in the normal mode, observing agency-mandated specific absorption rates and specific energy dose limits. Radiofrequency energy may be limited by using lower than normal radiofrequency flip and refocusing angles (eg, 125°), limiting the number of echoes per echo train (eg, 8 or less), and using long radiofrequency pulse modes. Exercising patient communication after every pulse sequence and performing MR imaging examinations under direct observation ensures patient well-being and early recognition of adverse effects.

IMPLANT MATERIALS AND SHAPES

The magnitude of artifact and visualization of the implant-tissue interface depends on its composition and shape. Metallic implants, ceramic components, and polyethylene liners lack mobile hydrogen atoms and are, therefore, devoid of signal.[13] Metallic orthopedic implants disturb the local field to varying degrees, with paramagnetic titanium producing the least susceptibility and

cobalt-chromium and stainless steel producing the greatest susceptibility.

Metal, Ceramic, and Polyethylene Components

In addition to titanium-based alloys and stainless steel, cobalt-chromium-molybdenum alloys are often used in orthopedic applications. Ferromagnetic and paramagnetic implants cause varying degrees of larger artifacts, whereas ceramic and polyethylene implants cause comparatively smaller artifacts.[14]

Orthopedic implants often contain cobalt, nickel, and chromium. Cobalt may cause distinctively large image artifacts that obscure critical periprosthetic structures.[15] Ceramic implants are used for hip replacements, whereas aluminum-based alloys have been used for knee replacements. Both alloy types are well-suited for postoperative MR imaging due to low magnetic susceptibility differences, resulting in smaller artifacts. The most commonly used total hip arthroplasty constructs are a ceramic head with titanium acetabular and femoral components. Ceramic-containing hip implants may feature ceramic-on-ceramic bearing surfaces, which have the benefits of good durability due to favorable wear-resistance and low degrees of immunologic host responses but may break and squeak.[16]

Implant Shape

Implant shape influences the resulting metallic artifacts on MR imaging. For example, the curved surface of acetabular components causes more field inhomogeneity than the more linear femoral component. Both B_0 and B_1 effects relate to implant shape.[17]

Magnetic Susceptibility

The magnitude of susceptibility increases in a linear relationship with B_0. Therefore, the native degree of metallic artifacts is lower at 1.5 T than 3.0 T. To reduce larger artifacts of 3.0 T, compressed sensing SEMAC affords higher numbers of artifact-reducing phase-encoding steps for potent metal artifact reduction within clinically acceptable acquisition times, resulting in substantial metal artifact reduction of metallic orthopedic osteosynthesis and arthroplasty implants.[18]

METAL ARTIFACT REDUCTION

Metallic artifact manifestations on MR imaging scans include distortions that occur in both in-plane and through-slice directions, signal voids,

Table 1
Basic metal artifact reduction protocol for postoperative MR imaging of large joints at 1.5 T field strength

Parameters	Coronal PD TSE	Coronal STIR TSE	Sagittal PD TSE	Sagittal STIR TSE	Axial PD TSE	Axial STIR TSE	Axial T1 TSE
Repetition time, ms	3800	3000	3800	3000	3800	3000	650
Echo time, ms	32	6.8	32	6.8	31	7	6.8
Receiver bandwidth, Hertz/pixel	500	500	500	500	500	500	500
Number of slices	31	25	31	25	35	31	25
Field-of-view, mm^2	270 × 270	300 × 300	270 × 270	300 × 300	230 × 230	230 × 230	300 × 300
Matrix	320 × 75%	256 × 75%	320 × 75%	256 × 75%	320 × 75%	256 × 75%	205 × 75%
Slice thickness, mm	3.5	4	3.5	4	4	4.5	5
Turbo factor	11	10	11	10	11	10	4
Acceleration factor	2	2	2	2	2	2	2
Acquisition time, min	3:31	3:44	3:31	3:56	2:45	2:56	2:45

Abbreviations: PD, proton-density–weighted; STIR, short tau inversion recovery; TSE, turbo spin echo.

and signal pile-up, resulting from static field inhomogeneities and B$_1$ effects.[17,19]

Spin Dephasing

Metallic orthopedic implants cause static magnetic field inhomogeneities, which result in accelerated dephasing of local spins and disproportionate signal loss. The radiofrequency-based spin refocusing of fast and turbo spin-echo pulse sequences minimizes spin dephasing effects, whereas gradient inversion-based spin refocusing of gradient-echo pulse sequences amplifies metal artifacts. Gradient-echo sequences are typically not used for routine metal artifact reduction MR imaging, although they may be used successfully for magnetic resonance angiography around metallic implants.[20]

Signal Displacement

Following the Larmor equation, disturbances of the local magnetic field gradient by metallic orthopedic implants result in erroneous local spin precession frequencies different from their expected gradient-defined values. The altered local spin precession frequencies result in erroneous spatial allocations and misregistration of MR signals in the frequency-encoded in-plane and through-plane directions. On MR imaging scans, the effects are complex composites of signal displacements

that include spatial misregistration, signal voids, summation (pile-up) artifacts, and geometric distortions.

Metal artifacts tend to be less prominent when the long axis is parallel to the B$_0$ field direction. Swapping the phase and frequency encoding directions may change the orientation of in-plane artifacts improving visualization of structures near curved or curvilinear prosthesis components. This technique rarely eliminates artifacts but can shift signal loss or pile-up artifacts to less anatomically important regions.

In-Plane Correction

Fast and turbo spin-echo pulse sequences with high receiver bandwidth are fundamental to almost any metal artifact reduction MR imaging technique (**Tables 1** and **2**). Increasing the receiver bandwidth in the receiver readout direction will apply more encoding frequencies per pixel, which results in less spatial signal displacement in the image domain. Increasing the receiver bandwidth will effectively confine the spread of a spectral distortion to a smaller number of adjacent pixels, resulting in small metal artifacts on the MR images (**Fig. 1**). Although image sharpness also increases, the trade-off with this technique is decreasing signal-to-noise ratios. In our practice, we use

Table 2
Basic metal artifact reduction protocol for postoperative MR imaging of small joints at 1.5 T field strength

Parameters	Sagittal PD TSE	Sagittal STIR TSE	Coronal PD TSE	Coronal STIR TSE	Axial PD TSE	Axial STIR TSE	Axial T1 TSE
Repetition time, ms	4350	4220	5040	4000	4500	4560	600
Echo time, ms	29	6.8	29	6.8	38	6.8	6.8
Receiver bandwidth, Hertz/pixel	500	500	500	500	500	500	500
Number of slices	35	28	35	28	45	37	41
Field-of-view, mm^2	160 × 160	200 × 200	160 × 160	200 × 200	160 × 160	200 × 200	160 × 160
Matrix	384 × 75%	320 × 75%	384 × 75%	320 × 75%	384 × 75%	320 × 75%	384 × 75%
Slice thickness, mm	3	4	3	4	4	5	4
Turbo factor	11	10	11	10	11	10	4
Parallel imaging factor	2	2	2	2	2	2	2
Acquisition time, min:s	4:13	4:33	4:32	4:41	4:04	4:55	3:55

Abbreviations: PD, proton-density–weighted; STIR, short tau inversion recovery; TSE, turbo spin echo.

receiver bandwidths of 500 Hz/pixel at 1.5 T and 600 to 700 Hz/pixel at 3.0 T.

VAT is a method to reduce in-plane distortions by applying an additional gradient in slice-encoding direction during signal readout. VAT assumes signal displacements occurring in 2 directions at a constant ratio, with the intent for slice displacements canceling in-plane displacements so that the in-plane displacements are subtracted. Applying VAT techniques results in sheared images that the observer sees the MR images at a tilted view angle. Although VAT reduces metallic artifacts, the main disadvantage is the introduction of blurring and loss of edge sharpness. The introduction of blurring can be mitigated by using high receiver bandwidth, as described previously. However, with receiver bandwidths of 500 to 700 Hz per pixel, the metal artifact reduction of VAT techniques is minimal and of limited practical usefulness.[13,21]

VAT does not resolve through-plane distortions by itself but pairs favorably with multispectral and multispatial techniques, such as SEMAC and MAVRIC, for resolving through-plane distortions.[22]

Through-Plane Correction

Most conventional metal artifact reduction MR imaging techniques affect in-plane–associated artifacts, whereas though-plane–associated artifacts remain largely unaffected. Among the basic methods, thinner slice thickness affects through-plane–associated signal displacement by indirectly increasing the bandwidth of the slice-encoding gradient. By effects similar to increasing the received readout bandwidth directly, using thinner slice sections increases the bandwidth of the slice-encoding gradients, which indirectly results in applying more encoding frequencies per slice section. The wider frequency encoding per slice translates to less spatial than spectral signal displacement. However, visible noise increases with tinner slice thickness, practically limiting slice thickness to no less than 3 mm within clinical MR imaging protocols.

Fat Suppression

STIR is generally preferred over spectral-based fat suppression for MR imaging around metallic implants. Spectral fat suppression often fails around implants due to local alterations of spin precession frequencies. Because the altered precession frequencies then fall outside the bandwidth of spectral fat suppression pulses, spectral fat suppression inevitably fails. Instead, STIR relies on the difference in T1 relaxation times of fat and water, which is unaffected by implant effects.

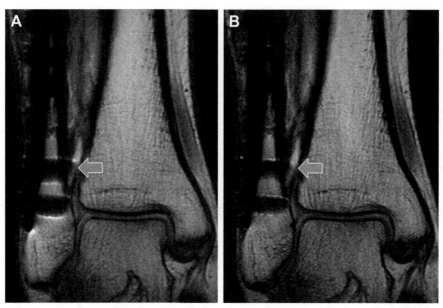

Fig. 1. Coronal proton-density–weighted turbo spin-echo 1.5 T MR imaging scans of the ankle with plate and screw osteosynthesis of the fibula. Low receiver bandwidth of 150 Hz per pixel results and larger artifacts (*A, arrow*) than higher receiver bandwidth of 400 Hz per pixel (*B, arrow*).

Dixon-based techniques may result in adequate fat suppression around implants with limited magnetic susceptibility differences to human tissue (**Fig. 2**).

Slice Encoding for Metal Artifact Correction and Multiacquisition Variable-Resonance Image Combination

Multispectral techniques, such as SEMAC and MAVRIC, directly address through-plane artifacts, thus enabling better visualization along implant-tissue interfaces.[14,20,23]

MAVRIC is a 3D acquisition technique that splits the metal-induced broad range of precession frequencies into discrete frequency bins and images each spectral bin separately. In this scheme, the off-resonance signal loss is minimized. SEMAC, on the other hand, is a 2D technique that resolves the through-place signal distortions through the excitation of multiple spatial bands. As such, MAVRIC may be referred to as multispectral, and SEMAC as multispatial imaging techniques. Some clinically available MAVRIC pulse sequences include SEMAC techniques.

SEMAC and MAVRIC have been shown to improve the detection of a broad spectrum of abnormalities around osteosynthesis and arthroplasty implants of the hip, knee, spine, and ankle.[13] However, these pulse sequences are time-consuming components of clinical metal artifact reduction protocols. Therefore, accelerated acquisition techniques resulting in faster total acquisition times are desirable in day-to-day clinical practice.

Similar to conventional fast and turbo spin-echo techniques, partial Fourier, parallel imaging, and echo train compaction using higher receiver bandwidths, turbo factors, faster gradients, and shorter radiofrequency pulses can substantially accelerate SEMAC and MAVRIC.[24,25]

Applied to SEMAC, echo train compaction and parallel imaging allow for flexible tissue contrasts, including T1, proton density, and T2 weighting. In addition, STIR fat suppression favorably combines with basic sequence acceleration (**Tables 3** and **4**).

Compressed sensing (CS) acceleration uses sparse undersampling patterns that can reduce the acquisition time of SEMAC pulse sequences with a high number of encoding steps by up to 70%.[26–28] CS-SEMAC techniques use sparsity-driven k-space undersampled data with subsequent iterative reconstruction to reconstruct part of the missing data. Commercially available CS SEMAC pulse sequences permit eightfold acceleration in clinical practice at 1.5 and 3.0 T, which can be applied to T1, proton density, and T2 contrasts. CS acceleration has also been applied to a MAVRIC prototype.[29]

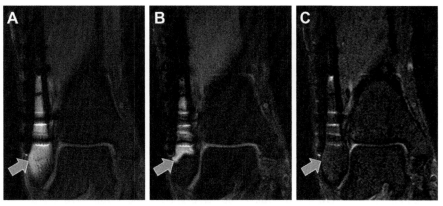

Fig. 2. Coronal short tau inversion recovery (STIR) turbo spin-echo 1.5 T MR imaging scans of the ankle with plate and screw osteosynthesis of the fibula. (*A*) Spectral fat suppression prominently fails (*arrow*) around the metallic implants. (*B*) Dixon water-only fat suppression results in less failed fat suppression (*arrow*). (*C*) STIR technique results in homogeneous fat suppression (*arrow*) around the metallic implants.

FIELD STRENGTH
Low-Field Magnets

As a function of the lower magnetic field strength, low-field MR systems may offer an advantage due to inherently smaller metal implant–related artifacts than 1.5 T and 3.0 T.[30] Low-field MR imaging scanners with a magnetic field strength of 1.0 T or less feature additional advantages of lower cost of ownership and permit open bore designs, which may be advantageous for patients with larger body sizes and claustrophobia. Low-field scanners have also been built as extremity units with

Table 3
Advanced metal artifact reduction protocol for postoperative MR imaging of large joints using SEMAC at 1.5 T field strength

Parameters	Coronal PD TSE	Coronal STIR TSE	Sagittal PD TSE	Sagittal STIR TSE	Axial PD TSE	Axial STIR TSE	Axial T1 TSE
Repetition time, ms	3910	3340	3980	3340	3900	4860	620
Echo time, ms	32	6.8	32	6.8	32	6.8	6.8
Number of SEMAC steps[a]	8	8	8	8	8	8	8
Receiver bandwidth, Hertz/pixel	500	500	500	500	500	500	500
Number of slices	29	25	33	25	35	35	27
Field-of-view, mm²	270 × 270	300 × 300	270 × 270	300 × 300	270 × 270	300 × 300	300 × 300
Matrix	320 × 75%	256 × 75%	320 × 75%	256 × 75%	320 × 75%	256 × 75%	192 × 75%
Slice thickness, mm	3.5	4	3.5	4	4	4	5
Turbo factor	11	10	11	10	11	10	4
Acceleration factor	3	3	3	3	3	3	3
Acquisition time, min:s	7:144	7:31	7:56	7:21	7:11	7:05	7:11

Abbreviations: PD, proton-density–weighted; SEMAC, slice encoding for metal artifact correction; STIR, short tau inversion recovery; TSE, turbo spin echo.
[a] The number of SEMAC-encoding steps may be increased for stronger metal artifact reduction.

Table 4
Advanced metal artifact reduction protocol for postoperative MR imaging of small joints using SEMAC at 1.5 T field strength

Parameters	Sagittal PD TSE	Sagittal STIR TSE	Coronal PD TSE	Coronal STIR TSE	Axial PD TSE	Axial T1TSE
Repetition time, ms	3920	3620	3340	3270	3440	580
Echo time, ms	31	7.6	29	7.6	29	7.6
SEMAC-encoding steps[a]	8	8	8	8	8	8
Receiver bandwidth, Hertz/ pixel	500	500	500	500	500	500
Number of slices	35	29	35	29	35	35
Field-of-view, mm^2	170 × 170	180 × 180	170 × 170	180 × 180	170 × 170	170 × 170
Matrix	320 × 75%	256 × 75%	320 × 75%	256 × 75%	320 × 75%	320 × 75%
Slice thickness, mm	3	4	3/0	4	4	4
Turbo factor	11	10	11	10	11	4
Parallel imaging factor	3	3	3	3	3	3
Acquisition time, min:s	6:15	6:55	5:21	5:45	5:50	5:15

Abbreviations: PD, proton-density–weighted; SEMAC, slice encoding for metal artifact correction; STIR, short tau inversion recovery; TSE, turbo spin echo.
[a] The number of SEMAC-encoding steps may be increased for stronger metal artifact reduction.

smaller form factors, requiring less space and shielding.

Promising results of low-field MR imaging scanners (0.3 T) have been described in patients with titanium volar wrist plating of distal radius fractures.[31] Although low magnetic field strength comes with the disadvantage of low signal-to-noise ratios, new generation low-field scanners at 0.55 T offer new possibilities for implant imaging, including improved visualization of bone-implant interfaces and superior metal artifact reduction in patients with cobalt-containing and metal-on-metal arthroplasty implants.[30]

High-Field Magnets

Attempts to apply artifact-reducing techniques in a clinical setting initially focused on 1.5 T MR imaging scanners, given that metal artifacts are amplified at higher field strength. However, because of the many advantages of 3.0 T field strength for musculoskeletal MR imaging,[18] the number of 1.5 T MR imaging systems is declining, creating a demand for effective metal artifact reduction at higher field strength. Several studies have shown the feasibility of using 2D fast spin-echo and 3D multispectral imaging sequences at 3.0 T.[32–34]

Compared with conventional 2D fast spin-echo, MAVRIC-selective (MAVRIC-SL) sequence, which possesses beneficial features of both SEMAC and MAVRIC techniques through retaining the slab selectivity of SEMAC by way of a Z gradient and higher SNR of MAVRIC using an overlapped spectral strategy with multiple frequency-selective

excitation, can significantly improve image quality and decreased image artifacts at 3.0 T in patients with various metallic implants.[34] A comparison of MAVRIC-SL at 1.5 and 3.0 T for MR imaging of hip arthroplasty implants showed larger artifacts, limited image quality, and worse fat saturation at 3.0 T.[33] However, the difference in metal artifact size did not significantly impact the visualization of anatomic structures and abnormalities.

INDICATIONS

Postoperative MR imaging can be indicated in various clinical settings in asymptomatic and symptomatic patient groups.[21] Asymptomatic patients may be imaged for routine implant integrity follow-up or surveillance for tumor recurrence. Symptomatic patients may present with pain or mechanical symptoms where postoperative complications, such as osseous abnormalities, implant instability, joint infection, periarticular adverse local tissue reactions, or soft tissue injury, may be causative.[35]

Failure of arthroplasty constructs can be broadly categorized into osseous abnormalities (eg, periprosthetic fractures), implant instability (eg, mechanical loosening, implant dislocation or component displacement), infection, component wear-induced synovitis and osteolysis, adverse local tissue reactions (ALTRs), and periarticular soft tissue injuries (eg, myotendinous and nerve injuries).[35,36]

Although ultrasound can play an important role in evaluating the postoperative joint, particularly for joint effusions and periarticular soft tissue abnormalities, this modality may be limited by various factors, such as operator experience and patient habitus. MR imaging is generally regarded as superior for detecting ALTRs and muscle abnormalities.[37]

CT using MAR techniques is superior to radiographs in the assessment of hip prosthesis loosening,[38] and can be superior to conventional metal artifact reduction MR imaging for evaluation of the bone-metal interface and detection of osteolysis for metallic implants with high magnetic susceptibility.[39] However, with the advent of newer metal suppression techniques, MR imaging can now demonstrate improved detail at the metal-osseous interface.[3] Furthermore, CT is less useful for evaluating pseudotumoral conditions, detecting fluid collections and myotendinous tears. Dual-energy CT-based virtual monoenergetic extrapolation and iterative metal artifact reduction may be combined,[40] resulting in an improved reduction of low- and high-density artifacts depending on the implant type and photon energy.[41] Metal artifact reduced CT datasets may be used to improve the image quality of cinematic rendering images in body regions with implants.[42,43]

A role for SPECT/CT has also been suggested in detecting impaired implant fixation in patients with painful hip arthroplasty; however, MR imaging remains superior in detecting soft tissue abnormalities.[44]

Arthroplasty Complications

Arthroplasty complications vary depending on the joint; however, component failure (**Fig. 3**), osseous stress reactions (**Fig. 4**), fractures (**Fig. 5**), and loosening apply to all implants. Following total knee and hip arthroplasty, more specific considerations include polyethylene liner wear, implant dissociation, instability (**Fig. 6**), and dislocation.[23]

Common modes of total knee arthroplasty failure include aseptic loosening, polyethylene wear–induced synovitis and osteolysis, periprosthetic joint infections, fracture, patellar clunk syndrome, recurrent hemarthrosis, arthrofibrosis, component malalignment, extensor mechanism injury, and instability.[20]

Implant Integrity, Integration, and Aseptic Loosening

Radiography and CT are the first-line modalities to assess the integrity of metallic implant components. Although metallic implant fractures can be visualized (see **Fig. 3**), MR imaging is best suited to evaluate the integrity of nonmetallic implant components, such as polyethylene inlays.[45] Aseptic loosening can occur as a result of implantation-associated suboptimal fixation, mechanical disruption, and secondary biologic fixation failure due to particle disease and osteolysis.

Loss of implant fixation, including initially bone resorption and osteolysis, characteristically manifests as a band of intermediate-to-high proton density and T2 signal intensity along the implant-bone interface (see **Fig. 4**). Subtle osteolysis and marrow edema are usually first identified near the bone implant or cement-bone interface and may be seen on MR imaging before radiographic changes occur. On further progression of loosening, defined as complete loss of implant fixation, trabecular microtrauma, disproportionate marrow edema, and periosteal edema may occur.

An important exception is the STIR hyperintensity of the marrow cavity after reaming and bone compaction during implantation, which may persist beyond 12 months postoperatively.[46]

Infection

Periprosthetic joint infection can be a challenging complication to identify. The clinical presentation is often nonspecific, with signs and symptoms overlapping with ALTRs, loosening, and soft tissue injury. Although preventive protocols have improved with an increasing number of joint replacements being performed, correspondingly, the overall number of infections have increased as well.[47] Despite a low incidence in total hip and knee arthroplasty (0.2%–2% of primary procedures),[1,48] periprosthetic joint infection represents the third leading cause of revision total hip arthroplasty in the United States.[49] A registry-based meta-analysis of causes for revision arthroplasty found that septic loosening was responsible for 9.8% of revisions of total ankle arthroplasty from 1993 to 2007, compared with 7.5% of revisions of total hip arthroplasty and 14.8% of revisions of total knee arthroplasty, both from 1979 to 2009.[50]

MR imaging findings of periprosthetic joint infection include joint effusions and synovitis, soft tissue findings such as periarticular edema, abscess formation, draining sinuses, and osseous changes such as marrow edema, periostitis, and bony destruction (**Fig. 7**). Lamellated synovial reaction and proliferation are frequently found.[23] Localized or diffuse enhancement may be present after intravenous gadolinium-based contrast.

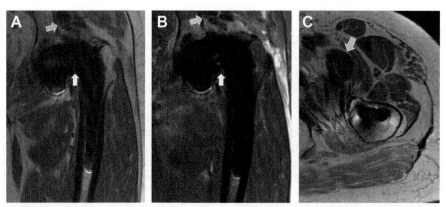

Fig. 3. A 76-year-old man with broken left total hip arthroplasty at the femoral head-neck junction. Metal artifact reduction MR imaging at 1.5 T including coronal proton-density–weighted SEMAC (A) STIR SEMAC (B), and axial proton-density high-bandwidth (C) turbo spin-echo pulse sequences. The coronal MR imaging scans (A and B) demonstrate varus angulation of the femoral head-neck junction (*white arrows*), indicating implant fracturing. The coronal (A and B) and axial (C) MR imaging scans demonstrate characteristically hypointense deposits (*gray arrows*) of macroscopic metallic deposits, characteristic of metallosis.

Myotendinous Injury

Tendinopathy and tendon tears around replaced joints show similar morphology and signal patterns to native joints. Common examples of affected tendons include the iliopsoas and adductor tendons after hip replacement,[14] the rotator cuff and long head bicep tendon after total shoulder arthroplasty and rotator cuff repair, the extensor mechanism (**Fig. 8**) and medial and lateral collateral ligament after total knee arthroplasty,[14] and the long flexor and peroneal tendons after ankle arthroplasty.[28]

Architectural distortion and fluid accumulation typify acute muscle, muscle-tendon junction, and muscle attachment injuries.[51] The grading of muscle tears is an important prognostic factor correlating with recovery time based on size and morphology. The degree of architectural disruption and overall length should be compared with that of the entire muscle. Hemorrhage may appear as ill-defined intramuscular blood products or a discrete hematoma with signal characteristics corresponding to those of hemorrhages elsewhere in the body. The longer-term sequelae of muscle trauma may also result in scarring, retraction, and atrophy.

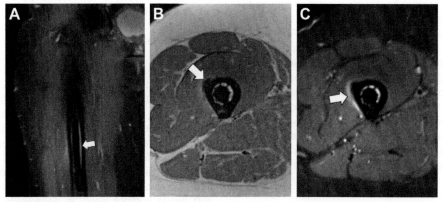

Fig. 4. A 60-year-old woman with right thigh pain after total hip arthroplasty. Metal artifact reduction MR imaging at 3.0 T including coronal STIR SEMAC (A), axial proton-density high-bandwidth (B), and axial proton-density high-bandwidth (C) turbo spin-echo pulse sequences. The coronal MR imaging scan (A) demonstrates STIR hyperintensity interposed between the femoral implant surface and host bone (*arrow*), indicating bone resorption with focal loss of fixation. The axial proton-density (B) and STIR (C) MR imaging scans show periosteal new bone formation (B, *arrow*) and periosteal edema (C, *arrow*) surrounding the native femoral cortex and new bone formation, indicating an osseous stress response without fracture.

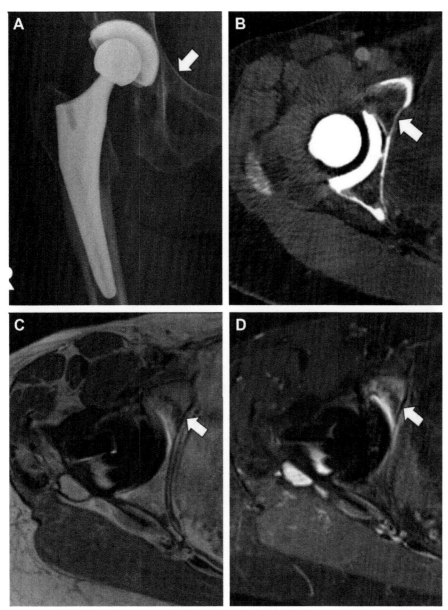

Fig. 5. A 62-year-old woman with right thigh pain after total hip arthroplasty. (*A*) Frontal radiograph demonstrates intact right hip arthroplasty implants with solid-appearing osseous fixation and intact periprosthetic bone (*arrow*). (*B*) Axial CT with iterative metal artifact reduction demonstrates intact periprosthetic bone without evidence of a fracture (*arrow*). Metal artifact reduction MR imaging at 3.0 T, including axial proton-density (*C*) and STIR (*D*) high-bandwidth turbo spin-echo pulse sequences. The axial MR imaging scans demonstrate a radiographically and CT-occult nondisplaced fracture along the anterior acetabulum with fracture line and surrounding bone marrow edema pattern (*arrows*).

Nerve Injury

Nerve injuries may occur at the time of surgery and may be seen as direct neural abnormalities or as secondary denervation or atrophic changes in the innervated musculature. The incidence of nerve injuries after total hip arthroplasty is 0.6% to 3.7%, which increases to 7.6% for revision arthroplasty (7.6%).[52] Dedicated metal artifact reduction MR imaging protocols yield high image quality and diagnostic accuracy for assessing lumbosacral nerve injuries and neuropathies in patients with metallic implants of the pelvis and hips (**Fig. 9**).[53]

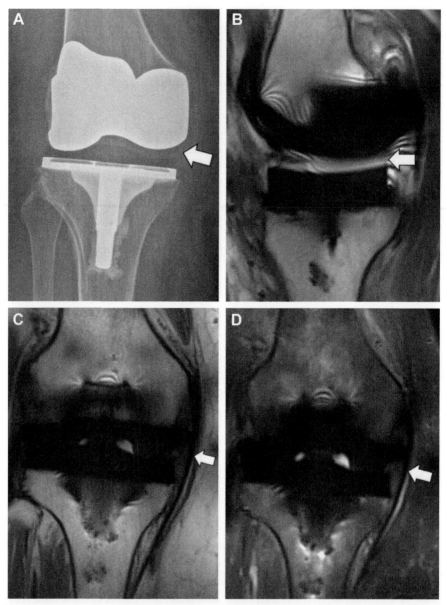

Fig. 6. A 68-year-old man with instability after right total knee arthroplasty. (*A*) Frontal radiograph demonstrates well-fixated knee arthroplasty implants in valgus alignment (*arrow*). Metal artifact reduction MR imaging at 1.5 T including sagittal proton-density SEMAC (*B*), coronal proton-density SEMAC (*C*), and coronal STIR SEMAC (*D*) turbo spin-echo pulse sequences. The sagittal MR imaging scan (*B*) demonstrates a gap (*arrow*) between the femoral implant component and tibial tray polyethylene component as an effect of medial valgus instability. The coronal proton-density (*C*) and STIR (*D*) MR imaging scans show an intact medial collateral ligament, providing useful information for balancing during revision surgery.

Adverse Local Tissue Reactions, Metallosis, and Particle Disease

ALTR refers to the tissue effects of immune responses to metal ions and corrosion products from metal-on-metal contact junctions of implants, which can result in aggressive synovitis with vascularized conglomerates and masses, resembling neoplastic tissue ("pseudotumor")[23] (**Fig. 10**). The term "metallosis" has been evolving, but is often used to describe tissue deposits of macroscopic metallic particles fretted from surfaces and junctions of metallic implants. On MR imaging scans, metallosis-associated synovial deposits are characteristically hypointense and demonstrate

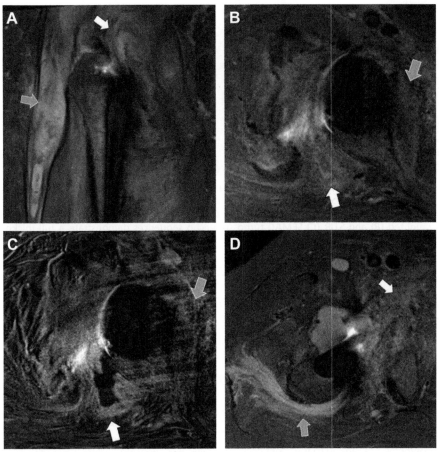

Fig. 7. A 62-year-old man with pain after right total hip arthroplasty. Metal artifact reduction MR imaging at 1.5 T including coronal STIR SEMAC (*A*), axial STIR SEMAC through the acetabular cup (*B*), axial contrast-enhanced T1-weighted SEMAC subtraction through the acetabular cup (*C*), and axial STIR SEMAC through the femoral stem (*D*) turbo spin-echo pulse sequences demonstrate findings of periprosthetic joint infection. (*A*) Coronal STIR SEMAC MR imaging scan shows edematous layered ("lamellated") synovitis (*white arrow*) and complex fluid in the greater trochanteric bursa (*gray arrow*). (*B* and *C*) Axial STIR (*B* and *D*) and contrast-enhanced T1-weighted (*C*) SEMAC subtraction MR imaging scans show edema and contrast enhancement of layered ("lamellated") synovitis (*white arrows*) and periarticular soft tissues (*gray arrow*).

varying degrees of dephasing and metal artifacts, reflective of metallic deposits (see **Fig. 3**).

Classic particle disease typically describes the effects of small worn polyethylene particles and tissue immune response. The term particle disease has also been applied to cement and larger metal tissue response debris. Early particle disease may be clinically occult, conspicuous only as effusions, irregular synovitis, and periarticular collections on fluid-sensitive MR imaging scans. More advanced particle disease characteristically demonstrates particulate synovitis with conglomerates and optional zones of geographic osteolysis filled with debris. Polyethylene-induced synovitic conglomerates and debris often have texture and signal intensity similar to muscle tissue

on proton-density–weighted MR imaging scans (see **Fig. 10**).

The group of metal-on-metal hip arthroplasty constructs deserve specific consideration. Within this group, metal-on-metal hip resurfacing arthroplasty implants have gained popularity as an alternative to total hip arthroplasty, particularly for active young patients due to favorable biomechanics and bone stock preservation. However, the cobalt-chromium bearings from which these are usually constructed may incite aggressive synovitis related to ALTR. As a result of widely recognized ALTR occurrences in patients with metal-on-metal hip arthroplasty implants, governmental authorities, including the FDA, have recommended metal artifact reduction MR imaging as part of routine postoperative surveillance.[54]

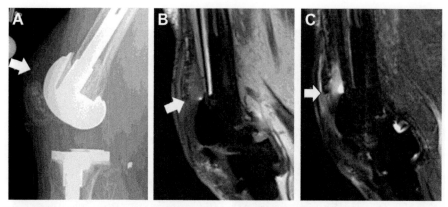

Fig. 8. A 70-year-old woman with anterior knee pain and weakness after total knee arthroplasty with distal quadriceps tendon allograft reconstruction. (*A*) Lateral radiograph demonstrating soft tissue swelling (*arrow*) over the anterior knee and patella baja. Metal artifact reduction MR imaging at 1.5 T including sagittal proton-density–weighted (*B*) and STIR (*C*) SEMAC turbo spin-echo sequences demonstrate a full-thickness tear of the distal quadriceps tendon allograft.

From a research perspective, synovial volume on MR imaging may be used as an ALTR marker in asymptomatic and symptomatic patients with metal-on-metal hip resurfacing arthroplasty implants.[55] Synovial thickening greater than 6 mm has been reported as an MR imaging finding with high sensitivity and specificity to predict ALTR in patients with metal-on-metal implants.[56]

Tumor Surveillance

Primary bone or soft tissue neoplasms in the vicinity of a hip prosthesis are rare, with the most common including undifferentiated pleomorphic sarcoma and osteosarcoma.[57,58] Metastatic disease, multiple myeloma, and locally recurrent disease are more common. Occasionally the morphologic appearances of neoplastic lesions may be similar to those of wear-induced osteolysis and immature heterotopic ossification.[35] Therefore, optimal metal artifact reduction MR imaging

in the postoperative surveillance setting is essential.

Limb salvage surgery with implantation of orthopedic tumor endoprosthesis has evolved into the preferred option for patients with malignant bone tumors of the extremities over traditional amputation.[59] Orthopedic tumor endoprostheses are typically larger than conventional arthroplasty implants, typically inducing significant metal-induced susceptibility artifacts. In an experimental model, substantial metal artifact reduction was achieved with a VAT-SEMAC pulse sequence in large-sized orthopedic tumor endoprostheses with demonstrable clinical benefits for assessing periprosthetic soft tissue abnormalities.[60] MAVRIC has also been shown to improve the image quality of tissues around tumor prostheses.[61]

FUTURE DIRECTIONS

With increased SNR, 7T MR imaging has the potential to contribute superior anatomic and

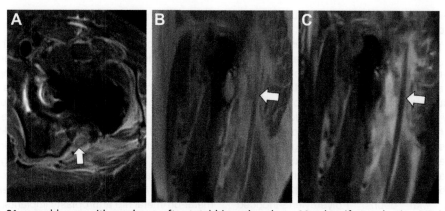

Fig. 9. An 81-year-old man with weakness after total hip arthroplasty. Metal artifact reduction MR imaging at 1.5 T including axial STIR high-bandwidth (*A*), sagittal proton-density–weighted SEMAC (*B*), and sagittal STIR SEMAC (*C*) turbo spin-echo pulse sequences demonstrate a segmentally STIR hyperintense (*A, arrow*), thickened (*A–C, arrows*), but continuous (*B and C, arrows*) sciatic nerve, indicating neuropathy.

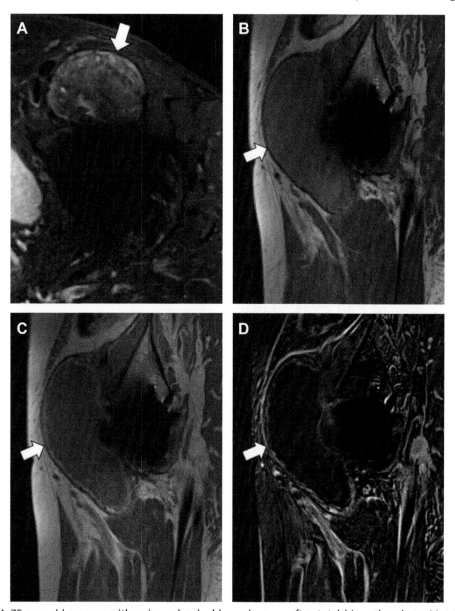

Fig. 10. A 75-year-old woman with pain and palpable groin mass after total hip arthroplasty. Metal artifact reduction MR imaging at 1.5 T including axial STIR high-bandwidth (*A*), sagittal T1-weighted high-bandwidth (*B*), sagittal contrast-enhanced T1-weighted high-bandwidth (*C*), and sagittal subtraction T1-weighted (*D*) high-bandwidth turbo spin-echo pulse sequences. Axial STIR high-bandwidth MR imaging scan demonstrates distended iliopsoas bursa filled with particulate synovitic debris (*arrow*). Sagittal T1-weighted high-bandwidth MR imaging scans show absent central and minimal peripheral contrast enhancement (*arrows*). Histopathological evaluation demonstrated mixed polyethylene wear–induced synovitis and adverse local tissue reaction due to trunnion corrosion.

pathologic information in the context of postoperative MR imaging of joints. However, safety concerns pertaining to metallic implants have restricted research advancement in this area. Few studies addressed the safety of orthopedic implants at 7T, including temperature rises, translational attraction, deflection angle, and torque.[62,63]

An evaluation of the MR imaging safety of 39 commonly used medical implants at 7T, including a cobalt-chromium Omnifit (La Mesa, CA) cemented head/neck long stem implant (6080–0530–200L, Stryker) with encouraging safety test results, showing a deflection angle of 15° and no torque or temperature change.[62] In contrast, another study investigating implants for magnetic field interactions at 7T demonstrated a deflection angle of 45° and moderate torque (the device aligned gradually to the magnetic field) of a Smith & Nephew (London, UK) Summit hip stem with a cobalt-chromium-molybdenum head, raising potential safety concerns for exposure to the 7T environment.[63] Therefore, although 7T MR imaging allows for higher spatial resolution, more larger-scale safety data are required to ensure participant safety.

SUMMARY

Postoperative joint MR imaging in the presence of metallic orthopedic implants is safe and now commonplace but remains challenging. Therefore, radiologists should be familiar with applying basic and advanced metal artifact reduction MR imaging techniques for improved detection of implant-related complications. With the broad clinical availability of advanced metal artifact reduction techniques, the ability to diagnose and treat arthroplasty-related complications has markedly improved.

CLINICS CARE POINTS

- Postoperative arthroplasty complications vary depending on the joint; however, component failure, osseous stress reactions, fractures, and loosening apply to all implants. More specific considerations after total knee and hip arthroplasty include polyethylene liner wear, implant dissociation, instability, and dislocation.

- Thorough evaluation of the postoperative joint is required to identify common complications, including prosthesis loosening, infection, adverse local tissue reaction, and periarticular soft tissue injuries.

- Ferromagnetic and paramagnetic implants cause greater artifacts compared with ceramic and polyethylene components.

- The radiologist should be familiar with basic and more advanced techniques for optimal metal artifact reduction.

- Fast and turbo spin-echo sequences, high transmit and receiver bandwidths, and thin slice thickness reflect basic metallic artifact reduction techniques. Fat suppression around metallic prostheses can be effectively achieved with bandwidth-adjusted STIR.

- SEMAC and MAVRIC represent more advanced metal artifact reduction techniques.

DISCLOSURE

J. Fritz received institutional research support from Siemens AG, BTG International Ltd., Zimmer Biomed, DePuy Synthes, QED, and SyntheticMR; is a scientific advisor for Siemens AG, SyntheticMR, GE Healthcare, QED, BTG, ImageBiopsy Lab, Boston Scientific, and Mirata Pharma; and has shared patents with Siemens Healthcare, Johns Hopkins University, and New York University. C.J. Burke and I. Khodarahmi have nothing to disclose.

REFERENCES

1. Kurtz S, Ong K, Lau E, et al. Projections of primary and revision hip and knee arthroplasty in the United States from 2005 to 2030. J Bone Joint Surg Am 2007;89(4):780–5.

2. Olsen RV, Munk PL, Lee MJ, et al. Metal artifact reduction sequence: early clinical applications. Radiographics 2000;20(3):699–712.

3. Talbot BS, Weinberg EP. MR imaging with metal-suppression sequences for evaluation of total joint arthroplasty. Radiographics 2016;36(1):209–25.

4. Kolind SH, MacKay AL, Munk PL, et al. Quantitative evaluation of metal artifact reduction techniques. J Magn Reson Imaging 2004;20(3):487–95.

5. Kumar NM, de Cesar Netto C, Schon LC, et al. Metal artifact reduction magnetic resonance imaging around arthroplasty implants: the negative effect of long echo trains on the implant-related artifact. Invest Radiol 2017;52(5):310–6.

6. Ariyanayagam T, Malcolm PN, Toms AP. Advances in metal artifact reduction techniques for periprosthetic soft tissue imaging. Semin Musculoskelet Radiol 2015;19(4):328–34.

7. Koff MF, Shah P, Potter HG. Clinical implementation of MRI of joint arthroplasty. Am J Roentgenol 2014; 203(1):154–61.

8. Khodarahmi I, Bonham LW, Weiss CR, et al. Needle heating during interventional magnetic resonance imaging at 1.5- and 3.0-T field strengths. Invest Radiol 2020;55(6):396–404.

9. Graf H, Steidle G, Schick F. Heating of metallic implants and instruments induced by gradient switching in a 1.5-Tesla whole-body unit. J Magn Reson Imaging 2007;26(5):1328–33.

10. Winter L, Seifert F, Zilberti L, et al. MRI-related heating of implants and devices: a review. J Magn Reson Imaging 2021;53(6):1646–65.

11. Khodarahmi I, Rajan S, Sterling R, et al. Heating of Hip Arthroplasty Implants During Metal Artifact Reduction MRI at 1.5- and 3.0-T Field Strengths. Invest Radiol 2021;56(4):232–43. https://doi.org/10.1097/RLI.0000000000000732. PMID: 33074932.

12. Tayton ER, Smith JO, Evans N, et al. Effects of setting bone cement on tissue-engineered bone graft: a potential barrier to clinical translation? J Bone Joint Surg Am 2013;95(8):736–43.

13. Khodarahmi I, Nittka M, Fritz J. Leaps in technology: advanced MR imaging after total hip arthroplasty. Semin Musculoskelet Radiol 2017;21(5): 604–15.

14. Fritz J, Lurie B, Miller TT. Imaging of hip arthroplasty. Semin Musculoskelet Radiol 2013;17(3):316–27.

15. Månsson S, Müller GM, Wellman F, et al. Phantom based qualitative and quantitative evaluation of artifacts in MR images of metallic hip prostheses. Phys Med 2015;31(2):173–8.

16. Jennings JM, Czuczman GJ, Johnson RM, et al. Metal Artifact Reduction Sequence Magnetic Resonance Imaging Abnormalities in Asymptomatic Patients with a Ceramic-on-Ceramic Total Hip Replacement. J Arthroplasty 2021;36(2):612–5. https://doi.org/10.1016/j.arth.2020.07.082. Epub 2020 Aug 6. PMID: 32950341.

17. Khodarahmi I, Kirsch J, Chang G, et al. Metal artifacts of hip arthroplasty implants at 1.5-T and 3.0-T: a closer look into the B1 effects. Skeletal Radiol 2021;50(5):1007–15.

18. Khodarahmi I, Fritz J. The value of 3 Tesla field strength for musculoskeletal magnetic resonance imaging. Invest Radiol 2021;56(11):749–63.

19. Hargreaves BA, Chen W, Lu W, et al. Accelerated slice encoding for metal artifact correction. J Magn Reson Imaging 2010;31(4):987–96.

20. Fritz J, Lurie B, Potter HG. MR imaging of knee arthroplasty implants. Radiographics 2015;35(5): 1483–501.

21. Khodarahmi I, Isaac A, Fishman EK, et al. Metal about the hip and artifact reduction techniques: from basic concepts to advanced imaging. Semin Musculoskelet Radiol 2019;23(3):e68–81.

22. Kretzschmar M, Nardo L, Han MM, et al. Metal artefact suppression at 3 T MRI: comparison of MAVRIC-SL with conventional fast spin echo sequences in patients with hip joint arthroplasty. Eur Radiol 2015; 25(8):2403–11.

23. Fritz J, Lurie B, Miller TT, et al. MR imaging of hip arthroplasty implants. Radiographics 2014;34(4): E106–32.

24. Del Grande F, Guggenberger R, Fritz J. Rapid musculoskeletal MRI in 2021: value and optimized use of widely accessible techniques. Am J Roentgenol 2021;216(3):704–17.

25. Fritz J, Guggenberger R, Del Grande F. Rapid musculoskeletal MRI in 2021: clinical application of advanced accelerated techniques. Am J Roentgenol 2021;216(3):718–33.

26. Fritz J, Ahlawat S, Demehri S, et al. Compressed sensing SEMAC: 8-fold accelerated high resolution metal artifact reduction MRI of cobalt-chromium knee arthroplasty implants. Invest Radiol 2016; 51(10):666–76.

27. Fritz J, Fritz B, Thawait GK, et al. Advanced metal artifact reduction MRI of metal-on-metal hip resurfacing arthroplasty implants: compressed sensing acceleration enables the time-neutral use of SEMAC. Skeletal Radiol 2016;45(10):1345–56.

28. de Cesar Netto C, Fonseca LF, Fritz B, et al. Metal artifact reduction MRI of total ankle arthroplasty implants. Eur Radiol 2018;28(5):2216–27.

29. Worters PW, Sung K, Stevens KJ, et al. Compressed-sensing multispectral imaging of the postoperative spine. J Magn Reson Imaging 2013; 37(1):243–8.

30. Runge VM, Heverhagen JT. Advocating the development of next-generation, advanced-design low-field magnetic resonance systems. Invest Radiol 2020;55(12):747–53.

31. Stecco A, Arioli R, Buemi F, et al. Overcoming metallic artefacts from orthopaedic wrist volar plating on a low-field MRI scanner. Radiol Med 2019;124(5):392–9.

32. Farrelly C, Davarpanah A, Brennan SA, et al. Imaging of soft tissues adjacent to orthopedic hardware: comparison of 3-T and 1.5-T MRI. Am J Roentgenol 2010;194(1):W60–4.

33. Nardo L, Han M, Kretzschmar M, et al. Metal artifact suppression at the hip: diagnostic performance at 3.0 T versus 1.5 Tesla. Skeletal Radiol 2015;44(11): 1609–16.

34. Gutierrez LB, Do BH, Gold GE, et al. MR imaging near metallic implants using MAVRIC SL: initial clinical experience at 3T. Acad Radiol 2015;22(3): 370–9.

35. Khodarahmi I, Fritz J. Advanced MR imaging after total hip arthroplasty: the clinical impact. Semin Musculoskelet Radiol 2017;21(5):616–29.

36. Deshmukh S, Omar IM. Imaging of hip arthroplasties: normal findings and hardware complications. Semin Musculoskelet Radiol 2019;23(2):162–76.

37. Siddiqui IA, Sabah SA, Satchithananda K, et al. A comparison of the diagnostic accuracy of MARS MRI and ultrasound of the painful metal-on-metal hip arthroplasty. Acta Orthop 2014;85(4): 375–82.

38. Gillet R, Teixeira P, Bonarelli C, et al. Comparison of radiographs, tomosynthesis and CT with metal artifact reduction for the detection of hip prosthetic loosening. Eur Radiol 2019;29(3):1258–66.

39. Robinson E, Henckel J, Sabah S, et al. Cross-sectional imaging of metal-on-metal hip arthroplasties. Can we substitute MARS MRI with CT? Acta Orthop 2014;85(6):577–84.

40. Ghodasara N, Yi PH, Clark K, et al. Postoperative spinal CT: what the radiologist needs to know. Radiographics 2019;39(6):1840–61.

41. Khodarahmi I, Haroun RR, Lee M, et al. Metal artifact reduction computed tomography of arthroplasty implants: effects of combined modeled iterative reconstruction and dual-energy virtual monoenergetic extrapolation at higher photon energies. Invest Radiol 2018;53(12):728–35.

42. Khodarahmi I, Fishman EK, Fritz J. Dedicated CT and MRI techniques for the evaluation of the postoperative knee. Semin Musculoskelet Radiol 2018; 22(4):444–56.

43. Rowe SP, Fritz J, Fishman EK. CT evaluation of musculoskeletal trauma: initial experience with cinematic rendering. Emerg Radiol 2018;25(1):93–101.

44. Bäcker HC, Steurer-Dober I, Beck M, et al. Magnetic resonance imaging (MRI) versus single photon emission computed tomography (SPECT/CT) in painful total hip arthroplasty: a comparative multi-institutional analysis. Br J Radiol 2020;93(1105): 20190738.

45. Li AE, Sneag DB, Miller TT, et al. MRI of polyethylene tibial inserts in total knee arthroplasty: normal and abnormal appearances. Am J Roentgenol 2016; 206(6):1264–71.

46. Germann C, Filli L, Jungmann PM, et al. Prospective and longitudinal evolution of post-operative periprosthetic findings on metal artifact-reduced MR imaging in asymptomatic patients after uncemented total hip arthroplasty. Skeletal Radiol 2021;50(6): 1177–88.

47. Porrino J, Wang A, Moats A, et al. Prosthetic joint infections: diagnosis, management, and complications of the two-stage replacement arthroplasty. Skeletal Radiol 2020;49(6):847–59.

48. Siljander MP, Sobh AH, Baker KC, et al. Multidrug-resistant organisms in the setting of periprosthetic joint infection-diagnosis, prevention, and treatment. J Arthroplasty 2018;33(1):185–94.

49. Bozic KJ, Kurtz SM, Lau E, et al. The epidemiology of revision total hip arthroplasty in the United States. J Bone Joint Surg Am 2009;91(1):128–33.

50. Sadoghi P, Liebensteiner M, Agreiter M, et al. Revision surgery after total joint arthroplasty: a complication-based analysis using worldwide arthroplasty registers. J Arthroplasty 2013;28(8): 1329–32.

51. Fritz B, Parkar AP, Cerezal L, et al. Sports imaging of team handball injuries. Semin Musculoskelet Radiol 2020;24(3):227–45.

52. Hasija R, Kelly JJ, Shah NV, et al. Nerve injuries associated with total hip arthroplasty. J Clin Orthop Trauma 2018;9(1):81–6.

53. Ahlawat S, Stern SE, Belzberg AJ, et al. High-resolution metal artifact reduction MR imaging of the lumbosacral plexus in patients with metallic implants. Skeletal Radiol 2017;46(7):897–908.

54. Farshad-Amacker NA, Nanz D, Thanbanbalasingam A, et al. 3-T MRI implant safety: heat induction with new dual-channel radiofrequency transmission technology. Eur Radiol Exp 2018;2(1):7.

55. Nawabi DH, Hayter CL, Su EP, et al. Magnetic resonance imaging findings in symptomatic versus asymptomatic subjects following metal-on-metal hip resurfacing arthroplasty. J Bone Joint Surg Am 2013;95(10):895–902.

56. Nawabi DH, Nassif NA, Do HT, et al. What causes unexplained pain in patients with metal-on metal hip devices? A retrieval, histologic, and imaging analysis. Clin Orthop Relat Res® 2014;472(2): 543–54.

57. Kavalar R, Fokter SK, Lamovec J. Total hip arthroplasty-related osteogenic osteosarcoma: case report and review of the literature. Eur J Med Res 2016;21:8.

58. Visuri T, Pulkkinen P, Paavolainen P. Malignant tumors at the site of total hip prosthesis. Analytic review of 46 cases. J Arthroplasty 2006;21(3):311–23.

59. Fritz J, Fishman EK, Corl F, et al. Imaging of limb salvage surgery. Am J Roentgenol 2012;198(3): 647–60.

60. Jungmann PM, Bensler S, Zingg P, et al. Improved visualization of juxtaprosthetic tissue using metal artifact reduction magnetic resonance imaging: experimental and clinical optimization of compressed sensing SEMAC. Invest Radiol 2019;54(1): 23–31.

61. Susa M, Oguro S, Kikuta K, et al. Novel MR imaging method–MAVRIC–for metal artifact suppression after joint replacement in musculoskeletal tumor patients. BMC Musculoskelet Disord 2015;16:377.

62. Feng DX, McCauley JP, Morgan-Curtis FK, et al. Evaluation of 39 medical implants at 7.0 T. Br J Radiol 2015;88(1056):20150633.

63. Dula AN, Virostko J, Shellock FG. Assessment of MRI issues at 7 T for 28 implants and other objects. Am J Roentgenol 2014;202(2):401–5.

Postoperative MRI of Shoulder Instability

Mohammad Samim, MD, MRCS[a],*, Soterios Gyftopoulos, MD, MBA, MSc[a,b]

KEYWORDS

- Anterior shoulder instability • Surgery • MRI • Bankart repair • Latarjet • Complications

KEY POINTS

- Most current treatment guidelines for anterior shoulder instability require preoperative imaging measurements of glenoid, humeral, and/or bipolar bone loss to determine surgical approach based on engaging and/or on- or off-track bipolar bone loss.
- Various surgical options, which are performed in isolation or combined, include Bankart repair, glenoid bone reconstruction, such as Latarjet procedure, remplissage, capsular shift/reefing, and ultimately, reverse shoulder arthroplasty.
- Patients with glenoid bone loss of less than 25% and anterior inferior labral tear are typically treated with Bankart labral repair, whereas those with glenoid bone loss greater than 25% are treated with glenoid bone augmentation procedure.
- The remplissage is typically performed for patients with engaging Hill-Sachs lesion with size greater than 20% of humeral head articular surface.
- Familiarity with various operative techniques and the normal postoperative imaging appearances and complications is essential for correct imaging interpretation.

INTRODUCTION

Glenohumeral instability is characterized as excessive motion of the humeral head over the glenoid, causing functional deficit.[1] Anterior shoulder dislocation is the most common form of traumatic shoulder instability, comprising 90% of all shoulder dislocations.[1] Although first time acute dislocation occurs usually as the result of a significant traumatic event, such as a fall on an outstretched arm with the arm in abduction and external rotation, recurrent multiple shoulder dislocations can recur following more minor traumatic events. This in part is owing to chronic shoulder joint laxity and instability resulting from repetitive and chronic injury to the static and/or dynamic joint stabilizers or osseous injuries to the glenohumeral joint.[2–4]

Surgical treatment options for shoulder instability and postoperative outcomes depend on the accurate preoperative assessment of the patient,

including the correct imaging characterization of the glenoid and humeral bone injuries.[5–8] Studies have shown that inaccurate and underestimated assessment of the extent of bone injury leading to inadequate treatment during surgery can result in higher risk of recurrent instability following surgery.[9,10] Therefore, most current treatment guidelines for anterior shoulder instability require preoperative imaging measurements of glenoid, humeral, and/or bipolar bone loss to help determine surgical approach based on whether the Hill-Sachs lesion is engaging and/or the bipolar bone loss is on or off track.[11,12]

Following shoulder instability surgery, patients may still present with recurrent instability even when the correct surgical option was performed. These patients may undergo imaging that highlights the necessity for radiologists to be able to assess the integrity of the repaired tissues, such as the repaired labrum, capsule, or tendon, and

[a] Department of Radiology, NYU Langone Medical Center, 301 East 17th Street, Room 600, New York, NY 10003, USA; [b] Department of Orthopedic Surgery, NYU Langone Orthopedic Center, 333 East 38th Street, New York, NY 10016, USA
* Corresponding author.
E-mail address: Mohammad.samim@nyulangone.org

Magn Reson Imaging Clin N Am 30 (2022) 601–615
https://doi.org/10.1016/j.mric.2022.02.003
1064-9689/22/© 2022 Elsevier Inc. All rights reserved.

orthopedic fixation hardware or grafts to evaluate for complications, such as loosening, fracture, or displacement of hardware or graft nonunion.

First, the authors provide an overview of the current treatment guidelines and options for the patient with anterior shoulder instability. Next, they review the normal and abnormal postoperative imaging appearances of the glenohumeral joint after treatment with the most common surgical stabilization techniques.

ANTERIOR SHOULDER INSTABILITY TREATMENT OPTION AND GUIDELINES

There are various factors that determine the optimal surgical option for a patient with anterior shoulder instability. Imaging, most notably MR imaging, has a key role in the preoperative evaluation of patients with traumatic anterior shoulder instability by demonstrating the typical soft tissue injuries, such as labral or capsular tears, and bone injuries, anterior glenoid bone loss, and Hill-Sachs impaction injuries. MR imaging, as well as computed tomography (CT), also allows for the accurate quantification of these bone injuries, referred to together as bipolar bone loss. The current biomechanical concepts determining surgical management of shoulder instability focus primarily on this bipolar bone loss quantification, which in turn determines if there is an engaging versus nonengaging Hill-Sachs injury or if the bipolar bone loss is considered "on-track" versus "off-track."[12,13]

In the "engaging and nonengaging" concept, the Hill-Sachs lesion is considered engaging if during dynamic intraoperative assessment the long axis of the humeral defect comes to lie parallel to and engages the anterior glenoid in a physiologic position of abduction and external rotation. In nonengaging lesions, the axis of the Hill-Sachs lesion remains nonparallel, and the lesion does not engage with the glenoid.[14] Arthroscopic repair is considered appropriate treatment for nonengaging lesions, whereas a capsular shift or bone graft may be required for engaging lesions.[13,14] The concept has become less popular recently because of various reasons, such as how most bipolar lesions can potentially engage if enough force is applied and/or the shoulder is placed in a nonphysiologic shoulder position during evaluation, which may lead to overdiagnosis of engagement.[15] In addition, if this assessment method is applied following Bankart repair to test if the preexisting engagement was eliminated, it would put the new repair at risk. Finally, this assessment method is purely a qualitative approach.[13]

The "on-track versus off-track" theory is based on a comparison between the Hill-Sachs interval and glenoid track, defined as the contact area between the humeral head and glenoid during shoulder abduction and external rotation and typically estimated as 83% of the glenoid width, that is used to predict recurrent instability.[12,16] If the Hill-Sachs interval is less than the glenoid track, the Hill-Sachs would maintain contact with the glenoid articular surface and is considered "on-track," which translates into less risk of engagement and instability. If the Hill-Sachs lesion is greater than the glenoid track, this would lead to reduced contact with the opposing glenoid articular surface. This is considered "off-track" and is thought to translate into increased risk of engagement and instability. This assessment can be performed on both CT and MR imaging.[12,17]

There are various surgical options available to treat anterior shoulder instability, which can be performed in isolation or combined. These include Bankart repair, glenoid bone reconstruction, such as Latarjet procedure, remplissage, capsular shift/reefing, and ultimately, reverse shoulder arthroplasty, which is usually reserved for elderly patients. Based on the glenoid track theory, a classification system has been proposed and accepted to guide surgical options.[12] The goal of surgery is essentially to convert the "off-track" lesions to "on-track." Patients with anterior shoulder instability are categorized into 4 groups with recommended treatment options for each (**Fig. 1**).[12] Surgeons may consider other factors as well to choose the appropriate surgery for their patients.

For instance, high-demand patients like professional athletes may undergo more advanced stabilization surgery relative to the size of their bone injuries, including open reduction and internal fixation for acute injuries or the Latarjet procedure variants for more chronic injuries, to decrease the chances of recurrent instability.[11,18]

In the next section, the authors review the surgical options for the patient with anterior shoulder instability and their typical postoperative appearances. The radiologist should be familiar with these surgical options and the treatment classifications/algorithms for this patient group in order to better understand and interpret postoperative shoulder instability imaging studies.

Bankart Labral Repair

Indication
Patients with anterior shoulder instability, glenoid bone loss of less than 25%, and anterior inferior labral tear are typically treated with Bankart labral

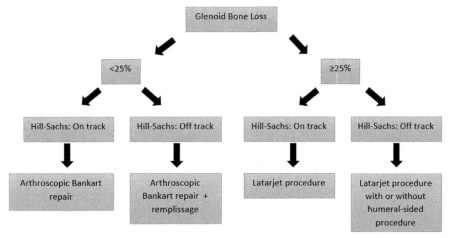

Fig. 1. The surgical treatment algorithm of anterior shoulder instability with bipolar bone lesion based on glenoid track status.

repair, with 0% to 7% rate of postoperative recurrent instability.[19–21]

Surgical technique

During Bankart labral repair, the torn and detached labrum is reattached surgically to the glenoid using anchor screws and sutures. If torn, the anteroinferior glenohumeral ligament may also be reattached to the glenoid.[8,22] Capsular shift plication surgery, which is essentially tightening of glenohumeral joint capsule after making a T-shaped incision and shifting of the capsule leaflets, is often performed with Bankart repair.[23] This procedure can be performed open or arthroscopically.

Postoperative imaging

MR arthrography is considered the ideal modality to evaluate the integrity of the labrum and capsule following Bankart repair.[24–27] On the postoperative MR imaging, intact repaired labrum and ligament should be present and reattached to the anteroinferior glenoid (**Fig. 2**).[28] The inhomogeneous signal and variable morphology of the repaired labrum or ligament, such as rounded, enlarged, or irregular frayed morphology, should be considered normal as long as the repaired tissue remains intact and continuous with the osseous attachments without gap.[28,29] If additional capsular shift plication surgery was performed, scar tissue formation with

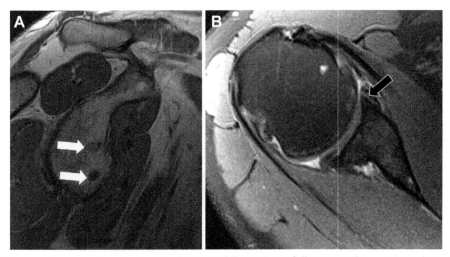

Fig. 2. A 59-year-old man with anterior shoulder instability 8 years following arthroscopic Bankart repair. (*A*) Sagittal T1-weighted and (*B*) axial T2-weighted with fat-suppression MR images show anterior glenoid suture anchors (*white arrows* in *A*) and intact anterior labrum at the region of the anchor (*black arrow* in *B*). Mild heterogeneity of the repaired labrum is an expected postoperative appearance.

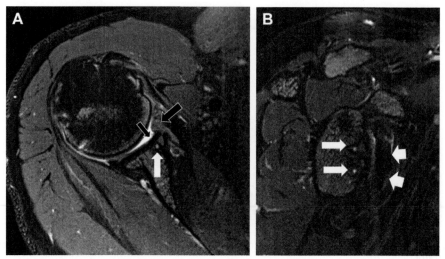

Fig. 3. A 43-year-old man with anterior shoulder instability 6 months following arthroscopic Bankart repair. (A) Axial T2-weighted with fat-suppression and (B) sagittal proton density with suppression MR images show suture anchors in the glenoid from Bankart repair (*white arrows*) and degenerated retear of the anterior labrum at the region of the anchor (*black arrow* in A). Note full-thickness anterior glenoid cartilage loss (*small black arrow* in A) and postsurgical thickening of the anterior capsule (*short arrows* in B).

thickening and heterogeneous signal along the anterior joint capsule with shortening of the axillary recess can be expected MR imaging findings.[28]

MR imaging findings indicative of recurrent tear of the repaired tissue following Bankart repair include detachment and fragmentation of the repaired labrum, presence of fluid signal in the labrum, or presence of gap between the labrum and the glenoid filled with fluid (**Figs. 3 and 4**). Findings suggestive of recurrent tear in MR arthrogram include imbibition of contrast material into the labrum and presence of gap between the labrum and the glenoid filled with contrast. Pooling of contrast material between the anteroinferior glenohumeral ligament and the glenoid at the site of surgical reattachment on MR arthrogram in the abduction external rotation position has been shown as a reliable secondary finding of retear of repaired anterior inferior labrum.[26]

The hardware used in Bankart repair, specifically anchor, screw, and suture material, should be assessed for loosening and displacement/dislodgment into the joint or surrounding soft tissues. Displacement of the hardware can also lead to mechanical impingement symptoms or cartilage damage if the hardware is found in the glenohumeral joint space (**Fig. 5**).[28,29] Chemical synovitis and foreign body reaction are known potential complications of using bioabsorbable screws and anchors.[30] Other possible complications of Bankart repair include infection, secondary osteoarthritis (see **Fig. 3**), and axillary nerve injury specifically after open stabilizing

procedure.[28] Following anterior capsular shift plication surgery, relative widening of the posterior capsule and posterior subluxation of the humeral head can be seen due to overtightening of the anterior joint capsule, whereas a large anterior capsular recess and rotator interval can be manifestations of insufficient capsular tightening.[28,31]

Assessment of osseous structures should be part of routine evaluation in all postoperative MR imaging examinations following shoulder instability surgery. In particular, the presence of osseous signs of recurrent anterior shoulder instability, including bone marrow edema pattern along the anterior glenoid and posterior humeral head or increased size of glenoid bone loss or Hill-Sachs lesion compared with preoperative imaging, should be highlighted.

Acute Reduction and Internal Fixation

Indication
In most patients, if the glenoid bone loss is greater than 25%, reduction and internal fixation may be the choice of treatment in the setting of acute glenoid fracture. A lower threshold to treat of less than 25% can be used in high-functional-demand patients, such as professional athletes. In these settings, the glenoid fracture ideally is not comminuted, making it easier to reattach to the anterior glenoid.

Surgical technique
Reduction and internal fixation can be performed via an open or arthroscopy approach. The fracture

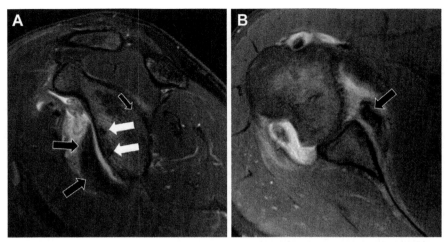

Fig. 4. A 29-year-old man with anterior shoulder instability 6 months following arthroscopic Bankart repair and remplissage. (*A*) Sagittal proton density with fat-suppression and (*B*) axial T2 with fat-suppression MR images show suture anchors in the glenoid from prior Bankart repair (*white arrows*) and retear of the anterior labrum with complete detachment of the thickened and scarred labrocapsular tissue (*black arrows*) with interposing fluid gap.

fragment is placed along the anterior glenoid in as close to an anatomic alignment as possible and fixed using screws.[11,32]

Postoperative imaging
The healing and alignment of the fracture can be assessed using serial radiographs or CT following surgery. With timely treatment, good fracture healing with restoration of the articular surface congruity of the glenoid can be expected.[28]

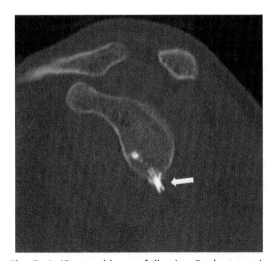

Fig. 5. A 43-year-old man following Bankart repair. Sagittal CT image shows a metallic anchor, which is partially extruded from anteroinferior glenoid (*arrow*).

Bristow and Latarjet Procedures

Indication
When chronic glenoid bone loss is greater than 25%, a glenoid bone augmentation procedure is typically indicated.[11] As mentioned previously, high-functional-demand patients maybe be indicated for glenoid bone augmentation in the presence of glenoid bone loss of less than 25%. In this population, bone augmentation can reduce the likelihood of postoperative recurrent anterior instability compared with Bankart repair.[13,33] The most commonly used glenoid augmentation procedures are the Bristow and Latarjet procedures.[34]

Surgical technique
Both Latarjet and Bristow procedures were originally described as open surgeries in 1954 and 1958, respectively,[35,36] with the arthroscopic approach becoming more popular in recent years.[37] Although both procedures have similarities, there are certain differences between the two. Hence, they should not be considered one procedure. In both procedures, using a surgical incision through the subscapularis muscle, the ipsilateral autologous coracoid bone block with attached conjoined tendon (biceps brachii and coracobrachialis) is harvested and attached to the anterior glenoid. The attached conjoined tendon acts as a dynamic stabilizer, which prevents anterior subluxation and simulates the function of the inferior glenohumeral ligament.[29,38]

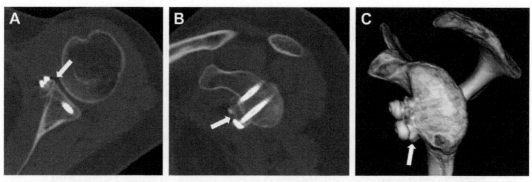

Fig. 6. A 29-year-old man with recurrent anterior shoulder instability underwent the Latarjet procedure. (*A*) Axial and (*B*) sagittal CT images show incorporated graft (*arrows*) with mature osseous bridging with the native glenoid and 2 screws with no signs of hardware failure. Notice the graft is flushed with the normal curvature of the glenoid on axial image. (*C*) Three-dimensional volume-rendered reconstructed CT image shows the position of the incorporated graft and the 2 associated screws.

There are, however, certain differences between the Bristow and Latarjet procedures. In the Bristow procedure, only the lateral tip of the coracoid process is transferred, and the graft is attached to the glenoid via its resected surface. During the Latarjet procedure, the entire horizontal coracoid pillar is transferred, and the graft is attached to the glenoid via inferior surface of the coracoid bone block and not the cut surface. As a result, the Bristow procedure's smaller coracoid bone block is typically fixed with a single screw, whereas the Latarjet procedure's larger coracoid bone block requires 2 screws for attachment to the glenoid. This larger bone block allows surgeons to reconstruct larger regions of glenoid bone loss and achieve more stability and successful union.[34]

The arthroscopic Latarjet procedure has been getting more attention in recent years. It is a technically demanding procedure that requires advanced arthroscopic skills. During the conventional arthroscopic approach, the anterior capsule is resected, whereas in the open Latarjet procedure, the anterior capsule is preserved and often reinforced.[29,34] Newer arthroscopic approaches, however, include anterior capsular reconstruction.[39] Regardless of their differences, efficacy of arthroscopic Latarjet in treating anterior shoulder instability in terms of recurrent instability rate is comparable to those of the open approach.[40,41]

There are alternative operative techniques for glenoid augmentation using other graft options, such as iliac crest autograft (Eden-Hybinette procedure), distal clavicle autograft, and cadaveric allograft.[42–45] These alternative procedures accomplish the primary goal of glenoid bone augmentation by replacing the glenoid bone defect. These techniques cannot provide the dynamic advantage of the Latarjet and Bristow procedure, which is the intact attached conjoined

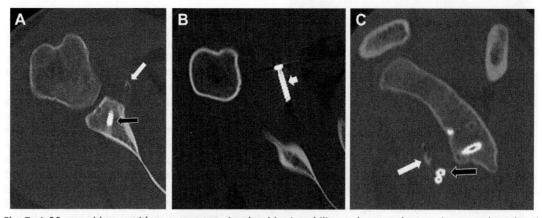

Fig. 7. A 26-year-old man with recurrent anterior shoulder instability underwent the Latarjet procedure. (*A, B*) Axial and (*C*) sagittal CT images show displaced nonunited coracoid graft (*white arrows*) with 1 broken screw (*black arrows*) and 1 screw completely dislodged into the anterior soft tissue (*short white arrow in B*).

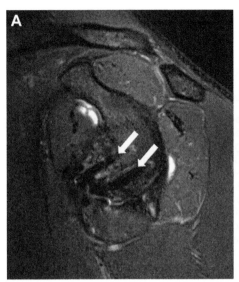
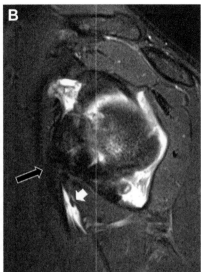

Fig. 8. A 24-year-old man with recurrent anterior shoulder instability underwent the Latarjet procedure. (*A, B*) Sequential sagittal proton density MR images with fat suppression show 2 screws (*white arrow*) transfixing the graft to the glenoid. The intact conjoined tendon attached to the coracoid graft (*black arrow*) has a role of dynamic stabilizer. There is a small adventitial bursa (*short white arrow* in *B*) formed between the graft and the conjoined tendon.

tendon to the coracoid graft.[29] In addition, these other autografts have additional postoperative morbidities mainly from the graft harvest site. Therefore, the Bristow and Latarjet procedures remain the first-line glenoid bone augmentation procedures.

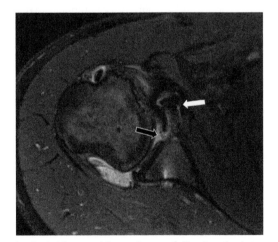

Fig. 9. A 36-year-old man 2 years following the Latarjet procedure with recurrent anterior shoulder instability. Axial proton density MR image with fat suppression shows partially dislodged screw with susceptibly artifact (*white arrow*). Note there is a fluid-filled cleft (*black arrow*) between the graft and the glenoid indicating nonunion. There is joint effusion and synovitis in the posterior joint recess.

Postoperative imaging

Radiographs and CT are the main imaging modalities to evaluate the graft status following Latarjet and Bristow procedures. The hardware position and the graft alignment and incorporation are routinely assessed with serial postoperative radiographs. Main potential complications of both procedures are the nonunion of the coracoid graft and hardware loosening or fracture. CT with new metal reduction technique allows optimal imaging assessment of healing and incorporation of the graft to the native glenoid and the integrity of the fixation screws (**Fig. 6**).[28] The fusion of the graft can be assessed qualitatively[46] or quantitatively[47] using CT. Although there is no certain definition of complete union in coracoid grafts, complete union has been suggested when there is fusion over more than 67% of its length.[47,48] It is important to know that not all patients with incomplete graft osseous union have postoperative pain or instability.[46] Fibrous union and delayed osseous union after many years have been shown in patients following Latarjet procedure with no signs of shoulder instability.[46,47] Therefore, union status of the graft should be interpreted within the clinical context considering patient symptoms after surgery.

Graft position is the most important factor determining technical success of the bone augmentation procedures[49] and should be evaluated on radiograph and CT. The ideal graft position should

Table 1
The surgical treatment algorithm of Hill-Sachs lesion based on the size of the lesion[61]

Hill-Sachs Lesion Size Involves % of Humeral Head Articular Surface	<20	20–40	>40
Treatment option	Nonoperative treatment	Smaller size lesions: remplissage, reduction Larger lesions: osteochondral allograft, partial arthroplasty Factors to consider: location and orientation of the lesion, glenoid bone loss, engagement, patient demand on joint, patient activity level, and age	Osteochondral allograft, partial arthroplasty, hemiarthroplasty

be flushed with the normal curvature of the native glenoid (see **Fig. 6**).[47] Complications can arise from suboptimal positioning of the graft, including nonunion (**Fig. 7**) and glenohumeral osteoarthritis when there is lateral positioning of the graft,[50] or recurrent instability with a medially positioned graft.[51] The graft position can be more accurately assessed using CT than radiography. The role of MR imaging has not been completely explored in the postoperative imaging assessment of Latarjet and Bristow procedures. Because of the presence of screws at the surgical site, images can be distorted from hardware artifact. Newer metal reduction techniques may allow improved image quality and assessment of the osseous fusion (**Figs. 8** and **9**).

Postoperative imaging evaluation should include search for other potential complications of Latarjet and Bristow procedure, including fracture of the graft, acute detachment of the subscapularis tendon, fatty degeneration of the subscapularis muscle in the chronic setting, infection, and secondary or accelerated osteoarthritis.[28,52,53]

OUTCOME

Systemic reviews have shown improved outcomes following Bankart repair in short- and long-term follow-up.[54,55] A recent systemic review of long-term outcomes of the arthroscopic Bankart repair at 10-year follow-up showed excellent long-term functional outcomes. Overall, 77.6% of athletes were able to return to sports postoperatively. The overall rate of recurrent instability was 31.2%, and the overall revision rate was

17.0%.[55] Almost 60% of patients had evidence of instability arthropathy with 10.5% of patients having moderate to severe arthropathy. Another recent meta-analysis comparing Bankart repair to Latarjet procedure showed that Bankart repair was associated with a higher risk of recurrent anterior shoulder instability and a lower risk of infection compared with Latarjet.[56]

Studies have confirmed significantly lower rates of recurrent instability for the common glenoid augmentation procedures (7.5% for Bristow and Latarjet procedures, 9.8% for Eden-Hybinette procedure) compared with the Bankart labral repair,[57] with a pronounced advantage for Latarjet from 6 to 10 years postoperatively in terms of recurrent shoulder instability.[56] The most important predictor of postoperative outcome has been shown to be the degree of glenoid bone loss. Recurrent instability following Bankart repair remains low (4%) for patients with insignificant glenoid bone loss, whereas it will increase substantially (35%–89%) in patients with significant glenoid bone loss (defined as engaging bone loss or when glenoid appeared as inverted pear during arthroscopy).[14] Rate of postoperative osteoarthritis development was not significantly different between the Bankart labral repair and glenoid augmentation procedures.[57]

MANAGEMENT OF HILL-SACHS LESION

Hill-Sachs lesions are present in 67% to 93% of first time anterior shoulder instability patients and can be seen in almost 100% of patients with recurrent anterior instability.[58,59] The Hill-Sachs impaction may vary in shape, depth, width, and

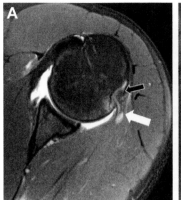 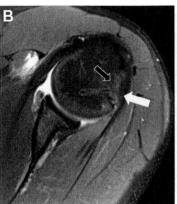 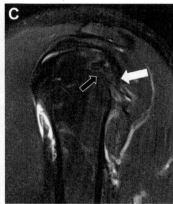

Fig. 10. A 29-year-old man with anterior shoulder instability 6 months following remplissage. (*A, B*) axial T2-weighted with fat suppression and (*C*) sagittal proton density with suppression MR images show changes related to infraspinatus tenodesis and remplissage (*white arrows*) fixed with an anchor in humeral head. There is complete filling of the defect by the intact remplissage soft tissue (*black arrows*) with no fluid pooling in the defect.

orientation with each presentation treated differently but not in isolation when concomitant labral tear and glenoid bone loss are present. It is still challenging to definitively determine which Hill-Sachs lesions are clinically significant, partly because there is no consensus on the method of evaluation of the size of defect that may cause recurrent instability.[59,60] Traditionally, Hill-Sachs lesions involving less than 25% of the humeral head surface are considered insignificant in isolation.[61] More recent studies, however, have shown that even a small Hill-Sachs lesion can become clinically significant in the presence of concomitant glenoid bone loss and cause engagement with the glenoid.[62] The importance and treatment options of the Hill-Sachs lesion can be assessed based on clinical evaluation, imaging characteristics such as percentage of humeral bone loss (Table1),[61] or most recently based on the glenoid track concept (see **Fig. 1**). Regardless of the method, in this section, the authors review the surgical treatment options of the Hill-Sachs lesion.

Remplissage

Indication
Remplissage is a French term that means "filling," and the remplissage procedure is the filling of the Hill-Sachs defect using joint capsule and infraspinatus tendon.[61] The remplissage is used for patients with engaging Hill-Sachs lesion with mild glenoid bone loss, and it is most typically

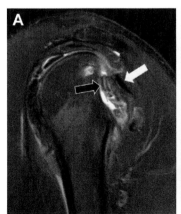 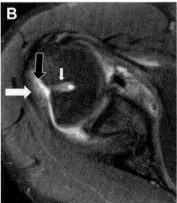 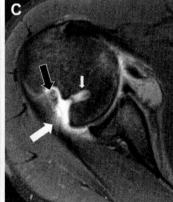

Fig. 11. A 29-year-old man with anterior shoulder instability 6 months following arthroscopic Bankart repair and remplissage (same patient as **Fig. 3**). (*A*) Sagittal proton density with fat-suppression, (*B, C*) axial T2-weighted with fat-suppression MR images show changes related to infraspinatus tenodesis and remplissage (*long white arrows*) with soft tissue only partially filling the large Hill-Sachs defect (*black arrows*). Fluid fills almost 50% of the defect compatible with grade 2 pooling indicating failure of the remplissage. Notice fluid and synovitis extends into the anchor tracts suggestive of loosening (*short white arrows*).

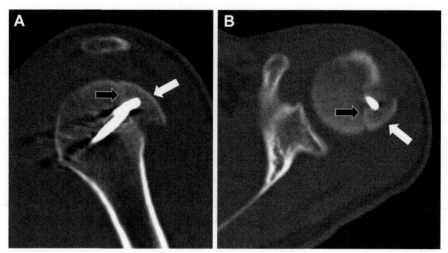

Fig. 12. A 20-year-old man with anterior shoulder instability 4 months following humeral head reconstruction using size-matched bulk allografts. (*A*) Sagittal and (*B*) axial CT images show size-matched bulk allograft being fitted in the chevron osteotomy in the Hill-Sachs defect (*white arrows*) transfixed with 2 screws. The graft is partially incorporated shown as areas of osseous bridging (*black arrows*).

performed in conjunction with an arthroscopic or open Bankart repair.[12]

Remplissage has been associated with lower recurrence rates of instability and improved outcome scores. The recurrence rates for a remplissage and concurrent Bankart repair range from 0% to 8%.[63,64] A potential disadvantage associated with remplissage is the anatomic alteration of rotator cuff muscles. As a result, there has been growing evidence demonstrating that

remplissage can lead to loss of internal-external range of motion and increase in joint stiffness.[65,66]

Surgical technique
This arthroscopic technique involves fixing the joint capsule (capsulodesis) and infraspinatus (tenodesis) with suture anchors along the humeral head defect.[62] The goal of this technique is to convert the Hill-Sachs defect from an intraarticular to an extraarticular defect, thus lowering the

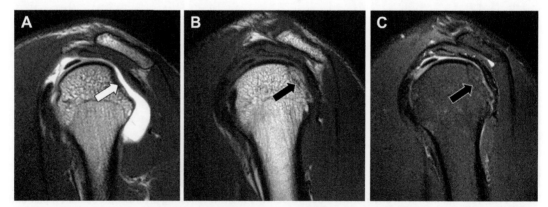

Fig. 13. A 24-year-old man with anterior shoulder instability before and 3 years following osteochondral allograft to the Hill-Sachs defect. (*A*) Coronal T1 arthrogram MR image shows large Hill-Sachs defect in the posterior superior humeral head (*white arrow*). (*B*) Coronal T1 and (*C*) coronal T2 fat-suppressed MR images 3 years after osteochondral allograft show fully incorporated graft filling the defect (*black arrow*) with mature osseous bridging and no marrow edema pattern or deep cystic changes.

chance of humeral head engagement along the glenoid rim, which can predispose to recurrent instability.[61]

Postoperative imaging

MR imaging of an intact remplissage procedure should demonstrate tenodesis of the infraspinatus tendon and the tendon and capsule closely filling the Hill-Sachs defect transfixed with suture anchors (**Fig. 10**).[29] Partial and complete dehiscence of soft tissue remplissage can manifest as the presence of joint fluid or contrast material pooling between the Hill-Sachs defect and the soft tissue. Rhee and colleagues[67] proposed an MR imaging grading system based on the filling index score of remplissage, which refers to the extent of contrast agent pooling in the Hill-Sachs defect on a 5-point scale on both axial and sagittal MR images:

- Grade 0: Filling failure with complete dehiscence when contrast agent pooling with complete separation of tenodesis and a large fluid gap
- Grade 1: Minimal filling with soft tissue with significant fluid level
- Grade 2: Partial filling with soft tissue with major defect and substantial contrast agent pooling in ≥50% of the whole length of the defect
- Grade 3: Partial filling with soft tissue with minor defect and minimal contrast agent pooling in less than 50% of the whole length of the defect
- Grade 4: Complete filling of the defect by soft tissue and no contrast agent pooling

The filling index score of remplissage grades 3 to 4 is indicative of an intact remplissage on a postoperative MR arthrogram, whereas grades 0 to 2 may indicate failed remplissage (**Fig. 11**). The investigators acknowledged that this grading system may not correlate with patient symptoms in short-term follow-up, and long-term follow-up studies are needed to validate the association of the status of the remplissage and patient outcomes.[67]

Humeral Head Reconstruction

Indication

Reconstruction of the humeral head is usually reserved for humeral bone loss greater than 40% of humeral head articular surface in young active patients.[11] For this purpose, cadaveric allograft or humeral head prosthetic cap has been used after matching the graft with the defect. There are 2 main cadaveric allograft options, osteochondral plug transfers and size-matched bulk grafts.[29]

The humeral head allograft reconstruction has been shown to restore joint biomechanics better than other procedures, including reduction and remplissage.[66,68] In a cohort study involving 18 patients who underwent open osteochondral allograft reconstruction, the investigators reported less favorable outcomes, such as osteoarthritis, partial graft collapse, and mild subluxation, although 89% of patients were able to return to work with no recurrent instability.[69] Snir and colleagues,[70] using a purely arthroscopic approach to osteochondral allograft reconstruction, were able to restore the native articular surface without compromising the shoulder's range of motion.

Surgical technique

For the osteochondral allograft reconstruction, the surgeon resects a cylindric-shaped osteochondral plug from a cadaver specimen and prepares the recipient humeral head by performing an osteotomy. The plug is subsequently trimmed to match the size and shape of the prepared osteotomy and is inserted into the osteotomy socket.[70,71] For the size-matched bulk allografts, the surgeon first performs a chevron osteotomy in the Hill-Sachs defect, and subsequently a size-matched cadaveric osteochondral allograft is made and transferred to fit the osteotomy. Allografts are usually fixed using fixation screws.

Postoperative imaging

Radiographs are routinely used to assess the graft status following surgery. Alignment of the graft should ideally be flushed or slightly above the native humeral head.[72] CT scan or MR imaging is usually done if patients remain or become symptomatic after surgery (**Figs. 12 and 13**). In early postoperative stages, sclerosis and marrow edema pattern of the graft can be expected on CT scan and MR imaging. In fact, bone marrow edema pattern in the graft and/or surrounding recipient bone can be present in 50% of asymptomatic patients and can persist for up to 3 years in a smaller subset of patients.[73] Joint effusion up to 2 years and small gaps at the bone-graft interface up to 3 years after surgery can be seen in asymptomatic patients before complete incorporation of the graft.[73] Signs suggestive of graft failure are graft motion or malalignment, worsening step-off, gradual increase in bone marrow edema pattern, collapse of the graft, osteonecrosis, and malalignment of the graft and progression of osteoarthritis.[72,73]

Hill-Sachs Reduction

There are multiple different techniques to fill or repair the Hill-Sachs defect. In a novel technique, surgeons tried to carefully raise the cortical surface of the humerus in small increments using bone tamp.[74] When the near normal articular congruity was achieved, the void was backfilled with injectable calcium phosphate bone cement through a separate tunnel. This technique has been shown to cause less shoulder stiffness and better range of motion after surgery compared with remplissage owing to its ability to preserve local anatomy while yielding similar results.[74]

SUMMARY

The selection of the most appropriate treatment option for the patient with anterior glenohumeral instability depends on several factors, such as extent of soft tissue injury and whether concomitant osseous injuries exist at the glenoid and humeral head. Familiarity with and understanding of the different operative techniques and their indications, the expected postoperative imaging appearances, and potential complications will help in the appropriate interpretation of these imaging studies.

CLINICS CARE POINTS

- Following Bankart repair, MR imaging or MR arthrogram should be evaluated for findings indicative of recurrent tear, including detachment and fragmentation of the repaired labrum, presence of fluid signal or contrast in the labrum, or fluid- or contrast-filled gap between the labrum and the glenoid. Inhomogeneous signal and variable morphology of the repaired labrum can be normal postoperative findings.

- presence of a bone marrow edema pattern along the anterior glenoid and posterior humeral head or increased size of glenoid bone loss or Hill-Sachs lesion compared with preoperative imaging is suggestive of recurrent shoulder instability.

- Imaging after Latarjet and Bristow procedures should be evaluated for nonunion of the coracoid graft and hardware loosening or fracture. However, because not all patients with incomplete graft osseous union have postoperative pain or instability, union status of the graft should be interpreted within the clinical context.

- Following remplissage, the presence of joint fluid or contrast material pooling between the Hill-Sachs defect and the infraspinatus soft tissue remplissage is concerning for partial and complete dehiscence of soft tissue.

DISCLOSURE

None of the authors have any pertinent disclosures.

REFERENCES

1. Shah AS, Karadsheh MS, Sekiya JK. Failure of operative treatment for glenohumeral instability: etiology and management. Arthroscopy 2011;27(5):681–94.
2. Porter DA, Birns M, Hobart SJ, et al. Arthroscopic treatment of osseous instability of the shoulder. HSS J 2017;13(3):292–301.
3. Demehri S, Hafezi-Nejad N, Fishman EK. Advanced imaging of glenohumeral instability: the role of MRI and MDCT in providing what clinicians need to know. Emerg Radiol 2017;24(1):95–103.
4. Murray IR, Goudie EB, Petrigliano FA, et al. Functional anatomy and biomechanics of shoulder stability in the athlete. Clin Sports Med 2013;32(4):607–24.
5. Provencher MT, Bhatia S, Ghodadra NS, et al. Recurrent shoulder instability: current concepts for evaluation and management of glenoid bone loss. J Bone Joint Surg Am 2010;92(Suppl 2):133–51.
6. Provencher MT, Ghodadra N, LeClere L, et al. Anatomic osteochondral glenoid reconstruction for recurrent glenohumeral instability with glenoid deficiency using a distal tibia allograft. Arthroscopy 2009;25(4):446–52.
7. Warner JJP, Gill TJ, O'hollerhan JD, et al. Anatomical glenoid reconstruction for recurrent anterior glenohumeral instability with glenoid deficiency using an autogenous tricortical iliac crest bone graft. Am J Sports Med 2006;34(2):205–12.
8. Piasecki DP, Verma NN, Romeo AA, et al. Glenoid bone deficiency in recurrent anterior shoulder instability: diagnosis and management. J Am Acad Orthop Surg 2009;17(8):482–93.
9. Crall TS, Bishop JA, Guttman D, et al. Cost-effectiveness analysis of primary arthroscopic stabilization versus nonoperative treatment for first-time anterior glenohumeral dislocations. Arthrosc J Arthrosc Relat Surg Off Publ Arthrosc Assoc N Am Int Arthrosc Assoc 2012;28(12):1755–65.
10. Owens BD, DeBerardino TM, Nelson BJ, et al. Long-term follow-up of acute arthroscopic Bankart repair for initial anterior shoulder dislocations in young athletes. Am J Sports Med 2009;37(4):669–73.
11. Ramhamadany E, Modi CS. Current concepts in the management of recurrent anterior gleno-humeral joint instability with bone loss. World J Orthop 2016;7(6):343–54.
12. Di Giacomo G, Itoi E, Burkhart SS. Evolving concept of bipolar bone loss and the Hill-Sachs lesion: from "engaging/non-engaging" lesion to "on-track/off-track" lesion. Arthrosc J Arthrosc Relat Surg Off

Publ Arthrosc Assoc N Am Int Arthrosc Assoc 2014; 30(1):90–8.

13. Gulati A, Dessouky R, Wadhwa V, et al. New concepts of radiologic preoperative evaluation of anterior shoulder instability: on-track and off-track lesions. Acta Radiol 2018;59(8):966–72.

14. Burkhart SS, De Beer JF. Traumatic glenohumeral bone defects and their relationship to failure of arthroscopic Bankart repairs: significance of the inverted-pear glenoid and the humeral engaging Hill-Sachs lesion. Arthrosc J Arthrosc Relat Surg Off Publ Arthrosc Assoc N Am Int Arthrosc Assoc 2000;16(7):677–94.

15. Kurokawa D, Yamamoto N, Nagamoto H, et al. The prevalence of a large Hill-Sachs lesion that needs to be treated. J Shoulder Elbow Surg 2013;22(9): 1285–9.

16. Yamamoto N, Itoi E, Abe H, et al. Contact between the glenoid and the humeral head in abduction, external rotation, and horizontal extension: a new concept of glenoid track. J Shoulder Elbow Surg 2007;16(5):649–56.

17. Gyftopoulos S, Beltran LS, Bookman J, et al. MRI evaluation of bipolar bone loss using the on-track off-track method: a feasibility study. AJR Am J Roentgenol 2015;205(4):848–52.

18. Dickens JF, Slaven SE, Cameron KL, et al. Prospective evaluation of glenoid bone loss after first-time and recurrent anterior glenohumeral instability events. Am J Sports Med 2019;47(5):1082–9.

19. Porcellini G, Campi F, Paladini P. Arthroscopic approach to acute bony Bankart lesion. Arthrosc J Arthrosc Relat Surg Off Publ Arthrosc Assoc N Am Int Arthrosc Assoc 2002;18(7):764–9.

20. Millett PJ, Horan MP, Martetschläger F. The "bony Bankart bridge" technique for restoration of anterior shoulder stability. Am J Sports Med 2013;41(3): 608–14.

21. Rowe CR, Patel D, Southmayd WW. The Bankart procedure: a long-term end-result study. J Bone Joint Surg Am 1978;60(1):1–16.

22. Harryman DT, Ballmer FP, Harris SL, et al. Arthroscopic labral repair to the glenoid rim. Arthrosc J Arthrosc Relat Surg Off Publ Arthrosc Assoc N Am Int Arthrosc Assoc 1994;10(1):20–30.

23. Neer CS, Foster CR. Inferior capsular shift for involuntary inferior and multidirectional instability of the shoulder. A preliminary report. J Bone Joint Surg Am 1980;62(6):897–908.

24. Palmer WE, Caslowitz PL. Anterior shoulder instability: diagnostic criteria determined from prospective analysis of 121 MR arthrograms. Radiology 1995;197(3):819–25.

25. Chandnani VP, Yeager TD, DeBerardino T, et al. Glenoid labral tears: prospective evaluation with MRI imaging, MR arthrography, and CT arthrography. AJR Am J Roentgenol 1993;161(6):1229–35.

26. Sugimoto H, Suzuki K, Mihara K, et al. MR arthrography of shoulders after suture-anchor Bankart repair. Radiology 2002;224(1):105–11.

27. Jana M, Srivastava DN, Sharma R, et al. Magnetic resonance arthrography for assessing severity of glenohumeral labroligamentous lesions. J Orthop Surg Hong Kong 2012;20(2):230–5.

28. Woertler K. Multimodality imaging of the postoperative shoulder. Eur Radiol 2007;17(12):3038–55.

29. Beltran LS, Duarte A, Bencardino JT. Postoperative imaging in anterior glenohumeral instability. AJR Am J Roentgenol 2018;211(3):528–37.

30. Burkhart SS. The evolution of clinical applications of biodegradable implants in arthroscopic surgery. Biomaterials 2000;21(24):2631–4.

31. Zlatkin MB. MRI of the postoperative shoulder. Skeletal Radiol 2002;31(2):63–80.

32. Cañete San Pastor P. Arthroscopic reduction and stable fixation of an anterior glenoid fracture with 4 Buttons. Arthrosc Tech 2020;9(9):e1349–55.

33. Rossi LA, Gorodischer T, Brandariz R, et al. High rate of return to sports and low recurrences with the Latarjet procedure in high-risk competitive athletes with glenohumeral instability and a glenoid bone loss <20. Arthrosc Sports Med Rehabil 2020; 2(6):e735–42.

34. Giles JW, Degen RM, Johnson JA, et al. The Bristow and Latarjet procedures: why these techniques should not be considered synonymous. J Bone Joint Surg Am 2014;96(16):1340–8.

35. Latarjet M. [Treatment of recurrent dislocation of the shoulder]. Lyon Chir 1954;49(8):994–7.

36. Helfet AJ. Coracoid transplantation for recurring dislocation of the shoulder. J Bone Joint Surg Br 1958;40-B(2):198–202.

37. Lafosse L, Lejeune E, Bouchard A, et al. The arthroscopic Latarjet procedure for the treatment of anterior shoulder instability. Arthrosc J Arthrosc Relat Surg Off Publ Arthrosc Assoc N Am Int Arthrosc Assoc 2007;23(11):1242.e1–5.

38. Arner JW, Peebles LA, Bradley JP, et al. Anterior shoulder instability management: indications, techniques, and outcomes. Arthrosc J Arthrosc Relat Surg Off Publ Arthrosc Assoc N Am Int Arthrosc Assoc 2020;36(11):2791–3.

39. Zhu YM, Jiang C, Song G, et al. Arthroscopic Latarjet procedure with anterior capsular reconstruction: clinical outcome and radiologic evaluation with a minimum 2-year follow-up. Arthrosc J Arthrosc Relat Surg Off Publ Arthrosc Assoc N Am Int Arthrosc Assoc 2017;33(12):2128–35.

40. Dumont GD, Fogerty S, Rosso C, et al. The arthroscopic Latarjet procedure for anterior shoulder instability: 5-year minimum follow-up. Am J Sports Med 2014;42(11):2560–6.

41. Wong SE, Friedman LGM, Garrigues GE. Arthroscopic Latarjet: indications, techniques, and results.

Arthrosc J Arthrosc Relat Surg Off Publ Arthrosc Assoc N Am Int Arthrosc Assoc 2020;36(8):2044–6.

42. Auffarth A, Kralinger F, Resch H. Anatomical glenoid reconstruction via a J-bone graft for recurrent post-traumatic anterior shoulder dislocation. Oper Orthopadie Traumatol 2011;23(5):453–61.

43. Scheibel M, Nikulka C, Dick A, et al. Autogenous bone grafting for chronic anteroinferior glenoid defects via a complete subscapularis tenotomy approach. Arch Orthop Trauma Surg 2008;128(11):1317–25.

44. Tokish JM, Fitzpatrick K, Cook JB, et al. Arthroscopic distal clavicular autograft for treating shoulder instability with glenoid bone loss. Arthrosc Tech 2014;3(4):e475–81.

45. Sayegh ET, Mascarenhas R, Chalmers PN, et al. Allograft reconstruction for glenoid bone loss in glenohumeral instability: a systematic review. Arthrosc J Arthrosc Relat Surg Off Publ Arthrosc Assoc N Am Int Arthrosc Assoc 2014;30(12):1642–9.

46. Shah AA, Butler RB, Romanowski J, et al. Short-term complications of the Latarjet procedure. JBJS 2012;94(6):495–501.

47. Samim M, Small KM, Higgins LD. Coracoid graft union: a quantitative assessment by computed tomography in primary and revision Latarjet procedure. J Shoulder Elbow Surg 2018;27(8):1475–82.

48. Jones CP, Coughlin MJ, Shurnas PS. Prospective CT scan evaluation of hindfoot nonunions treated with revision surgery and low-intensity ultrasound stimulation. Foot Ankle Int 2006;27(4):229–35.

49. Marion B, Klouche S, Deranlot J, et al. A prospective comparative study of arthroscopic versus mini-open Latarjet procedure with a minimum 2-year follow-up. Arthrosc J Arthrosc Relat Surg 2017;33(2):269–77.

50. Hovelius L, Sandström B, Olofsson A, et al. The effect of capsular repair, bone block healing, and position on the results of the Bristow-Latarjet procedure (study III): long-term follow-up in 319 shoulders. J Shoulder Elbow Surg 2012;21(5):647–60.

51. Lunn JV, Castellano-Rosa J, Walch G. Recurrent anterior dislocation after the Latarjet procedure: outcome after revision using a modified Eden-Hybinette operation. J Shoulder Elbow Surg 2008;17(5):744–50.

52. Scheibel M, Tsynman A, Magosch P, et al. Postoperative subscapularis muscle insufficiency after primary and revision open shoulder stabilization. Am J Sports Med 2006;34(10):1586–93.

53. Millett PJ, Clavert P, Warner JJP. Open operative treatment for anterior shoulder instability: when and why? J Bone Joint Surg Am 2005;87(2):419–32.

54. Gao B, DeFroda S, Bokshan S, et al. Arthroscopic versus open bankart repairs in recurrent anterior shoulder instability: a systematic review of the association between publication date and postoperative

recurrent instability in systematic reviews. Arthroscopy 2020;36(3):862–71.

55. Murphy AI, Hurley ET, Hurley DJ, et al. Long-term outcomes of the arthroscopic Bankart repair: a systematic review of studies at 10-year follow-up. J Shoulder Elbow Surg 2019;28(11):2084–9.

56. Imam MA, Shehata MSA, Martin A, et al. Bankart repair versus Latarjet procedure for recurrent anterior shoulder instability: a systematic review and meta-analysis of 3275 shoulders. Am J Sports Med 2021;49(7):1945–53.

57. Longo UG, Loppini M, Rizzello G, et al. Latarjet, Bristow, and Eden-Hybinette procedures for anterior shoulder dislocation: systematic review and quantitative synthesis of the literature. Arthrosc J Arthrosc Relat Surg Off Publ Arthrosc Assoc N Am Int Arthrosc Assoc 2014;30(9):1184–211.

58. Rowe CR, Zarins B, Ciullo JV. Recurrent anterior dislocation of the shoulder after surgical repair. Apparent causes of failure and treatment. J Bone Joint Surg Am 1984;66(2):159–68.

59. Welsh MF, Willing RT, Giles JW, et al. A rigid body model for the assessment of glenohumeral joint mechanics: influence of osseous defects on range of motion and dislocation. J Biomech 2016;49(4):514–9.

60. Randelli P, Ragone V, Carminati S, et al. Risk factors for recurrence after Bankart repair a systematic review. Knee Surg Sports Traumatol Arthrosc Off J ESSKA 2012;20(11):2129–38.

61. Fox JA, Sanchez A, Zajac TJ, et al. Understanding the Hill-Sachs lesion in its role in patients with recurrent anterior shoulder instability. Curr Rev Musculoskelet Med 2017;10(4):469–79.

62. Provencher MT, Frank RM, Leclere LE, et al. The Hill-Sachs lesion: diagnosis, classification, and management. J Am Acad Orthop Surg 2012;20(4):242–52.

63. Boileau P, O'Shea K, Vargas P, et al. Anatomical and functional results after arthroscopic Hill-Sachs remplissage. J Bone Joint Surg Am 2012;94(7):618–26.

64. Wolf EM, Arianjam A. Hill-Sachs remplissage, an arthroscopic solution for the engaging Hill-Sachs lesion: 2- to 10-year follow-up and incidence of recurrence. J Shoulder Elbow Surg 2014;23(6):814–20.

65. Elkinson I, Giles JW, Faber KJ, et al. The effect of the remplissage procedure on shoulder stability and range of motion: an in vitro biomechanical assessment. J Bone Joint Surg Am 2012;94(11):1003–12.

66. Giles JW, Elkinson I, Ferreira LM, et al. Moderate to large engaging Hill-Sachs defects: an in vitro biomechanical comparison of the remplissage procedure, allograft humeral head reconstruction, and partial resurfacing arthroplasty. J Shoulder Elbow Surg 2012;21(9):1142–51.

67. Rhee YG, Cho NS, Yoo JH, et al. Filling Index Score of Remplissage (FISOR): a useful measurement tool to evaluate structural outcome after remplissage. J Shoulder Elbow Surg 2015;24(4):613–20.

68. Sekiya JK, Wickwire AC, Stehle JH, et al. Hill-Sachs defects and repair using osteoarticular allograft transplantation: biomechanical analysis using a joint compression model. Am J Sports Med 2009;37(12): 2459–66.

69. Miniaci A, Gish MW. Management of anterior glenohumeral instability associated with large Hill–Sachs defects. Tech Shoulder Elb Surg 2004;5(3):170–5.

70. Snir N, Wolfson TS, Hamula MJ, et al. Arthroscopic anatomic humeral head reconstruction with osteochondral allograft transplantation for large Hill-Sachs lesions. Arthrosc Tech 2013;2(3):e289–.

71. Saltzman BM, Riboh JC, Cole BJ, et al. Humeral head reconstruction with osteochondral allograft transplantation. Arthrosc J Arthrosc Relat Surg Off Publ Arthrosc Assoc N Am Int Arthrosc Assoc 2015;31(9):1827–34.

72. Favinger JL, Ha AS, Brage ME, et al. Osteoarticular transplantation: recognizing expected postsurgical appearances and complications. Radiogr Rev Publ Radiol Soc N Am Inc 2015;35(3):780–92.

73. Link TM, Mischung J, Wörtler K, et al. Normal and pathological MR findings in osteochondral autografts with longitudinal follow-up. Eur Radiol 2006; 16(1):88–96.

74. Garcia GH, Degen RM, Bui CNH, et al. Biomechanical comparison of acute Hill-Sachs reduction with remplissage to treat complex anterior instability. J Shoulder Elbow Surg 2017;26(6):1088–96.

Postoperative MR Imaging of the Rotator Cuff

Mohammad A. Alfaqih, MD, DABR®[a],*, William B. Morrison, MD[b]

KEYWORDS

- Postoperative • MR imaging • Complication • Shoulder • Rotator cuff • Repair • Acromioplasty

KEY POINTS

- Thorough understanding of the anatomic rotator cuff repair and the other surgical options for irreparable cuff tears, expected normal postoperative findings, and potential complications is essential for better MR imaging interpretation.
- During the first year after rotator cuff anatomic repair, the appearance of the repaired tendon is variable and does not correlate with clinical prognosis.
- One of the most common complications after rotator cuff repair is retear.

INTRODUCTION

Shoulder pain represents a remarkable burden of disease. It is the third most common musculoskeletal condition for which patients seek medical attention, following low back pain and knee pain. Self-reported estimates of shoulder pain range between 16% and 26% in the general population. In patients with shoulder pain, rotator cuff tears are the most common pathology, representing 65% to 70% of patients.[1]

In symptomatic rotator cuff tears that do not respond to conservative therapy, surgical intervention may be recommended.[2,3] Around 25% of patients may experience persistent or new pain and functional limitation after rotator cuff tendon surgery.[4] The most common etiologies to consider in symptomatic patients after rotator cuff surgery are rotator cuff retear, hardware dislodgement, and postoperative synovitis.[4] Despite advancements in surgical treatments for rotator cuff tears, postoperative retear continues to be a challenge for both reparable and irreparable rotator cuff tears.[5,6] The literature reports a wide range of rotator cuff retear incidence, ranging from 9% to 94%.[4] Predictive factors for rotator cuff repair outcome include the size of the tear at the time

of surgery, the degree of muscle atrophy and fatty infiltration, and the quality of the tendon tissue itself.[7]

Treatment options for symptomatic full-thickness rotator cuff tears include physical therapy, surgical anatomic repair, or reconstructive procedures. Shoulder arthroplasty may be an appropriate option if there is rotator cuff arthropathy. The primary parameters that influence the appropriate treatment choices for symptomatic full-thickness rotator cuff tears are the tear size, rotator cuff muscle atrophy and fatty infiltration, symptom severity, acuity of symptoms, and response to previous conservative treatment.[3] Rotator cuff tears are categorized according to their maximum dimension as small (1 cm), medium (1–3 cm), large (3–5 cm), or massive (equal or greater than 5 cm). Moderate to severe rotator cuff fatty infiltration and muscle atrophy are associated with rotator cuff retear and unfavorable clinical outcomes.[2]

Massive rotator cuff tears are characterized as tears that exceed 5 cm in width or involve 2 or more torn tendons. Massive rotator cuff tears are not always irreparable, because many massive tears may be repaired with advanced surgical techniques. After primary repair of large to

Funded by: SAUARALETR.
[a] King Saud University, College of Medicine, Riyadh 12372, Saudi Arabia; [b] Thomas Jefferson University Hospital, 111 South 11th Street Suite 3350, Philadelphia, PA 19107, USA
* Corresponding author.
E-mail address: MAlfaqih1@ksu.edu.sa

Magn Reson Imaging Clin N Am 30 (2022) 617–627
https://doi.org/10.1016/j.mric.2022.02.004

massive tears, structural failure can develop in up to 25% to 94% of patients within 2 years. Irreparable rotator cuff tears are typically large in size, proximally retracted, have poor tendon quality, and have advanced cuff muscle atrophy and fatty infiltration. Joint preserving options are preferable whenever possible in younger patients without secondary glenohumeral arthritis, advanced acromiohumeral pseudoarthrosis, or pseudoparalysis. Nonsurgical treatment and reverse total shoulder arthroplasty have been established as preferred treatment options for symptomatic rotator cuff arthropathy with relatively sedentary demands, providing acceptable pain and function improvements. Surgical options for irreparable cuff tears include superior capsular reconstruction, graft augmentation, tendon transfer, and subacromial balloon spacer.[8]

The purpose of this article is to demonstrate both normal and abnormal postoperative MR imaging findings of the anatomic rotator cuff repair and the other surgical options for irreparable cuff tears.

NORMAL ANATOMY AND BIOMECHANICS OF NATIVE ROTATOR CUFF

The rotator cuff is a group of 4 muscles that originate from the scapula and insert to the greater and lesser tuberosities of the humerus. The subscapularis muscle originates from the subscapular fossa on the anterior aspect of the scapula and its tendon inserts into the lesser tuberosity. The supraspinatus muscle originates from the supraspinous fossa on the posterior aspect of the scapula and its tendon inserts into the superior facet of the greater tuberosity. The infraspinatus muscle originates from the infraspinous fossa on the posterior aspect of the scapula and its tendon inserts into the middle facet along the posterolateral aspect of the greater tuberosity. The teres minor muscle originates from the lower portion of the infraspinous fossa on the posterior aspect of the scapula and its tendon inserts into the inferior facet of the greater tuberosity. Contrary to popular belief, the supraspinatus footprint is smaller in size, more anteriorly placed, and shared with the infraspinatus, whereas the infraspinatus footprint is substantially bigger than previously assumed.[9]

The force couples of the shoulder are a crucial concept to understand the pathoanatomy of superior humeral migration which occurs with rotator cuff pathology. In an oversimplified view, there are coronal and transverse force couples. In the coronal force couple, the elevator force (deltoid and supraspinatus) must be balanced by the depressor force (infraspinatus, teres minor, and subscapularis). In the transverse force couple, the posterior force (infraspinatus and teres minor) must be balanced by the anterior force (subscapularis). These force couples must work in a precisely coordinated synchronized balance to preserve the geometric center of the glenohumeral joint during static and dynamic status without humeral head translation. The force coupling concept is crucial in the treatment of irreparable rotator cuff tears in which the purpose of the surgery is not necessarily to repair the rotator cuff but rather to balance the force couples.[10–12]

IMAGING MODALITIES AND TECHNIQUES

Radiography is the preferred first imaging modality for post-operative rotator cuff repair.[1] Radiographs are useful to assess the presence of degenerative changes of the glenohumeral joint, superior migration of the humeral head, the extent of previous subacromial decompression, and presence of acromioclavicular (AC) joint disease or os acromiale.[13]

MR imaging is crucial in the evaluation of symptomatic patients who have undergone rotator cuff surgery. In most cases, MR imaging is used to examine the integrity of the rotator cuff and assess for complications such as tendon retear or suture anchor displacement.[13] However, magnetic susceptibility artifacts from screws, metallic anchors, and metallic shavings continue to be an issue in postoperative MR imaging. Metal anchor artifacts are often modest enough that there is no need to alter the MR imaging protocol. If the inhomogeneity of the local magnetic field causes a distortion of the MR image that decreases the accuracy of rotator cuff retear detection, there are protocol modifications that can be useful. These MR imaging protocol modifications include using a lower magnetic field strength, increase receiver bandwidth, using short tau inversion recovery for fluid sensitivity, switching the phase and frequency-encoding directions, avoiding frequency-selective fat suppression sequences, avoiding gradient-echo sequences, using a larger matrix size, thinner slices, and reducing the voxel size.[14] In addition, specific MR imaging metal artifact reduction sequences are now available commercially to acquire fluid-sensitive images with a high signal-to-noise ratio and minimize susceptibility artifacts, such as multiple acquisition with variable-resonance image combination (MAVRIC) and slice encoding for metal artifact correction (SEMAC) sequences.[15]

Direct MR imaging arthrography may enhance diagnostic accuracy in postoperative shoulders owing to joint distention.[14] Direct MR imaging arthrography is the most sensitive and specific method for diagnosing full-thickness and partial-thickness retears, with sensitivity ranging from 86% to 100% and specificity ranging from 59% to 100%.[5] However, direct MR imaging arthrography has been shown to reveal a high number of false-positive retears in patients who have undergone rotator cuff repair,[13] because watertight repair is not necessary for optimal clinical outcome.[5]

Ultrasound images are not significantly degraded by metal artifact, possess high spatial resolution, and allow dynamic evaluation in real time, and therefore are useful for evaluation of the postoperative rotator cuff especially when MR imaging is contraindicated. However, ultrasound is highly operator dependent. In comparison to MR imaging, ultrasound showed lower interobserver agreement in the evaluation of tear size, tendon retraction, and muscle atrophy.[4]

Computed tomography (CT) arthrography is often indicated for patients who have a contraindication to MR imaging, significant metal artifact, or severe rotator cuff arthropathy and need osseous evaluation for shoulder arthroplasty.[8]

IMAGING FINDINGS AND PATHOLOGY
Primary Anatomic Repair of the Rotator Cuff

Overview
Primary anatomic repair is indicated for patients with symptomatic small to medium full-thickness rotator cuff tears. The initial recommendations for rotator cuff injury treatment from the American Academy of Orthopedic Surgeons (AAOS) evidence-based 2010 Clinical Practice Guideline (CPG) stated that "Rotator cuff repair is an option for patients with chronic, symptomatic full-thickness tears" because the existing literature at the time only provided a weak recommendation for repair. The updated 2019 CPG recommendations for rotator cuff injury treatment stated that "strong evidence supports that both physical therapy and surgical management resulted in a notable improvement in patient reported outcome for patients with symptomatic small to medium full-thickness rotator cuff tears." In addition, the current updated CPG recommendations stated that "Moderate evidence supports that healed rotator cuff repairs show improved patient-reported and functional outcomes compared with physical therapy and unhealed rotator cuff repairs."

There is compelling evidence that physical therapy alone improves patient-reported outcomes in symptomatic individuals with full-thickness rotator cuff tears. However, with nonoperative treatment, the size of the rotator cuff tear, muscle atrophy, and fatty infiltration may worsen over a 5- to 10-year time frame. In patients with high-grade partial-thickness rotator cuff tears who have failed conservative therapy, strong evidence supports either conversion to full-thickness or transtendinous/in situ repair as a reasonable approach.[3] There is no long-term difference between open and arthroscopic repairs in terms of patient-reported outcome or cuff healing rates. However, short-term postoperative recovery and pain management are better with arthroscopic repair.[3] The purpose of surgical anatomic repair is to reattach the torn rotator cuff tendon to its footprint on the tuberosity in a near anatomic form, using minimum tension to restore optimal rotator cuff muscle balance. Contrary to popular belief, there is no compelling evidence that double-row rotator cuff repair constructs improve patient-reported outcomes when compared with single-row vertical mattress repair constructs. However, double-row vertical mattress repair has a lower rate of retear than single-row vertical mattress repair while assessing for both partial and full thickness retears.[3]

Normal postoperative findings
Even though most orthopedic hardware currently used is made of a bioabsorbable material and creates little susceptibility artifact, in some patients, image quality may be degraded as a result of artifact from metallic orthopedic hardware.[16] During the first year after rotator cuff surgery, the appearance of the repaired tendon is variable and does not correlate with clinical prognosis. This variability depends on the degree and duration of the rotator cuff disease process, as well as the period between repair and imaging.[17]

Rotator cuff tendons that have been repaired may look thinner or thicker than normal tendons, depending on the residual preoperative tendon thickness.[14] Increased intrasubstance T2 signal intensity is observed in the great majority of rotator cuff repairs, which can persist for several months to years (**Fig. 1**). This increased intrasubstance T2 signal intensity can be ascribed to preexisting tendinosis, postoperative granulation tissue, scarring, or an artifact attributable to the suture material.[5,18] It is also worth noting that after a rotator cuff repair, a part of the torn tendon may be intentionally left unrepaired. This is frequently due to poor tissue quality and should not be regarded as a recurring tear.[16] Thus, a thorough comparison with the preoperative MR imaging scan and correlation with the operative report, if available, should be undertaken.

After rotator cuff repair, expected bone marrow edema-like signal changes in the greater

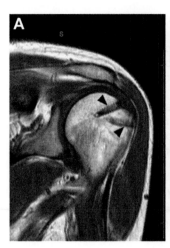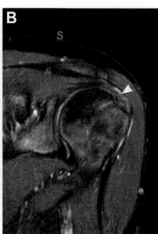

Fig. 1. Intact rotator cuff repair 4 years after surgery in a 53-year-old female. (*A*) Oblique coronal T1-weighted MR image of the shoulder shows proximal and distal suture anchors (*arrowheads*) in the greater tuberosity related to double-row technique for rotator cuff repair. (*B*) Oblique coronal fat-suppressed T2-weighted MR image shows expected intermediate signal (*arrowhead*) within the distal supraspinatus tendon at the site of repair.

tuberosity occur as a result of normal response to anchors (**Fig. 2**). Suture anchors embedded in bone absorb water and undergo hydrolysis; hence, focal edema-like signal can be detected near suture anchors for up to 2 years after surgery, until they are eventually replaced by bone.[18]

Complications

Although most patients have a positive outcome after rotator cuff surgery, around 6% to 25% of patients continue to be symptomatic, experiencing pain and dysfunction.[13,18] Patients with this condition, known as failed rotator cuff syndrome, pose a diagnostic and therapeutic challenge to the treating physician.[13]

Complications of rotator cuff repair include retear, displaced or broken anchors or sutures, nerve injury, muscle atrophy and fatty infiltration, recurrent subacromial spur, deltoid muscle dehiscence after open surgery, stiffness and adhesive capsulitis, glenohumeral osteoarthritis, chondrolysis, and infection.[19]

One of the most common complications after rotator cuff repair is retear (**Figs. 3–6**). The literature reports a wide range of rotator cuff retear incidence, ranging from 9% to 94%.[4] Rotator cuff retears are not necessarily symptomatic.[13] Most rotator cuff retears are thought to be caused by insufficient tendon healing due to poor tissue quality[13] or by fixation failure at the bone due to anchor withdrawal or suture breakdown.[18]

Conventional MR imaging is accurate in identifying rotator cuff full-thickness retears with reported sensitivity and specificity of 84% and 91%, respectively, and a sensitivity and specificity of 83% for partial tears.[5] However, Motamedi and colleagues reported a sensitivity of 91% but a poor specificity of 25%.[20] Nonetheless, conventional MR imaging is rather imprecise in identifying tear

size, with a proclivity toward overdiagnosis of retears.[13]

Rotator cuff retears exhibit similar MR imaging findings as preoperative rotator cuff tears, including fluid or contrast signal intensity extending into or through the repaired tendon with an accompanying tendon gap in the repaired tendon.[18] The presence of intermediate signal intensity scar and granulation tissue may give the impression of a partial-thickness retear, leading to an exaggeration of the degree of retear. MR arthrography may aid in distinguishing retear from granulation tissue when contrast fills in the tear but not the granulation tissue.[5]

The Sugaya classification is an MR imaging–based classification system that was introduced for determining the thickness and discontinuity of repaired cuff tendons (**Table 1**). This classification has a strong correlation with the patient's functional outcomes with good intraobserver and interobserver reliability.[16,21]

Ultimately, if the mechanics of repair are understood, diagnosis of recurrent tear on MR imaging becomes easier; the suture anchor is composed of an anchor component that is driven into the bone, and a suture that is sewn into the tendon. Anchors are typically nonmetallic, such as PEEK (polyether ether ketone); the suture is composed of variable materials and is faintly visible as a low signal on MR imaging sequences, often with slight susceptibility artifact. Failure of repair can be related to rupture of the suture or migration of the anchor. The most important sign of breakdown is uncovering of the anchor site (see **Figs. 4** and **5**). As noted earlier, full-thickness communication can be a normal postoperative finding. However, if there is a full-thickness (or undersurface partial-thickness defect) in the cuff tendon at the anchor site, with fluid signal overlying the anchor head,

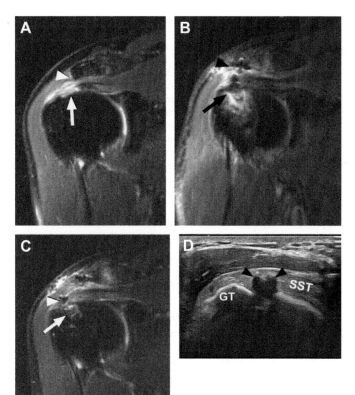

Fig. 2. Rotator cuff repair in a 48-year-old male with expected outcome. (*A*) Preoperative oblique coronal fat-suppressed T2-weighted MR image of the shoulder shows a full-thickness tear of the supraspinatus tendon (*arrow*). Note small subacromial spur (*arrowhead*). (*B*) Oblique coronal fat-suppressed T2-weighted MR image of the same patient 2 weeks after acromioplasty (*arrowhead*) and rotator cuff repair. Note bone marrow edema (*arrow*) around the anchor related to a recent surgery. (*C*) Oblique coronal fat-suppressed T2-weighted MR image of the same patient 8 weeks later showing resolution of bone marrow edema around the anchor (*arrow*). Note slight artifact within the distal supraspinatus tendon (*arrowhead*) caused by the suture in its normal position. (*D*) Ultrasound image in the longitudinal plane of the same patient showing shadowing from the suture in place (*arrowheads*) within the intact supraspinatus tendon (SST). GT, greater tuberosity.

this is highly specific for recurrent tear. Another sign of repair failure is retraction of a suture. If a linear or curved focus of low signal is seen within a tendon next to the repair site, this suggests rupture of the suture. Finally, migration of the anchor from its predrilled site is diagnostic of failure (see **Fig. 6**). Nonmetallic anchors create no artifact and displacement is easily detected on MR imaging. The presence of osteolysis around the loosening anchor before its dislodgement can be detected as a focal T2 high signal intensity that is thicker than expected postoperative surgical hydrolysis of the anchor[5] (see **Figs. 3, 5, 6**).

Infections of the superficial and deep wounds were observed to be more prevalent in individuals after open rotator cuff surgery than arthroscopic

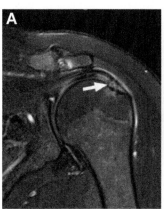

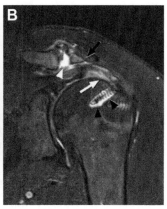

Fig. 3. Preoperative and postoperative rotator cuff surgery with failure of repair in a 63-year-old female. (*A*) Preoperative oblique coronal fat-suppressed T2-weighted MR image of the shoulder shows undersurface partial thickness tear (*arrow*) of the supraspinatus tendon at its footprint. (*B*) Oblique coronal fat-suppressed T2-weighted MR image of the same patient 5 years after surgery shows recurrent tear of the supraspinatus tendon with discontinuity of fibers (*white arrow*). Note linear fluid signal surrounding the bioabsorbable anchor (*black arrowheads*), which can be a sign of loosening. There has been acromioplasty (*black arrow*) with disruption of the inferior capsule of the acromioclavicular joint (*white arrowhead*).

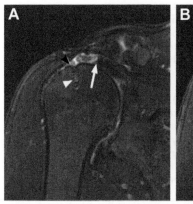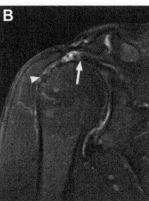

Fig. 4. Breakdown of rotator cuff repair in a 70-year-old male. (*A*) Oblique coronal fat-suppressed T2-weighted MR image of the shoulder 10 years after surgery shows recurrent full-thickness supraspinatus tear with retraction of fibers (*arrow*). Note proximal anchor in the humerus (*white arrowhead*) with fluid signal over the hub (*black arrowhead*) related to breakdown of repair. (*B*) Adjacent oblique coronal fat-suppressed T2-weighted MR image shows uncovering of the distal anchor (*white arrowhead*), which is protruding slightly from the cortical margin. Note retracted supraspinatus tendon (*arrow*).

repair.[16] Deep shoulder infections are uncommon after arthroscopic repair, occurring in between 0.3% and 1.9% of cases.[5]

Subacromial Decompression

Overview

Subacromial decompression may be performed as a concomitant treatment for patients with small- to medium-sized full-thickness rotator cuff tears and existing chronic extrinsic impingement of the rotator cuff tendon by degenerative productive changes of the AC joint, enthesopathy of the acromial insertion site of the coracoacromial ligament, or by developmental predisposition such as os acromiale or a hooked acromion. Acromioplasty, distal clavicle resection (Mumford procedure), and resection of the os acromiale are all

treatments that can be used to decompress the subacromial space[15] (**Figs. 7 and 8**).

The updated 2019 AAOS CPG recommendations stated that "Moderate strength evidence does not support the routine use of acromioplasty as a concomitant treatment compared with arthroscopic repair alone for patients with small-to medium-sized full-thickness rotator cuff tears" and also stated that "Moderate strength evidence supports the use of distal clavicle resection as a concomitant treatment to arthroscopic repair for patients with full-thickness rotator cuff tears and symptomatic acromioclavicular joints." Decompression of the subacromial space can be accomplished either arthroscopically or by open surgery. Acromioplasty is a burr shaving of the undersurface of the acromion, where the spur is present. The subacromial bursa may be debrided. The

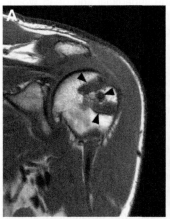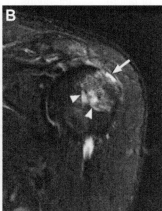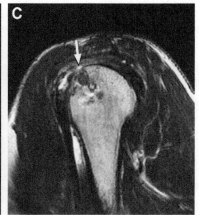

Fig. 5. Failure of rotator cuff repair in a 69-year-old male 3 years after surgery. (*A*) Oblique coronal T1-weighted MR image of the shoulder shows multiple anchors (*arrowheads*) within the greater tuberosity, with poorly defined margins. (*B*) Oblique coronal fat-suppressed T2-weighted MR image shows bone marrow edema (*arrowheads*) surrounding the anchors. Fluid signal is present at the tendon footprint (*arrow*). (*C*) Oblique sagittal T2-weighted MR image shows uncovering of the anchor hub (*arrow*), which should be covered by tendon tissue, consistent with recurrent full-thickness tear.

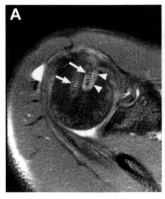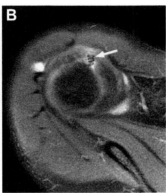

Fig. 6. Failure of rotator cuff repair in a 48-year-old male, 2 years after surgery. (*A*) Axial fat-suppressed proton density MR image of the shoulder shows 2 anchors (*arrows*) within the humeral head. Hyperintensity surrounds one of the anchors (*arrowheads*), which can be associated with loosening. (*B*) Adjacent axial fat-suppressed proton density MR image shows displaced anchor fragment (*arrow*) within the distal supraspinatus tendon.

coracoacromial ligament is usually preserved to keep the humeral head from superior migration. The Mumford procedure entails partial surgical excision of the distal clavicle articulating with the AC joint and is usually performed in the presence of painful AC joint arthritis.[14]

Normal postoperative findings
Following acromioplasty, bone burring may cause mild magnetic susceptibility artifact on postoperative MR imaging. However, this normally does not impact rotator cuff assessment.

Flattening of the undersurface of the acromion and discrete defect along the anterior acromion are characteristic imaging findings on postoperative MR images (see **Figs. 3** and **7**). In addition, intermediate signal intensity granulation tissue is formed in the space of the excised subacromial/subdeltoid bursa.[14]

Following a Mumford procedure, there is usually no significant susceptibility artifact on postoperative MR imaging (see **Fig. 8**). Blunting of the distal clavicle and apparent widening of the AC joint space are characteristic imaging findings on postoperative MR images.[15]

Complications
Excessive acromioplasty including excision of the coracoacromial ligament can lead to instability and superior humeral migration.[14] Excessive acromial resection can result in fractures or disruption of the AC joint capsule (see **Fig. 3**). Following acromioplasty, AC joint osteoarthritis progression and scarring of the subacromial space may occur.[18]

Superior Capsular Reconstruction

Overview
Superior capsular reconstruction is a relatively new surgical technique, best suited for young patients with irreparable massive rotator cuff tear and no significant glenohumeral arthritis. Superior capsular reconstruction is accomplished by reconstructing the superior capsule as a static restraint, thereby preventing superior humeral translation and preserving the glenohumeral joint's native geometric center. Initially, fascia lata autografts have shown promising early results, but dermal allografts have gained popularity in recent years because of concerns of donor site morbidity. This technique involves graft fixation by anchors into the superior glenoid and greater tuberosity to reconstruct the superior capsule. Surgical technique modification of superior capsular reconstruction includes the incorporation of the

Table 1
Sugaya classification, MR T2-weighted imaging–based classification system for thickness and discontinuity of repaired cuff tendons

Classification	Repaired Tendon Thickness Compared with Normal Rotator Cuff Tendon
Type I	Sufficient thickness with homogeneous low signal intensity
Type II	Sufficient thickness with high signal intensity
Type III	Insufficient thickness (less than half the thickness) without discontinuity
Type IV	Presence of a minor discontinuity (only 1 or 2 slices on both oblique coronal and sagittal images)
Type V	Presence of a major discontinuity (more than 2 slices on both oblique coronal and sagittal images)

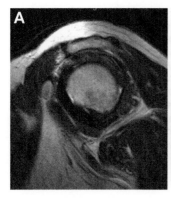
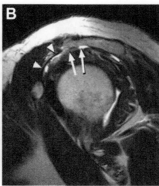

Fig. 7. Acromioplasty in a 58-year-old male. (*A*) Preoperative sagittal T2-weighted MR image through the acromion. (*B*) Postoperative sagittal T2-weighted MR image following acromioplasty shows shaving of bone from the undersurface of the anterior acromion (*arrows*). Note preservation of the coracoacromial ligament (*arrowheads*).

residual cuff over the graft and the installation of subacromial spacer.[22]

Normal postoperative findings

The expected postoperative MR imaging findings of superior capsular reconstruction is a taut graft covering the superior humeral head demonstrating low signal intensity with no fluid signal discontinuity throughout its length. Small sutures holes in the graft material along the medial and lateral edges should not be mistaken for tears[5].

Complications

The postoperative superior humeral translation is a reasonable indicator of superior capsule reconstruction graft failure. Complete or partial tear of the superior capsule reconstruction graft often occurs along the medial (glenoid) or lateral (humeral) attachment. Tears at the side-to-side attachment of the graft to the remaining rotator cuff tendon should be investigated because tears at this location may be the sole postoperative finding of partial graft failure. It is critical to review the operative report to verify that side-to-side attachment was performed, as this is not always done, which might result in a misleading diagnosis of side-to-side tear.[23]

Patch Graft Augmentation and Bridging

Overview

The purpose of patch graft is to bridge the gap between the irreparable torn rotator cuff edge and the footprint to alleviate the tension on the repair and preserve shoulder function. Grafts may be used to augment reparable partial and full-thickness tears when there are concerns about the primary repair's healing and strength.[23,24] Various graft materials have been used, including autograft biceps tendon and fascia lata, allograft acellular human dermal graft, xenograft porcine dermis, and synthetic poly-L-lactide acid grafts.

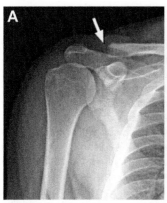
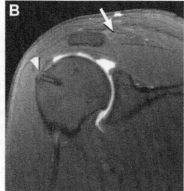
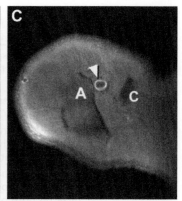

Fig. 8. Mumford procedure in a 40-year-old male. (*A*) Anteroposterior radiograph of the shoulder following Mumford procedure shows resection of the distal clavicle (*arrow*). (*B*) Oblique coronal T1-weighted fat-suppressed MR arthrogram. Note absence of the distal clavicle (*arrow*) and bioabsorbable suture anchor (*arrowhead*) related to rotator cuff repair. (*C*) Axial T1-weighted fat-suppressed MR image shows widening of the distance between the acromion (labeled "A") and the clavicle (labeled "C") with metallic artifact (*arrowhead*) related to surgical resection.

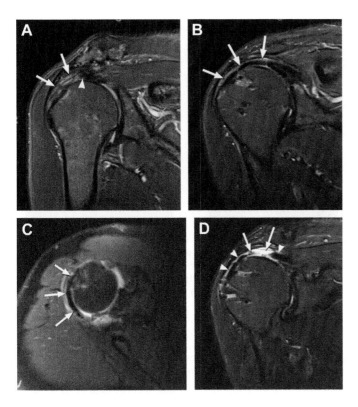

Fig. 9. Rotator cuff repair with patch graft in a 71-year-old male. (*A*) Preoperative oblique coronal fat-suppressed T2-weighted MR image of the shoulder shows a large full-thickness tear of the supraspinatus tendon (*arrows*) with retracted tendon (*arrowhead*). (*B, C*) Oblique coronal (*B*) and axial (*C*) fat-suppressed fluid-sensitive MR images 1 year after surgery show intact low signal patch graft (*arrows*). (*D*) Oblique coronal fat-suppressed T2-weighted MR image of the same patient an additional 3 years later shows remnants of the patch graft (*arrowheads*) with fluid signal at the site of graft failure (*arrows*).

Clinical outcomes are influenced by the graft material; human dermal extracellular matrix grafts showed significant lower postoperative retears, whereas porcine grafts did not.[5]

Normal postoperative findings

MR imaging is the imaging modality of choice for postoperative evaluation of rotator cuff graft augmentation and graft bridging surgery (**Fig. 9**). The postoperative appearance is expected to be low signal in the graft and the augmentation material with no fluid-filled defect.[23]

Complications

Sugaya classification can be used to classify the MR imaging appearance and integrity of the reconstructed tendon, with type IV and V tendons considered full-thickness retears (see **Table 1**). A recurrent tear should be considered if there is a full-thickness fluid cleft in the graft.[23] Graft material and spacers can also become displaced into the recesses of the bursa or joint (**Fig. 10**).

Tendon Transfers

Overview

Tendon transfer is one of the options for young patients with irreparable massive rotator cuff tear and no significant glenohumeral arthritis. The purpose of tendon transfer is to restore the glenohumeral joint force couples for better pain relief and potential functional improvement. The donor tendon is chosen based on the location of the rotator cuff deficiency. The irreparable posterosuperior rotator cuff tear is often reconstructed with latissimus dorsi transfer when the subscapularis is intact. Trapezius tendon transfer is recently considered another alternative option in patients with irreparable posterosuperior rotator cuff tears. The irreparable anterosuperior rotator cuff tear (mainly subscapularis) is often reconstructed with pectoralis major transfer. Transfers of the latissimus dorsi and pectoralis major tendons have demonstrated reliable pain relief, but the functional improvement is uncertain.

The harvested latissimus dorsi tendon is often detached from the humeral attachment, passed via surgical plane created deep to the deltoid and posterior to the teres minor, brought superior to the humeral head, and attached to the supraspinatus footprint.

The harvested pectoralis major tendon is commonly detached from the insertion of the sternal head portion at the proximal humeral diaphysis and reattached to the lesser tuberosity to function as the native subscapularis tendon. The location of the harvested pectoralis major tendon in reference to the coracoid process varies depending on the surgical techniques.[11,23,25]

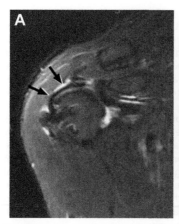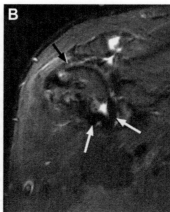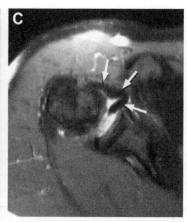

Fig. 10. Failure and displacement of patch graft in a 62-year-old male. (*A*) Oblique coronal fat-suppressed T2-weighted MR image of the shoulder 1 year after surgery shows intact low signal patch graft in place (*arrows*). (*B*) Oblique coronal fat-suppressed T2-weighted MR image of the same patient 2 years later shows fluid signal at the site of previous graft (*black arrow*). Graft is displaced into the axillary recess (*white arrows*). (*C*) Axial fat-suppressed proton density MR image from the same examination as (*B*) shows displaced patch graft in the axillary recess (*arrows*).

Normal postoperative findings

On postoperative MR imaging, the transferred tendon is expected to demonstrate a heterogeneous low to intermediate signal intensity without any fluid gap defect. Owing to scar formation, the unaffected preserved tendon portion of the latissimus dorsi tendon may remain intermediate in signal intensity at its humeral insertion.[23]

Complications

The potential complications of tendon transfer include tears of the tendon graft, denervation of the transferred muscle as a result of iatrogenic nerve damage, infection, hematoma, and injury to the neurovascular structures.[23]

- One of the most common complications after rotator cuff repair is retear.

- In superior capsular reconstruction, small sutures holes in the graft material along the medial and lateral edges should not be mistaken for tears.

- In patch graft augmentation, a recurrent tear should be considered if there is a full-thickness fluid cleft in the graft.

- In tendon transfer, potential complications include muscle denervation of the transferred muscle as a result of iatrogenic nerve damage.

SUMMARY

MR imaging is critical in the evaluation of symptomatic patients who have undergone rotator cuff surgery. A thorough understanding of common and new evolving advanced surgical techniques, expected normal postoperative findings, and potential complications is essential for better MR imaging interpretation.

CLINICS CARE POINTS

- During the first year after rotator cuff anatomic repair, the appearance of tendons is variable and does not correlate with clinical prognosis.

DISCLOSURE

The authors have nothing to disclose.

REFERENCES

1. Nazarian LN, Jacobson JA, Benson CB, et al. Imaging algorithms for evaluating suspected rotator cuff disease: Society of Radiologists in Ultrasound consensus conference statement. Radiology 2013; 267(2):589–95.
2. Morag Y, Jacobson JA, Miller B, et al. MR Imaging of Rotator Cuff Injury: What the Clinician Needs to Know. RadioGraphics 2006;26(4):1045–65.
3. Weber S, Chahal J. Management of Rotator Cuff Injuries. J Am Acad Orthop Surg 2020;28(5):e193.
4. Lee SC, Williams D, Endo Y. The Repaired Rotator Cuff: MRI and Ultrasound Evaluation. Curr Rev Musculoskelet Med 2018;11(1):92–101.

5. Samim M, Beltran L. The Postoperative Rotator Cuff. Magn Reson Imaging Clin N Am 2020;28(2):181–94.

6. Xu B, Chen L, Zou J, et al. The Clinical Effect of Arthroscopic Rotator Cuff Repair techniques: A Network Meta-Analysis and Systematic Review. Sci Rep 2019;9(1):4143.

7. Adler RS. Postoperative rotator cuff. Semin Musculoskelet Radiol 2013;17(1):12–9.

8. Cvetanovich GL, Waterman BR, Verma NN, et al. Management of the Irreparable Rotator Cuff Tear. J Am Acad Orthop Surg 2019;27(24):909–17.

9. Huang BK, Resnick D. Novel Anatomic Concepts in Magnetic Resonance Imaging of the Rotator Cuff Tendons and the Footprint. Magn Reson Imaging Clin N Am 2012;20(2):163–72.

10. Mura N, O'Driscoll SW, Zobitz ME, et al. The effect of infraspinatus disruption on glenohumeral torque and superior migration of the humeral head: A biomechanical study. J Shoulder Elbow Surg 2003;12(2):179–84.

11. Omid R, Lee B. Tendon transfers for irreparable rotator cuff tears. J Am Acad Orthop Surg 2013;21(8):492–501.

12. Burkhart SS. Arthroscopic treatment of massive rotator cuff tears. Clinical results and biomechanical rationale. Clin Orthop 1991;(267):45–56.

13. Strauss EJ, McCormack RA, Onyekwelu I, et al. Management of failed arthroscopic rotator cuff repair. J Am Acad Orthop Surg 2012;20(5):301–9.

14. McMenamin D, Koulouris G, Morrison WB. Imaging of the shoulder after surgery. Eur J Radiol 2008;68(1):106–19.

15. Beltran LS, Bencardino JT, Steinbach LS. Postoperative MRI of the shoulder: Postoperative MRI of Shoulder. J Magn Reson Imaging 2014;40(6):1280–97.

16. Kalia V, Freehill MT, Miller BS, et al. Multimodality Imaging Review of Normal Appearance and Complications of the Postoperative Rotator Cuff. Am J Roentgenol 2018;211(3):538–47.

17. Crim J, Burks R, Manaster BJ, et al. Temporal evolution of MRI findings after arthroscopic rotator cuff repair. AJR Am J Roentgenol 2010;195(6):1361–6.

18. Pierce JL, Nacey NC, Jones S, et al. Postoperative Shoulder Imaging: Rotator Cuff, Labrum, and Biceps Tendon. RadioGraphics 2016;36(6):1648–71.

19. Mohana-Borges AVR, Chung CB, Resnick D. MR Imaging and MR Arthrography of the Postoperative Shoulder: Spectrum of Normal and Abnormal Findings. RadioGraphics 2004;24(1):69–85.

20. Motamedi AR, Urrea LH, Hancock RE, et al. Accuracy of magnetic resonance imaging in determining the presence and size of recurrent rotator cuff tears. J Shoulder Elbow Surg 2002;11(1):6–10.

21. Sugaya H, Maeda K, Matsuki K, et al. Functional and Structural Outcome After Arthroscopic Full-Thickness Rotator Cuff Repair: Single-Row Versus Dual-Row Fixation. Arthroscopy 2005;21(11):1307–16.

22. Tokish JM, Makovicka JL. The Superior Capsular Reconstruction: Lessons Learned and Future Directions. J Am Acad Orthop Surg 2020;28(13):528–37.

23. Samim M, Walsh P, Gyftopoulos S, et al. Postoperative MRI of Massive Rotator Cuff Tears. Am J Roentgenol 2018;211(1):146–54.

24. Sunwoo JY, Murrell GAC. Interposition Graft Repair of Irreparable Rotator Cuff Tears: A Review of Biomechanics and Clinical Outcomes. J Am Acad Orthop Surg 2020;28(19):e829–38.

25. Elhassan BT, Cox RM, Shukla DR, et al. Management of Failed Rotator Cuff Repair in Young Patients. J Am Acad Orthop Surg 2017;25(11):e261–71.

Postoperative MR Imaging of the Elbow

Lawrence Lo, MD[a], Toluwalase Ashimolowo, MD[b], Luis S. Beltran, MD[c],*

KEYWORDS

• Elbow • MR imaging • Postoperative • Complications • Sports • Surgical techniques

KEY POINTS

• MR imaging for the postoperative elbow is challenging because of the rare nature of premorbid injuries and lack of imaging before revision.
• MR imaging findings are confounding because of an increased sensitivity for signal changes of postoperative structures.
• Knowledge of different operative approaches is essential to evaluate for postoperative complications.

INTRODUCTION

Elbow injuries are a growing problem particularly among overhead athletes, because more children and adolescents are participating in sporting activities.[1] Understanding the biomechanical forces involved is key to appropriate treatment and successful return to play. The goal of surgical management of elbow injuries is to restore the capsuloligamentous and osseous contributions to stability as much as possible.[2] However, postoperative MR imaging evaluation is difficult because of the variety of surgical techniques available, and the lack of postoperative MR imaging for suspected complications because many are diagnosed clinically and a revision may be performed without imaging. This article reviews some of the commonly performed surgical techniques for select elbow injuries. Postoperative MR imaging findings and complications are discussed with integration of the current literature available.

MR IMAGING TECHNIQUE

MR imaging is the modality of choice for evaluating graft integrity following elbow surgery. It is also useful for following postoperative soft tissue and osseous changes until complete healing from surgery. Several considerations should be taken when interpreting postoperative MR imaging for elbow injuries. Because of the sensitive nature of MR imaging, graft degeneration in certain cases cannot be reliably distinguished from graft tear, because they can have similar signal characteristics and appearance. Depending on the fixation hardware, metallic artifacts can impede accurate postoperative assessment at the suture/anchor sites.[3,4] Hence, many contemporary MR imaging techniques are developed to address concerns of metallic artifacts, signal to noise ratio, homogeneous fat suppression, and image resolution to improved visualization of postoperative anatomy and pathology.[3,5]

OSTEOCHONDRAL GRAFT RECONSTRUCTION IN CAPITELLAR OSTEOCHONDRITIS DISSECANS

Osteochondritis dissecans (OCD) of the capitellum most commonly affects young overhead athletes, such as baseball players and gymnasts, with approximately 60% of the compressive forces generated at the elbow during axial loading activities transmitted to the capitellum.[6] The cause remains unknown and is likely multifactorial

a Hospital of the University of Pennsylvania, Penn Medicine University City, 3737 Market Street, 6th Floor, Mailbox 4, Philadelphia, PA 19104, USA; b Summit Radiology, 770 Cady Way, Atlanta, GA 39316, USA; c Department of Radiology, Brigham and Women's Hospital, 75 Francis Street, Boston, MA 02115, USA
* Corresponding author.
E-mail address: lbeltran@bwh.harvard.edu

Magn Reson Imaging Clin N Am 30 (2022) 629–643
https://doi.org/10.1016/j.mric.2022.02.001
1064-9689/22/© 2022 Elsevier Inc. All rights reserved.

including altered biomechanics, repetitive trauma, localized ischemia, and genetic factors.[7] Treatment depends on the stability of the capitellar OCD. Although there is no consensus on MR imaging classification of capitellar OCD, several classifications based on MR imaging findings have been proposed.[8] The presence of T2-hyperintense rim or fracture line, multiple or large surrounding cysts, and fluid-filled osteochondral defects are highly sensitive for unstable lesions proven on surgery in a study by Jans and colleagues.[9]

Surgical Technique

Operative management is appropriate for failed conservative management, unstable lesions, intra-articular loose bodies, and pain affecting daily activities. Potential surgical interventions include removal of loose bodies, cartilage reparative techniques including microfracture, and osteochondral autograft transplantation (OAT). Here, we focus on OAT because it is widely performed with excellent results.[10] Surgical approach depends on the lesion location and surgeon's preference.[11] The posterior anconeus-split approach from Iwasaki and colleagues[12] involves posterior exposure of the radiocapitellar joint by splitting the anconeus muscle and incising the joint capsule. The capitellar OCD lesion is then directly assessed followed by removal of the unstable fragment. Small cylindrical osteochondral autografts harvested from the knee or ribs are trimmed to match the recipient site at the bed of the OCD lesion. Several tubular tunnels approximately 2-mm deeper than the length of the grafts are created at the recipient site through the underlying healthy bone. The cylindrical autografts are then transplanted perpendicular to the articular surface into the prepared tunnels. For OCD lesions more anteriorly located on the capitellum, lateral elbow surgical approaches are used. The Kocher approach is the classic lateral elbow approach, where the fascia between the extensor carpi ulnaris and the anconeus muscles is incised, followed by incision of the radiocapitellar capsule and the annular ligament.[13] Two key structures that are at high risk of injury for lateral surgical approaches are the lateral collateral ligament and the posterior interosseous nerve (PIN). Alternatives to the Kocher lateral elbow approach, including a lateral midaxial approach by Schrumpf and colleagues,[14] are developed to address these concerns.

Postoperative Imaging

Appearance of the transplanted osteochondral autografts depends on the timing from surgery. Graft incorporation and healing is seen as early as 3 months following surgery (**Fig. 1**).[15] On MR imaging, grafted cartilage may appear thicker than the adjacent native cartilage with or without complete osseous union. When multiple osteochondral cylinders are used, the periphery of the grafted cartilage may be thicker than the central portion by design.[12] Once completely incorporated, the osteochondral graft should demonstrate full-thickness integration with the adjacent native cartilage and marrow characteristics of the surrounding healthy bone.[16]

Although results are generally excellent with osteochondral autografts, complications can occur mainly in the setting of pain and delayed return to competitive activity.[16–18] In addition to poor graft incorporation, heterogeneous T1 signal intensity of the bone part of the osteochondral graft may indicate poor vascularization and osteonecrosis.[15] Regarding necrotic subchondral bone, Yamamoto and colleagues[18] found that these can heal in the early postoperative period. Incongruent articular surface with subchondral cysts and edema is seen in graft degeneration, which may not correlate with clinical outcome.[16] Loose or unstable cartilaginous lesions, incomplete osseous fusion, and hypertrophic bone remodeling are additional abnormal findings seen in OAT. If a lateral surgical approach is used, including the Kocher approach and its variations, the lateral collateral ligament should be investigated for injury with attention given to the lateral epicondylar attachment where a subperiosteal release is performed. Iatrogenic injury to the PIN may occur during surgical dissection of the overlying intermuscular fascia to access the radiocapitellar joint. Therefore, the PIN nerve should be thoroughly investigated along its proximal course from the radial nerve bifurcation.[14]

DISTAL BICEPS BRACHII TENDON REPAIR

Distal biceps tendon rupture, although a uncommon injury, typically affects middle-aged men.[19] Patients often report a popping sensation with pain and swelling after eccentric extension force loaded on a flexed elbow. Most distal biceps tendon ruptures are repaired surgically to restore supination and flexion strength.[20]

Surgical Technique

Contemporary techniques for distal biceps tendon repair are performed through either a single anterior incision, or a double incision via the posterior approach. In the single incision anterior approach, the incision is made between the pronator teres and brachioradialis muscles beginning at the

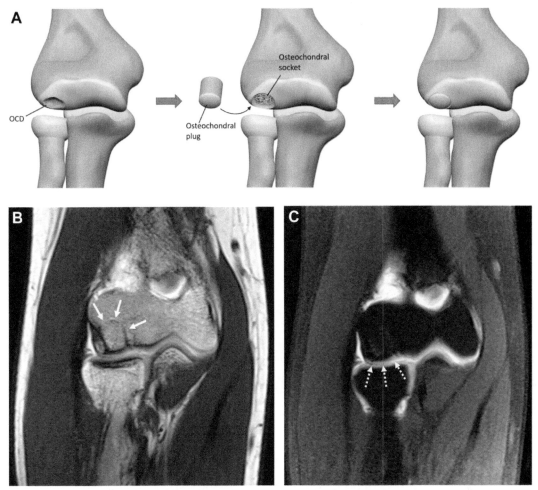

Fig. 1. A 16-year-old female gymnast with prior unstable osteochondritis dissecans of the capitellum. (*A*) Illustration of normal osteochondral autograft transfer at the capitellum. (*B*) Coronal T1 image shows good incorporation of the osteochondral autograft transfer (*arrows*) to the native surrounding bone at the capitellum. (*C*) Coronal T2FS image shows mild heterogeneity of the overlying cartilage (*arrows*) without full-thickness defects or deep fissuring. FS, fat saturated.

antecubital fossa.[20] The lateral antebrachial cutaneous nerve is identified and protected throughout the procedure. The torn tendon is located, and the adhesions are released. Two suture anchors are placed approximately 1 cm apart into the ulnar aspect of the bicipital tuberosity. Finally, the located torn tendon is reattached onto the bicipital tuberosity. For the double incision posterior approach, a transverse incision is made anteriorly at the antecubital fossa, followed by a second posterolateral muscle-splitting incision through the common extensor and the supinator muscles to expose the bicipital tuberosity.[21] In the posterior approach, the forearm is held in protonation to protect the PIN during muscle dissection. Many options exist for tendon reattachment at the bicipital tuberosity, including bone tunnels, suture anchors, interference screw, and cortical buttons,

all of which seem to be sufficient for securing the tendon to bone during the healing phase.[22]

Postoperative Imaging

Evaluation of the distal biceps tendon after reattachment is difficult with MR imaging. For the first year after reattachment, the biceps tendon may exhibit heterogeneity and signal intensity that lags behind functional recovery (**Fig. 2**).[23] Fixation artifacts and partial volume averaging because of the oblique course of the tendon at the reattachment site may preclude accurate evaluation at the radial tuberosity. In addition, the biceps tendon may not normalize to its native appearance for up to 6 years after surgery.[24] Intratendinous ossification can also occur without correlation to function outcome.[25]

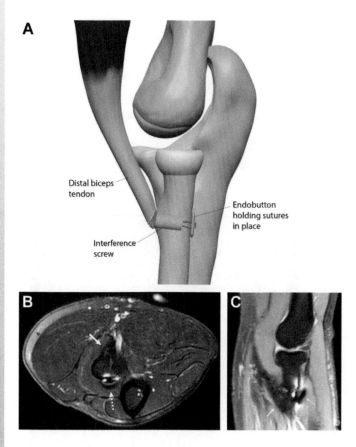

A

Distal biceps tendon

Endobutton holding sutures in place

Interference screw

B

C

Fig. 2. A 72-year-old man with prior rupture of biceps tendon postrepair. (*A*) Illustration showing normal biceps tendon repair with bone tunnel, interference screw, and cortical button at the radial tuberosity. Axial T2FS (*B*) and sagittal PDFS (*C*) images show an intact distal biceps tendon (*solid arrow*) fixed to the radial tuberosity with a cortical button (*dotted arrow*). PDFS, proton density fat saturated.

The total complication rate for bicep tendon reattachment is estimated to be around 15% to 35%.[26] The PIN and lateral antebrachial cutaneous nerve may be injured during surgery, which are more frequently seen with the single incision technique.[27] Heterotopic ossification and proximal radioulnar synostosis are more frequently associated with the double incision technique, and the location and extent should be described for excision planning in symptomatic patients.[26] Certain fixation devices are predisposed to bicipital tuberosity osteolysis, particularly with interference screws.[28] Rerupture of the distal bicep tendon usually occurs in the early postoperatively period (**Fig. 3**), although MR imaging is limited in differentiating rerupture from tendinosis and postoperative scarring (**Fig. 4**) because both would demonstrate tendon heterogeneity.[29] Although guidelines are lacking for interpretation of MR imaging findings after surgery, a study by Rashid and colleagues[30] showed that a gap between the distal end of the tendon and its footprint at the radial tuberosity can indicate failure of repair, because these tendons were not directly in contact with the radial tuberosity but instead bridged by a friable fibrous tissue found on revision surgery.

ULNAR COLLATERAL LIGAMENT RECONSTRUCTION

Ulnar collateral ligament (UCL) injury is common in overhead athletes, such as baseball pitchers. During the late cocking and early acceleration phases of the throwing biomechanics, valgus stress on the UCL is often sufficient to cause a tear. The primary indication for surgery is failure of nonoperative management, which includes rest from pitching and subsequent physical therapy, coupled with the desire to return to competitive sports activity.[31]

Surgical Technique

The original technique described by Jobe and colleagues[32] in 1986 involved a palmaris longus tendon autograft, the complete detachment of the flexor-pronator mass from the medial epicondyle, and submuscular transposition of the ulnar nerve. The tendon graft is pulled through the ulnar and humeral tunnels to form a figure-of-eight configuration and then sutured onto itself. Because of the high rate of ulnar nerve paresthesia, the original technique was modified by Jobe using a flexor-pronator muscle splitting

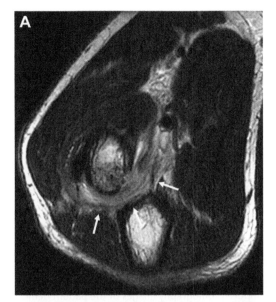

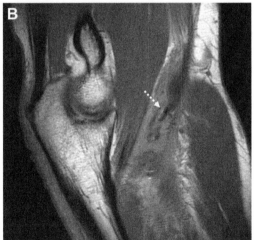

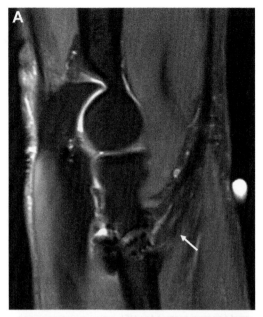

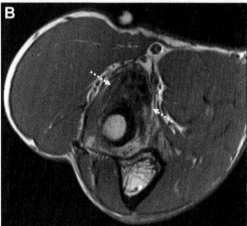

Fig. 3. A 36-year-old man with clinical concern of re-ruptured biceps tendon repair. (*A*) Axial T2 image shows a diffusely heterogeneous distal biceps tendon near the radial attachment (*arrows*). (*B*) Sagittal PD image demonstrates what seems to be a retracted end of a torn tendon (*arrow*). However, the biceps tendon was found to be in continuity with the radial tuberosity at exploratory surgery with intact supination on traction, leading to no repair or revision performed. PD, proton density.

Fig. 4. A 58-year-old man with elbow pain and paresthesia status post biceps tendon repair performed 1 year prior. (*A*) Sagittal PDFS image demonstrates mildly hyperintense signal within the distal biceps tendon (*arrow*) without fluid clefts. (*B*) Axial PD image demonstrates diffuse thickening and intermediate signal of the distal biceps tendon, suggesting moderate tendinosis (*dotted arrows*).

approach to access the UCL without ulnar nerve transposition.[33] Additional concerns regarding graft fixation and tensioning from the original Jobe technique led to the development of a docking technique first described by Rohrbough and colleagues.[34] Similar to the modified Jobe technique, the docking technique used a muscle-splitting approach without ulnar nerve transposition, but instead "docks" the free ends of the tendon graft in the humerus through a single humeral tunnel with sutures tied over a bone bridge. Other variations of the original Jobe technique have been described, with differences in the treatment of ulnar nerve and graft configuration, but no studies have indicated a clear benefit of one technique over another.[35]

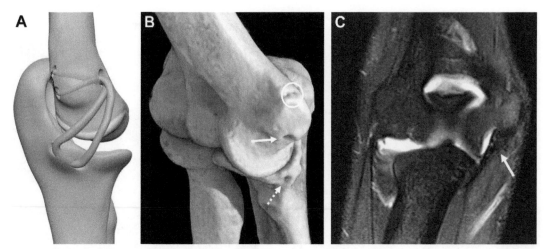

Fig. 5. A 22-year-old man, right hand–dominant baseball pitcher, with normal UCL reconstruction performed 2 years prior. (*A*) Illustration showing normal UCL reconstruction with intact graft threaded through humeral and ulnar bone tunnels using a figure-of-eight configuration with sutures tying the ends of the graft together. (*B*) Three-dimensional global illumination rendering from computed tomography images of the patient demonstrates important surgical landmarks including a bone bridge (*circle*), a humeral tunnel (*solid arrow*), and an ulnar tunnel (*dotted arrow*) for UCL reconstruction via the Tommy John surgery. (*C*) Coronal T2FS image demonstrates an intact UCL reconstruction graft with homogeneously hypointense signal (*arrow*).

Postoperative Imaging

Expected MR imaging appearance after UCL reconstruction depends on the surgical technique and time since surgery. The UCL graft should be thicker than the native UCL and remain taut without redundancy. Most normal grafts demonstrate low T1 and T2 signal, whereas approximately 20% of normal grafts demonstrate intermediate T1 and T2 signal commonly seen proximally (**Fig. 5**).[36] In patients with ulnar nerve transposition, the ulnar nerve, which is transposed anterior to the medial epicondyle, can appear prominent and mildly hyperintense on T2-weighted imaging without focal caliber change.[37]

Intra-articular contrast on MR arthrogram extending between the distal UCL graft and the sublime tubercle, known as the well-recognized "T-sign" for partial tear in the native UCL, is often seen in normal distal graft insertion because the ulnar graft tunnels are approximately 3 to 4 mm distal to the articular surface.[38]

Overall complication rate for UCL reconstructions are estimated to be around 10%, and graft tears in about 2% of cases.[35,39] MR arthrogram in this setting is more sensitive for evaluating partial graft tears from adjacent granulation tissue and serves to distend the elbow joint to better differentiate adjacent medial structures.[38] Graft

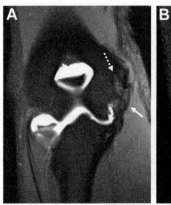 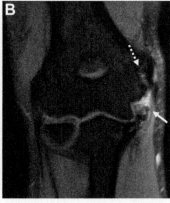

Fig. 6. UCL reconstruction complications. (*A*) A 21-year-old male baseball pitcher with elbow pain status post UCL reconstruction performed 3 years prior. Coronal T1FS image demonstrates diffuse thickening and intermediate signal of the reconstructed UCL (*solid arrow*), which suggests graft degeneration. Note the intact humeral tunnel (*dotted arrow*). (*B*) A 25-year-old man with elbow pain on pitching and prior UCL reconstruction 2 years prior. Coronal PDFS image demonstrates fluid gap between the retracted UCL graft (*solid arrow*) and the humeral tunnel (*dotted arrow*) at the medial epicondyle. Rerupture of the UCL graft was found on revision Tommy John surgery.

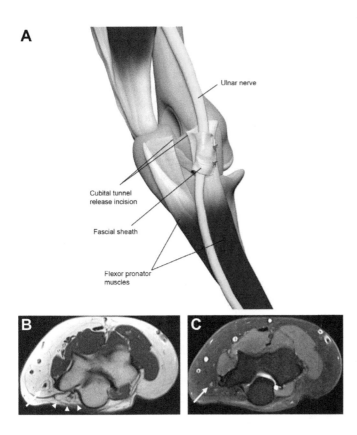

A

Ulnar nerve

Cubital tunnel
release incision

Fascial sheath

Flexor pronator
muscles

Fig. 7. A 51-year-old woman with paresthesia of the ring and pinky fingers status post ulnar nerve transposition 3 years prior. (*A*) Illustration showing cubital tunnel release in ulnar nerve decompression and transposition. Axial PD (*B*) and axial PDFS (*C*) images demonstrate normal signal and caliber of the ulnar nerve (*arrow*) outside of the unroofed cubital tunnel (*arrowheads*).

degeneration is evidenced by diffuse intermediate T1 and mildly hyperintense T2 signal with graft thickening and loss of discernible UCL graft fibers (**Fig. 6**A). Larger tears demonstrate disruption of graft fibers and fluid signal on T2-weighted imaging (**Fig. 6**B), with or without intra-articular contrast imbibition through the tear on T1-weighted imaging depending on whether there is extension to the articular surface. In smaller partial tears, there is subtle increased signal on T1-weighted imaging without discrete disruption of fibers on MR arthrogram caused by subtle intra-articular contrast imbibition into the torn fibers. Redundancy or waviness of the graft can also suggest possible interstitial tear. Regarding symptomatic ulnar neuritis after ulnar nerve transposition in UCL reconstruction, little has been published correlating to imaging findings, although the ulnar nerve should be carefully evaluated as in all cases of ulnar neuritis (see later). Lastly, postoperative ossification within the UCL graft adjacent to the medial epicondyle can become symptomatic.

ULNAR NERVE DECOMPRESSION IN CUBITAL TUNNEL SYNDROME

Cubital tunnel syndrome is the most common compressive neuropathy at the elbow, resulting from compression and traction of the ulnar nerve. Timely surgical treatment is important because chronic nerve compression can result in permanent neuropathy and muscle weakness. In the United States, the rate of surgical management has increased by 47% in recent decades.[40] Ulnar nerve transposition remains one of the most commonly performed surgeries in the setting of failed conservative management and is widely used in revision surgery.[41]

Surgical Technique

The most common surgical interventions for cubital tunnel syndrome are in situ or simple decompression, medial epicondylectomy with decompression, and anterior transposition. For simple decompression, the ulnar nerve is released at the level of the medical epicondyle by transection of the cubital tunnel retinaculum also termed the Osborne ligament, and distally by transection of the fascia between the two heads of the flexor carpi ulnaris muscle. Proximal release of the fascia between the medial triceps muscle and medial intermuscular septum, and the arcade of Struthers if present, may be performed if indicated. Circumferential dissection of the ulnar nerve is not performed to minimize devascularization and to

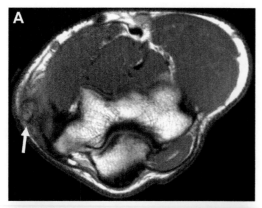

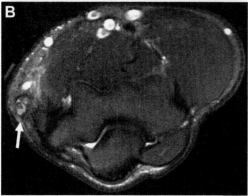

Fig. 8. A 49-year-old man with persistent ulnar neuropathy status post subcutaneous transposition of the ulnar nerve 1 year prior. Axial PD (*A*) and axial T2FS (*B*) images demonstrate diffuse thickening and edema of the ulnar nerve (*arrow*). Surrounding ill-defined intermediate soft tissue signal likely representing perineural scar tissue in the region of the fascial sling. Note the loss of fascicular architecture of the transposed ulnar nerve.

avoid creating hypermobility of the nerve.[42] Medial epicondylectomy, another option for surgical management, is often performed with simple decompression. The nerve is first released similar to simple decompression, then the medial epicondyle is exposed by subperiosteal dissection of the flexor-pronator or the common flexor origin. An oblique osteotomy is performed to remove normal bone or excessive osteophytes posteriorly while preserving the origin of the UCL, thereby increasing the space available for the cubital tunnel. The cut surface of the bone is then contoured, and the common flexor origin reconstructed.[43] For symptoms caused by ulnar nerve subluxation or dislocation at the medical epicondyle, anterior transposition of the ulnar nerve can increase stability. There are two main types of anterior transposition: subcutaneous and submuscular. In subcutaneous anterior transposition, the ulnar

nerve is released as in simple decompression and circumferentially dissected, then anteriorly transposed to a position medial to the medical epicondyle into a subcutaneous fascial sling. Submuscular anterior transposition has similar initial technique as subcutaneous transposition, with the ulnar nerve anterior transposed superficial to the brachialis muscle and deep to the flex-pronator muscle. Submuscular transposition requires the release of the flexor-pronator mass, which increases the surgical time and involves a greater risk of surgical morbidity.[42] There has been no consensus on the most appropriate surgical technique for cubital tunnel syndrome, because most studies demonstrate similar results in terms of surgical outcomes.[44]

Postoperative Imaging

Normal postoperative appearance of cubital tunnel release depends on the surgical technique (**Fig. 7**). In simple decompression, the ulnar nerve can appear prominent with increased T2 signal and mild surrounding soft tissue edema for asymptomatic patients. The cubital tunnel retinaculum may also appear thickened, whereas portions of it may appear diminutive. Expected changes of medial epicondylectomy include mild marrow edema in the medial epicondyle and increased signal of the common flexor tendon at the epicondylar origin in addition to changes of simple decompression. Similar to other surgical techniques for cubital tunnel release, little is published on the postoperative appearance of anterior ulnar nerve transposition. In subcutaneous transposition there is absence of the cubital tunnel with anterior course of the ulnar nerve in the subcutaneous fat where the nerve courses anteriorly deep to flexor-pronator musculature in submuscular decompression. Signal and caliber changes of the ulnar nerve with surround soft tissue edema and atrophy of the flexor ulnaris muscle is seen in both types of anterior transposition, whereas postoperative thickening of the common flexor tendon is seen with submuscular transposition.[45]

Many factors may contribute to failure of ulnar nerve decompressive surgery, including unrecognized dynamic nerve instability, incomplete decompression, kinking at a proximal or distal structure, postoperative seroma or hematoma, and perineural fibrosis.[41,45] In all cases of ulnar neuritis, the following characteristics of the ulnar nerve should be carefully evaluated: course, caliber, signal, fascicular architecture, and perineural fat.[37] Of note, none of these characteristics were definitively predictive of postoperative symptom recurrence.[46] In simple decompression, focal

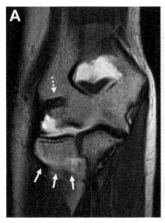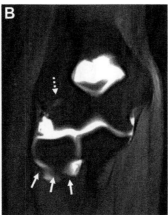

Fig. 9. A 17-year-old girl with LUCL repair 4 years prior. Coronal PD (*A*) and coronal T1FS (*B*) demonstrate suture anchor (*dotted arrow*) at the lateral epicondyle. The repaired LUCL appears intact (*solid arrows*) to the distal attachment at the supinator crest of ulna.

changes in ulnar nerve caliber and morphology may suggest nerve entrapment (**Fig. 8**). Focal kinking or angulation in the area of the Osborne ligament or the intermuscular septum is suggestive of incomplete decompression.[41] Medial epicondylectomy commonly demonstrates marrow and soft tissue edema in asymptomatic patients. Because the common flexor tendon is reconstructed at the osteotomized medial epicondyle, partial tearing at the attachment can occur. Attention should be also given to the anterior band of the UCL because injury can occur perioperatively caused by the close proximity to the flex-pronator origin. Subluxation and instability of the ulnar nerve in anterior subcutaneous transposition may be present but missed before surgery, or secondary to suboptimal anchoring of the ulnar nerve in the subcutaneous sling. In addition, perineural fibrosis is a common occurrence in failed anterior transposition.[43] A dense rind of scarring about the nerve with obliteration of the perineural fat may be helpful to differentiate the true impingement cases in the region of the flexor-pronator mass, especially when associated with focal nerve caliber, course, or signal changes.

LATERAL COLLATERAL LIGAMENTOUS COMPLEX RECONSTRUCTION

The lateral collateral ligament complex is composed of the lateral ulnar collateral ligament (LUCL), radial collateral ligament, and annular ligament, with the LUCL serving as the primary stabilizer against varus and posterolateral rotatory instability.[47] Lateral collateral ligament complex insufficiency and consequently posterolateral rotatory instability typically results from a fall onto outstretched hand, which generates a combination of axial, valgus, and external rotatory forces of the forearm. Biomechanically, isolated

reconstruction of the LUCL approximately restores posterolateral rotatory and varus stability.[47–49]

Surgical Technique

Several surgical techniques and fixation modalities are available for LUCL reconstruction, including the single bundle technique or the docking technique. The Kocher lateral elbow approach is used to expose and detach the injured LUCL from its origins. In the single bundle technique, two drill holes are created, one at the supinator crest and another at the isometric point on the lateral epicondyle. A tendon autograft or allograft is tightly fixed to the ulnar and humerus with interference screws or cortical buttons.[50] In the docking technique, an osseous tunnel connecting two drill holes is created at the supinator crest. Another tunnel is created at the isometric point of the humerus with two puncture holes.[51,52] The graft is then woven through the ulnar tunnel and securely docked into the humeral tunnel with sutures from the graft exiting through the two puncture holes and tied over a bone bridge after adequate graft tensioning. Some have described a dual-reconstruction approach where the reconstruction graft is passed through the annular ligament in a biomechanical configuration similar to the native radial collateral ligament and the LCUL.[53]

Postoperative Imaging

Literature is scant on postoperative appearance of LUCL reconstruction. In a study by Kim and colleagues,[54] complete tendon-to-bone healing is seen at 3 months postoperatively where the graft reconstruction demonstrates homogeneous T2-hypointense signal (**Fig. 9**). In the same study, one case demonstrated incomplete healing with graft heterogeneity on T2-weighted imaging near the humeral attachment and associated widening of the radiocapitellar joint space of unknown clinical significance. Surgical outcome is favorable for LUCL reconstruction, with low complication rate and up to 90% achieving postoperative elbow stability.[47] Distal humerus fracture initiated through the bone tunnel has been reported as a complication, in addition to recurrent instability and graft failure (**Fig. 10**).[50]

COMMON FLEXOR AND EXTENSOR TENDON REPAIR

Lateral epicondylitis, also known as "tennis elbow," is a frequent cause of lateral elbow pain and is classically associated with tennis in which repetitive supination and protonation of the forearm on an extended elbow results in degeneration of the common extensor tendon at the lateral epicondylar attachment.[55] Medial epicondylitis, also known as "golfer's elbow," which occurs much less frequently than lateral epicondylitis, is a result of flexor-pronator muscle overuse in repetitive forearm protonation and wrist flexion seen in golfers and baseball pitchers among other sports.[56] Nonsurgical treatment is the mainstay of care for medial and lateral epicondylitis, and surgical management is considered in setting of failed conservative treatment and tendon disruption in high-level athletes.

Surgical Technique

The extensor carpi radialis brevis (ECRB) tendon is the most commonly affected contribution of the common extensor tendon in lateral epicondylitis.[57] The suture technique described and popularized by Nirschl and colleagues has provided excellent long-term results.[58,59] The extensor carpi radialis longus tendon is retracted anteromedially to expose the ECRB tendon. The degenerated portion of the ECRB tendon is then identified and excised while leaving the normal tendon intact. A single drill hole is made to the anterior lateral epicondyle to enhance vascular supply and healing. Lastly, closure over the ECRB is performed by suturing the extensor carpi radialis longus tendon to the extensor aponeurosis. Surgical approach for medial epicondylitis is similar in concept, with excision of the pathologic tendon and reattachment back to the medial epicondyle.[56] Considerations are taken to protect the medial antebrachial cutaneous nerve, the ulnar nerve, and the UCL during surgical dissection. Reattachment options differ depending on the extent of the tendinosis and tearing. A side-to-side tendon repair may be performed for small lesions of the common flexor tendon.[60] In more extensive

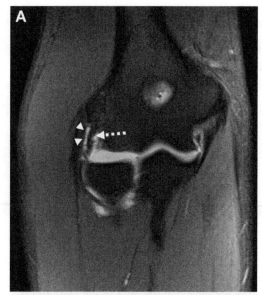

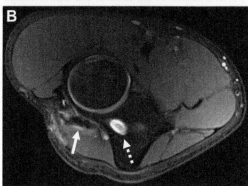

Fig. 10. A 20-year-old wrestler with history of LUCL reconstruction 10 months prior. (A) Coronal T1FS image demonstrates intra-articular contrast imbibition between the LUCL graft and the common extensor tendon (*arrowheads*). The LUCL reconstruction graft (*arrow*) appears diffusely heterogeneous with widening of the radiocapitellar articulation, suggesting a full-thickness tear. (B) Axial PDFS image demonstrates diffuse thickening of the LUCL graft (*solid arrow*) and surrounding soft tissue edema. Note suture anchor at the proximal ulna (*dotted arrow*).

lesions of the common flexor tendon, a flexor-pronator mass incision is commonly performed to excise the pathologic portion, and the medial epicondyle is prepared with multiple small drill holes before reattachment of the flexor-pronator origin.

Postoperative Imaging

There is limited literature on the postoperative imaging appearance of the common flexor and extensor tendon repair. MR imaging is not commonly performed for postoperative

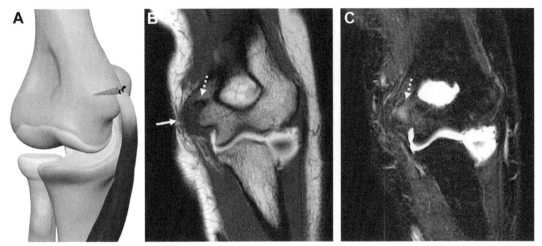

Fig. 11. A 21-year-old female hockey player with common flex tendon repair 1 year prior. (A) Illustration showing repair of the common flexor tendon with suture anchor at the medial humeral epicondyle. (B) Coronal T1 image demonstrates suture anchor (*dotted arrow*) at the medial epicondyle and diffusely heterogeneous signal of the common flexor tendon (*solid arrow*), suggesting moderate tendinosis. (C) Coronal T2FS image demonstrates marrow edema (*arrow*) at the medial epicondyle, which may be stress related or reactive changes.

epicondylitis because complications are rare and are usually diagnosed clinically.[56,61] Correlation with preoperative MR imaging is helpful because the flexor and extensor tendons may demonstrate similar increased signal or defect on T2-weighted imaging in setting of tendon degeneration and granulation postoperatively (**Fig. 11**).[62,63] In medial epicondylitis, a concurrent ulnar nerve transposition may be performed depending on clinical symptoms of ulnar neuritis. The anterior band of

the UCL is just deep to the common flexor origin, and it may be reconstructed during the same surgery for preexisting injury, or it can sustain iatrogenic injury during common flexor tendon repair.[60]

DISTAL TRICEPS TENDON REPAIR

Distal triceps tendon ruptures are extremely rare, accounting for less than 1% of all tendon ruptures.[64] Complete rupture of the triceps tendon

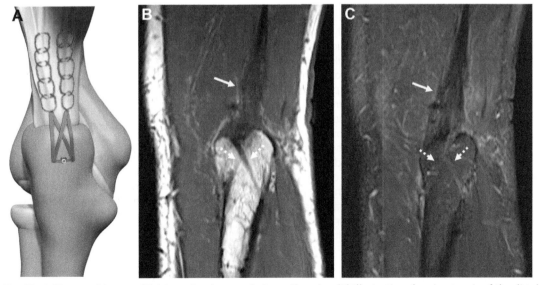

Fig. 12. A 29-year-old man with triceps tendon repair 4 months prior. (A) Illustration showing repair of the distal triceps tendon onto the olecranon. Coronal T1 (B) and coronal T2FS (C) images demonstrate two suture tunnels in a cruciate configuration (*dotted arrows*). The repaired distal tendon (*solid arrow*) is intact.

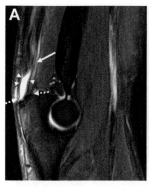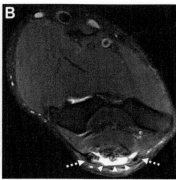

Fig. 13. A 24-year-old lacrosse player with history of triceps tendon repair 1 year prior. Sagittal PDFS image (*A*) and axial PDFS image (*B*) demonstrate high-grade partial retear of the repaired triceps tendon. Retracted tendon stump appears heterogeneous with intermedia signal (*solid arrow*). Some tendon fibers remain attached to the olecranon (*dotted arrows*) and a large fluid gap between the torn fibers (*arrowheads*).

typically occurs in the setting of forceful eccentric load against a contracting triceps muscle, most commonly seen in the athletic world among football players and body builders.[65] Acute partial or complete rupture of the triceps tendon are best managed by surgical reattachment within 3 weeks of injury.[66]

Surgical Technique

Many surgical techniques for distal triceps tendon repair have been reported, with no clear superiority of one technique over another in terms of clinical outcome.[64] The transosseous cruciate bone-tunnel technique is the historical standard for repair, using a Krackow-type suture passed through the distal triceps tendon and two small bone tunnels at the olecranon tied over a bone bridge (**Fig. 12**).[67,68] Other modified techniques have recently become popular to restore the native anatomic footprint and improve mechanical strength. The transosseous-equivalent (also termed anatomic double row) technique described by Yeh and colleagues[69] showed significantly greater repair strength compared with the traditional bone tunnel or suture anchor techniques. A Krakow stitch is first used to secure and prepare the torn central triceps tendon. Two suture anchors are positioned in the proximal olecranon with sutures from these anchors passed through the tendon creating horizontal mattress stitches. Suture ends from the anchors and the Krachow-type stitch are secured to additional two anchors placed more distally on the dorsal aspect of the ulna.[64,66,70] This configuration compresses the entire width of the tendon against the prepared bone bed underneath, better recreating the native anatomic footprint. Lastly, depending on the chronicity of injury, graft augmentation may be performed.[66]

Postoperative Imaging

Complications after triceps tendon repair are rare, some of which include olecranon bursitis, flexion contracture, extension weakness, and rerupture.[70] Among cases with complications, rerupture has been reported in up to 25% of cases particularly in professional athletes or high-demand patients.[71,72] Similar to preoperative evaluation, MR imaging obtained in the setting of suspected reinjury can localize the tear and quantify how much of it is torn and retracted (**Fig. 13**).[73] Additional potential complications include iatrogenic injury of the ulnar nerve medially and the radial nerve proximally during surgical dissection and tendon mobilization.[74] Thus, the ulnar and radial nerves should be investigated along their entire course on postoperative MR imaging. Degree of enthesophyte formation after bone-to-tendon healing should be reported, because it is thought to be a contributing factor to triceps tendon abnormalities and potentially rupture.[75] For patients with olecranon enthesophyte excision and primary distal triceps tendon repair, subsequent tendon thickening, scar formation, calcification, and insertional enthesophyte may contribute to greater surgical site morbidity.[75,76]

SUMMARY

MR imaging for the postoperative elbow is challenging because of the rare nature of premorbid injuries, postoperative complications that are evaluated clinically without additional imaging for revision, and lack of consensus and long-term data for varying surgical techniques. Knowledge of different operative approaches is essential to evaluate for postoperative complications of tendon repair, ligamentous reconstruction, osteochondral grafting, and nerve transposition on MR imaging, which can help guide postoperative treatment for the referring clinicians.

DISCLOSURE AND CONFLICT OF INTEREST

The authors declare that they have no conflict of interest or relevant disclosures.

CLINICS CARE POINTS

- In postoperative MR imaging of the elbow, signal changes of the repaired structure must be interpreted with patient's clinical symptoms to avoid overdiagnosing of complications.

- In the postoperative elbow, be mindful of the timing from surgery because normal findings can have varied appearance, particularly in the short-term postoperative period (3 months).

- For repaired tendons and ligaments, normal postoperative appearance can mimic pathology that is similar-appearing to their abnormal native counterparts (eg, T-sign in native UCL tear is a normal postoperative appearance for repaired UCL).

- If possible, every MR image should be interpreted with the surgical approach and technique in mind to look for other complications related to the surgery.

DISCLOSURE

The authors have nothing to disclose.

REFERENCES

1. Hoang QB, Mortazavi M. Pediatric overuse injuries in sports. Adv Pediatr 2012;59:359–83.
2. Ring D, Jupiter JB. Reconstruction of posttraumatic elbow instability. Clin Orthop 2000;370:44–56.
3. Johnson D, Stevens KJ, Riley G, et al. Approach to MR imaging of the elbow and wrist. Magn Reson Imaging Clin N Am 2015;23:355–66.
4. Hargreaves BA, Worters PW, Pauly KB, et al. Metal-induced artifacts in MRI. Am J Roentgenol 2011; 197:547–55.
5. Jungmann PM, Agten CA, Pfirrmann CW, et al. Advances in MRI around metal. J Magn Reson Imaging 2017;46:972–91.
6. Tis JE, Edmonds EW, Bastrom T, et al. Short-term results of arthroscopic treatment of osteochondritis dissecans in skeletally immature patients. J Pediatr Orthop 2012;32:226–31.
7. Shea KG, Jacobs JC, Carey JL, et al. Osteochondritis dissecans knee histology studies have variable findings and theories of etiology. Clin Orthop 2013; 471:1127–36.
8. Bexkens R, Simeone FJ, Eygendaal D, et al. Interobserver reliability of the classification of capitellar osteochondritis dissecans using magnetic resonance imaging. Shoulder Elb 2020;12:284–93.
9. Jans LBO, Ditchfield M, Anna G, et al. MR imaging findings and MR criteria for instability in osteochondritis dissecans of the elbow in children. Eur J Radiol 2012;81:1306–10.
10. Logli AL, Bernard CD, O'Driscoll SW, et al. Osteochondritis dissecans lesions of the capitellum in overhead athletes: a review of current evidence and proposed treatment algorithm. Curr Rev Musculoskelet Med 2019;12:1–12.
11. Johnson CC, Roberts SM, Mintz D, et al. A matched quantitative computed tomography analysis of 3 surgical approaches for osteochondral reconstruction of the capitellum. J Shoulder Elbow Surg 2018;27: 1762–9.
12. Iwasaki N, Kato H, Funakoshi T, et al. Autologous osteochondral mosaicplasty for osteochondritis dissecans of the elbow in teenage athletes. J Bone Joint Surg Am 2009;91:2359–66.
13. Cutler HS, Kelly D, Gross B, et al. Increased articular exposure of the lateral elbow joint with the anconeus approach compared to the Kocher approach: a cadaver study. Arch Orthop Trauma Surg 2021; 141:917–23.
14. Schrumpf M, Daluiski A, Richards J, et al. The mid-axial (universal) approach to the lateral elbow. Elb Surg 2011;12:6–11.
15. Shimada K, Tanaka H, Matsumoto T, et al. Cylindrical costal osteochondral autograft for reconstruction of large defects of the capitellum due to osteochondritis dissecans. J Bone Joint Surg Am 2012;94: 992–1002.
16. Weigelt L, Siebenlist S, Hensler D, et al. Treatment of osteochondral lesions in the elbow: results after autologous osteochondral transplantation. Arch Orthop Trauma Surg 2015;135:627–34.
17. Kirsch JM, Thomas J, Bedi A, et al. Current concepts: osteochondritis dissecans of the capitellum and the role of osteochondral autograft transplantation. Hand 2016;11:396–402.
18. Yamamoto Y, Ishibashi Y, Tsuda E, et al. Osteochondral autograft transplantation for osteochondritis dissecans of the elbow in juvenile baseball players: minimum 2-year follow-up. Am J Sports Med 2006; 34:714–20.
19. Kelly MP, Perkinson SG, Ablove RH, et al. Distal biceps tendon ruptures: an epidemiological analysis using a large population database. Am J Sports Med 2015;43:2012–7.
20. Srinivasan RC, Pederson WC, Morrey BF. Distal biceps tendon repair and reconstruction. J Hand Surg 2020;45:48–56.
21. Grewal R, Athwal GS, MacDermid JC, et al. Surgical technique for single and double-incision method of acute distal biceps tendon repair. JBJS Essent Surg Tech 2012;2:e22.

22. Mazzocca AD, Burton KJ, Romeo AA, et al. Biomechanical evaluation of 4 techniques of distal biceps brachii tendon repair. Am J Sports Med 2007;35: 252–8.

23. Hechtman KS, Thorpe M, Gampel B, et al. Effectiveness of MRI to assess the integrity of distal biceps tendon repair during the first year postoperatively. Curr Orthop Pract 2014;25:563–7.

24. Schmidt CC, Styron JF, Lin EA, et al. Distal biceps tendon anatomic repair. JBJS Essent Surg Tech 2017;7:e32.

25. Alemann G, Dietsch E, Gallinet D, et al. Repair of distal biceps brachii tendon assessed with 3-T magnetic resonance imaging and correlation with functional outcome. Skeletal Radiol 2015;44:629–39.

26. Garon MT, Greenberg JA. Complications of distal biceps repair. Orthop Clin North Am 2016;47:435–44.

27. Amin NH, Volpi A, Lynch TS, et al. Complications of distal biceps tendon repair: a meta-analysis of single-incision versus double-incision surgical technique. Orthop J Sports Med 2016;4:1–5.

28. Amarasooriya M, Bain GI, Roper T, et al. Complications after distal biceps tendon repair: a systematic review. Am J Sports Med 2020;48:3103–11.

29. Prokuski V, Leung NL, Leslie BM. Diagnosis, etiology and outcomes of revision distal biceps tendon reattachment. J Hand Surg 2020;45:156.e1–9.

30. Rashid A, Copas D, Watts AC. Failure of distal biceps repair by gapping. Shoulder Elb 2016;8:192–6.

31. Erickson BJ, Harris JD, Chalmers PN, et al. Ulnar collateral ligament reconstruction: anatomy, indications, techniques, and outcomes. Sports Health 2015;7:511–7.

32. Jobe FW, Stark H, Lombardo SJ. Reconstruction of the ulnar collateral ligament in athletes. J Bone Joint Surg Am 1986;68:1158–63.

33. Thompson WH, Jobe FW, Yocum LA, et al. Ulnar collateral ligament reconstruction in athletes: muscle-splitting approach without transposition of the ulnar nerve. J Shoulder Elbow Surg 2001;10: 152–7.

34. Rohrbough JT, Altchek DW, Hyman J, et al. Medial collateral ligament reconstruction of the elbow using the docking technique. Am J Sports Med 2002;30: 541–8.

35. Vitale MA, Ahmad CS. The outcome of elbow ulnar collateral ligament reconstruction in overhead athletes: a systematic review. Am J Sports Med 2008; 36:1193–205.

36. Daniels SP, Mintz DN, Endo Y, et al. Imaging of the post-operative medial elbow in the overhead thrower: common and abnormal findings after ulnar collateral ligament reconstruction and ulnar nerve transposition. Skeletal Radiol 2019;48:1843–60.

37. Bucknor MD, Stevens KJ, Steinbach LS. Elbow imaging in sport: sports imaging series. Radiology 2016;279:12–28.

38. Wear SA, Thornton DD, Schwartz ML, et al. MRI of the reconstructed ulnar collateral ligament. Am J Roentgenol 2011;197:1198–204.

39. Dines JS, Yocum LA, Frank JB, et al. Revision surgery for failed elbow medial collateral ligament reconstruction. Am J Sports Med 2008;36:1061–5.

40. Soltani AM, Best MJ, Francis CS, et al. Trends in the surgical treatment of cubital tunnel syndrome: an analysis of the national survey of ambulatory surgery database. J Hand Surg 2013;38:1551–6.

41. Chadwick N, Morag Y, Smith BW, et al. Imaging appearance following surgical decompression of the ulnar nerve. Br J Radiol 2019;92:1–6.

42. Staples JR, Calfee R. Cubital tunnel syndrome: current concepts. J Am Acad Orthop Surg 2017;25: e215–24.

43. Osei DA, Padegimas EM, Calfee RP, et al. Outcomes following modified oblique medial epicondylectomy for treatment of cubital tunnel syndrome. J Hand Surg 2013;38:336–43.

44. Caliandro P, La Torre G, Padua R, et al. Treatment for ulnar neuropathy at the elbow. Cochrane Database Syst Rev 2016;11:1–47.

45. Rhodes NG, Howe BM, Frick MA, et al. MR imaging of the postsurgical cubital tunnel: an imaging review of the cubital tunnel, cubital tunnel syndrome, and associated surgical techniques. Skeletal Radiol 2019;48:1541–54.

46. Sivakumaran T, Sneag DB, Lin B, et al. MRI of the ulnar nerve pre- and post-transposition: imaging features and rater agreement. Skeletal Radiol 2021; 50:559–70.

47. Fares A, Kusnezov N, Dunn JC. Lateral ulnar collateral ligament reconstruction for posterolateral rotatory instability of the elbow: a systematic review. Hand 2020;00:e1–7.

48. De Giorgi S, Vicenti G, Bizzoca D, et al. Lateral collateral ulnar ligament reconstruction techniques in posterolateral rotatory instability of the elbow: a systematic review. Injury 2020;15:e1–5.

49. Badhrinarayanan S, Desai A, Watson JJ, et al. Indications, outcomes, and complications of lateral ulnar collateral ligament reconstruction of the elbow for chronic posterolateral rotatory instability: a systematic review. Am J Sports Med 2021;49:830–7.

50. Conti Mica M, Caekebeke P, van Riet R. Lateral collateral ligament injuries of the elbow: chronic posterolateral rotatory instability (PLRI). EFORT Open Rev 2016;1:461–8.

51. Sanchez-Sotelo J, Morrey BF, O'Driscoll SW. Ligamentous repair and reconstruction for posterolateral rotatory instability of the elbow. J Bone Joint Surg Br 2005;87:54–61.

52. Jones KJ, Dodson CC, Osbahr DC, et al. The docking technique for lateral ulnar collateral ligament reconstruction: surgical technique and clinical outcomes. J Shoulder Elbow Surg 2012;21:389–95.

53. Rhyou IH, Park MJ. Dual reconstruction of the radial collateral ligament and lateral ulnar collateral ligament in posterolateral rotator instability of the elbow. Knee Surg Sports Traumatol Arthrosc 2011;19: 1009–12.

54. Kim JW, Yi Y, Kim TK, et al. Arthroscopic lateral collateral ligament repair. J Bone Joint Surg Am 2016;98:1268–76.

55. Ahmad Z, Siddiqui N, Malik SS, et al. Lateral epicondylitis: a review of pathology and management. Bone Joint J 2013;95:1158–64.

56. Ciccotti MC, Schwartz MA, Ciccotti MG. Diagnosis and treatment of medial epicondylitis of the elbow. Clin Sports Med 2004;23:693–705.

57. Inagaki K. Current concepts of elbow-joint disorders and their treatment. J Orthop Sci 2013;18:1–7.

58. Dunn JH, Kim JJ, Davis L, et al. Ten- to 14-year follow-up of the Nirschl surgical technique for lateral epicondylitis. Am J Sports Med 2008;36:261–6.

59. Organ SW, Nirschl RP, Kraushaar BS, et al. Salvage surgery for lateral tennis elbow. Am J Sports Med 1997;25:746–50.

60. Amin NH, Kumar NS, Schickendantz MS. Medial epicondylitis: evaluation and management. J Am Acad Orthop Surg 2015;23:348–55.

61. Cohen M, da Rocha Motta Filho G. Lateral epicondylitis of the elbow. Rev Bras Ortop 2012;47:414–20.

62. Wada T, Moriya T, Iba K, et al. Functional outcomes after arthroscopic treatment of lateral epicondylitis. J Orthop Sci 2009;14:167–74.

63. Yoon JP, Chung SW, Yi JH, et al. Prognostic factors of arthroscopic extensor carpi radialis brevis release for lateral epicondylitis. Arthrosc J Arthrosc Relat Surg 2015;31:1232–7.

64. Walker CM, Noonan TJ. Distal triceps tendon injuries. Clin Sports Med 2020;39:673–85.

65. Thomas JR, Lawton JN. Biceps and triceps ruptures in athletes. Hand Clin 2017;33:35–46.

66. Marinello PG, Peers S, Sraj S, et al. A treatment algorithm for the management of distal triceps ruptures. Tech Hand Up Extrem Surg 2015;19:73–80.

67. Dunn JC, Kusnezov N, Fares A, et al. Triceps tendon ruptures: a systematic review. Hand 2017;12:431–8.

68. Scheiderer B, Imhoff FB, Morikawa D, et al. The V-shaped distal triceps tendon repair: a comparative biomechanical analysis. Am J Sports Med 2018;46:1952–8.

69. Yeh PC, Stephens KT, Solovyova O, et al. The distal triceps tendon footprint and a biomechanical analysis of 3 repair techniques. Am J Sports Med 2010;38:1025–33.

70. Keener JD, Sethi PM. Distal triceps tendon injuries. Hand Clin 2015;31:641–50.

71. Mirzayan R, Acevedo DC, Sodl JF, et al. Operative management of acute triceps tendon ruptures: review of 184 cases. Am J Sports Med 2018;46: 1451–8.

72. Giannicola G, Bullitta G, Rotini R, et al. Results of primary repair of distal triceps tendon ruptures in a general population: a multicentre study. Bone Joint J 2018;100:610–6.

73. Mair SD, Isbell WM, Gill TJ, et al. Triceps tendon ruptures in professional football players. Am J Sports Med 2004;32:431–4.

74. Edelman D, Ilyas A. Triceps tendon anatomic repair utilizing the "suture bridge" technique. J Hand Microsurg 2018;10:166–71.

75. Waterman BR, Dean RS, Veera S, et al. Surgical repair of distal triceps tendon injuries: short-term to midterm clinical outcomes and risk factors for perioperative complications. Orthop J Sports Med 2019;7:1–6.

76. Alvi HM, Kalainov DM, Biswas D, et al. Surgical management of symptomatic olecranon traction spurs. Orthop J Sports Med 2014;2:1–5.

Postoperative Imaging of the Wrist and Hand

Eva Llopis, MD[a],*, Luis Cerezal, MD, PhD[b], Rocio Auban, MD[c], Luis Aguilella, PhD[d], Francisco del Piñal, PhD[e]

KEYWORDS

- Scaphoid fracture • Distal radius fractures • Fibrocartilage • Scapholunate ligament
- Carpal tunnel release • Trapeziometacarpal joint surgery techniques • Tendon sutures • Arthrodesis

KEY POINTS

- Knowledge of surgical techniques is essential to understand posttreatment complications.
- Wrist plain films are still the first imaging technique for pretreatment and posttreatment.
- CT and MR protocols should be tailored if metal artifacts are present

Abbreviations	
CRPS	Complex regional pain syndrome
TFCC	Triangular fibrocartilage complex
SLL	Scapholunate ligament
LTL	Lunotriquetral ligament
CRPP	Closed reduction with percutaneous pinning
ORIF	Open reduction with internal fixation

INTRODUCTION

There is a wide range of different surgical procedures performed in the wrist and hand from congenital to tumoral lesions, and a significant number of them will develop postsurgical pain. Unfortunately, there are a limited number of publications on radiological complications of wrist surgeries, most based on anecdotal evidence through personal experiences rather than randomized series. Surgeons have based their postsurgical evaluation on clinical examinations and plain films. However, as patients have become more functionally demanding such as with increased involvement in recreational sports and exercise in the general population, imaging has become important to rule out complications.

The first step is to understand the different surgical approaches that might differ from open surgery, microsurgery, and arthroscopy. It is essential to know the normal anatomy after surgery to be able to distinguish pathologic findings.

This article reviews a selection of the most frequent and important surgical procedures, normal postoperative anatomy, and their complications.

a Department of Radiology, Hospital de la Ribera, IMSKE, km 1, Ctra Corbera, 46600 Alzira, Valencia, Spain; b Diagnostico medico Cantabria, C de Castilla, 6, 39002 Santander, Cantabria, Spain; c Department of Radiology, Hospital de Manises, Av de la Generalitat Valenciana, 50, 46940 Manises, Valencia, Spain; d Department of Orthopedics, Hospital de la Ribera, km 1, Ctra Corbera, 46600 Alzira, Valencia, Spain; e Instituto de cirugía plástica y de la mano, Hospital de la Lux, Madrid y Hospital Mutua Montañesa, C de Serrano, 58, 28001 Madrid, Spain
* Corresponding author.
E-mail address: Evallopis@gmail.com

Magn Reson Imaging Clin N Am 30 (2022) 645–671
https://doi.org/10.1016/j.mric.2022.03.004
1064-9689/22/© 2022 Elsevier Inc. All rights reserved.

IMAGING TECHNIQUES
Radiographs

The first and most important imaging technique after wrist surgery is plain film radiography. Despite the limitations of radiographs including overlap of different structures and the limitations for soft tissue assessment, they still provide a useful neutral position image, allowing to assess alignment and bone structures and to easily compare with preoperative images. Initial plain films should include posteroanterior and lateral neutral views. Additional projections can be useful to evaluate certain structures, such as clenched posteroanterior and oblique at 30° for dorsal ulnar wrist or ulnar deviation.[1,2]

Computed Tomography

Computed tomography (CT) has an important role in the evaluation of the postoperative wrist, especially after fracture reconstructions, allowing multiplanar reconstructions to evaluate the location of the fixation devices and follow the fracture healing process. Metal devices can cause excessive beam attenuation and image degradation. These artifacts can be decreased by traditional methods such as optimizing patients' position, decreasing the speed of rotation and increasing the kVol and mAs to increase the number of photons that reach the detector, and using soft tissue kernel reconstructions to decrease the visual artifact seen with bone reconstructions. Advanced iterative reconstructions minimize scatter and edge effects by using correction algorithms.

Metal reduction algorithms are used to improve CT quality, based on in-painting, frequency splitting, or a combination of these techniques. Dual-energy CT offers reduction through the implementation of energy-specific postprocessing; whereas the high-energy beam has less attenuation, the low-energy beam provides superior soft tissue contrast improving the image quality by creating a virtual monochromatic image.[3–7]

Magnetic Resonance Imaging (MRI)

High-resolution MR imaging is essential to evaluate small wrist structures. The authors favor the use of small dedicated surface coils with the patient in the superman position, or if the patient cannot tolerate that position, the wrist is placed on the side of the patient with the palm down in the pronated position. It is important to avoid lateral position of the wrist with the palm supinated, because this makes evaluation of the ulnar side of the wrist and hand and the first carpal row more difficult. High-resolution small-field-of-view images ranging from 8 to 12 cm are essential. To improve quality and reduce surgical metal artifacts, some measures should be taken including increased bandwidth, decreased echo timing, avoiding gradient echo- and frequency-selective fat saturation images, and instead using inversion recovery, short T1 inversion recovery (STIR) images, DIXON protocols, or specific new metal artifact reduction protocols such as multiadquisition variable resonance image combination (MAVRIC).[8–10]

GENERAL COMPLICATIONS
Infections

Postoperative infection in the hand and wrist is rare, occurring in 1% to 2% of cases.[1] The incidence increases in the high-risk population and depends on several factors such as the type of surgery, presence of open wound, and timing of surgery. Nevertheless, for most wrist and hand surgery involving soft tissue structures, the risk of infection is very low, and therefore antibiotic prophylaxis is not recommended. However, for surgeries involving osseous structures, where the risk increases, prophylaxis is recommended.[11]

For infections that occur at the surgery site, depending on the surgery location, the spread of the infection will be different. Fixation devices such as pins, screws, or plates might develop infections along their track. Infection at the pin site insertion of distal radial fracture surgery has been reported to occur in 25.8% of external fixations[12] (Fig. 1). The knowledge of the history of the patient together with the anatomic spaces in which the infection spreads is essential for early detection and management of these patients.[13] Infections might affect the subcutaneous tissue, deep structures, tendon sheaths and bursae, as well as joints and bones (Fig. 2).

Flexor tendons are surrounded by a close synovial sheath from the head of the metacarpal level to the distal interphalangeal joint. At the palmar side of the wrist, the flexor tendons have 2 distinct superficial bursas: the radial bursa, a continuation of the flexor pollicis longus tendon sheath, and the ulnar bursa, a continuation of the tendon sheath of the fifth flexor tendon that proximally overlaps with the fourth, third, and second flexor tendon sheaths. The radial and ulnar bursa frequently communicate. Deep to these bursae are the volar deep subfascial spaces, which can be divided into thenar, midpalmar, and hypothenar, and are separated by the midpalmar septum and the hypothenar septum. Proximally, the space of Parona in the forearm is located between the pronator

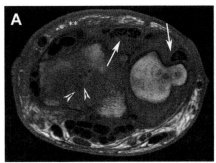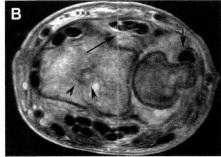

Fig. 1. Infection in a distal radius fracture at site of fixation pins. (A) Axial FSE T1 and (B) axial FSE T2 fat saturation MR images demonstrating osteomyelitis (*arrowheads*), effusion, tenosynovitis of the extensor compartments (second, third, fourth, fifth, and sixth) (*arrows*), and cellulitis in the subcutaneous tissues (*asterisks*). FSE, fast spin echo.

quadratus muscle and the sheath of the flexor digitorum profundus, and communicates distally with the midpalmar spaces. If there is a rupture of the superficial ulnar or radial bursa in the wrist, an infection can spread into these deep spaces and proximally into the forearm.

The extensor tendons have 6 extensor compartments that extend from the radiocarpal joint to the carpal metacarpal joint below the dorsal carpal ligament. The dorsal spaces are superficially the dorsal subcutaneous space, deeply the dorsal subaponeurotic space, and distally the interdigital web spaces. Dorsal infections spread easily because there are no physical barriers (see Fig. 2).[13]

Usually, an infection begins with cellulitis that might progress to an abscess and spread into the tendon sheaths, bursae, and deep spaces and through the space of Parona extend proximally to the forearm.

Plain film can be useful to rule out bone abnormalities and some soft tissue edema with or without gas; however, ultrasonography (US) and MR, especially MR after gadolinium intravenous injection, are more specific in differentiating cellulitis from noninfectious soft tissue edema; ruling out abscesses, septic arthritis, or osteomyelitis; and in the ability to delineate extension into deeper spaces[13] (see **Figs. 1** and **2**).

Complex Regional Pain Syndrome, Sympathetic Dystrophy, or Sudech Dystrophy, Complex Regional Pain Syndrome Type I

The first step to diagnose sympathetic dystrophy following surgery is to rule out other potential complications of the surgery. After ruling out other causes, sympathetic dystrophy, complex regional pain syndrome (CRPS) type I, has been specifically described after carpal tunnel surgery, wrist fractures, and fasciectomy for Dupuytren contracture. This condition should be differentiated from a clinically similar condition secondary to neuropathic pain after trauma to a peripheral nerve, CRPS type II. The Budapest consensus in 2003 established the clinical criteria for CRPS type I as pain disproportionate to the injury, edema, changes in skin blood flow, trophic changes, and sweating changes, and ruled out other causes that explain signs and symptoms.[14,15] Radiological findings

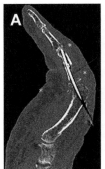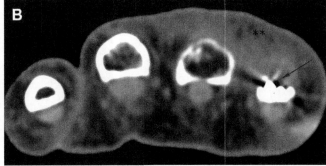

Fig. 2. Infection in a proximal phalanx treated with intramedullary nail. (A) Sagittal MPR reconstruction and (B) axial CT images show bone osteolysis of the proximal phalanx on its dorsal side (*arrow*) and soft tissue edema in the surrounding structures (*asterisks*). MPR, multiplanar reconstruction.

are inconsistent and nonspecific, and therefore its diagnosis should remain clinical and reports should be very cautious when suggesting CPRS because the radiologists' main role is to rule out other causes of pain.[16] Radiographs might show osseous demineralization and soft tissue edema (**Fig. 3**). In early stages, MR can show skin thickening, soft tissue edema, and periarticular enhancement after intravenous contrast. Contrast enhancement decreases in late stages when muscle atrophy can be seen.[17] Bone marrow edema can also be seen, with subcortical enhancement and periosteal enhancement; however, up to 50% of cases of CRPS do not show postcontrast enhancement. US has been used to distinguish neuropathic from nonneuropathic CRPS, thanks to the ability of US to depict myoglobular distortion, which neuropathic CRPS does not show.[18]

Healing Assessment

The bone healing process has several stages including acute fracture, hematoma formation, inflammation, proliferation, differentiation, ossification, and remodeling. Healing of any fracture has a primary or direct healing component occurring where the fracture surfaces are rigidly in contact referred to as intramembranous healing and secondary or indirect healing component with callus formation around the fracture surfaces. Direct healing requires complete stability of the fracture without movement, whereas in indirect healing, interfragmentary movement stimulates inflammation and callus formation, followed by woven bone, which remodels into lamellar bone.

Radiographs remain the best first-line tool for assessment of bone healing. In the tibia and femur, healing criteria have been established, referred to as the radiographic union score for hip fractures (RUSH) and radiographic union scale in tibial fractures (RUST) score systems, which are based on the callus formation and the visibility of the fracture line. However, in the wrist and hand, no accepted criteria have been accepted.

CT is superior to radiography with higher sensitivity and specificity and thus performed when radiography is equivocal in assessment of healing. Early signs of healing are blurring of fracture margins and external callus. CT limitations are the beam artifact of metal fixation devices despite the improvement of new techniques and algorithms.[19]

PET with fludeoxyglucose F 18 could potentially play an important role in the assessment of fracture healing due to its ability to monitor metabolic activity of fracture repair; however, for wrist and hand fractures, due to the small and peripheral location of the hand its assessment is difficult and has not been accepted as a valid method.[19]

Complications Related with Arthroscopy Approach

The utilization and indications of wrist arthroscopy have increased in the last several years and can be used as the only approach for treatment or adjunctively to open surgery. The most common indications for wrist arthroscopy are surgery of the triangular fibrocartilage complex (TFCC), instability and ligament surgeries, dorsal ganglia, and

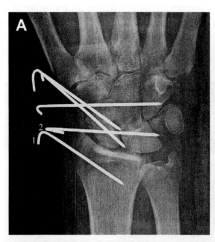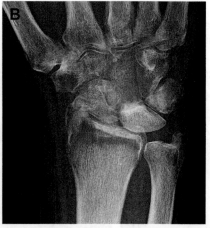

Fig. 3. Distal radius fracture and scapholunate acute tear treated with Kirschner wires. (*A*) Posteroanterior (PA) wrist film shows the wires crossing the distal radius lateral fracture (1) and a wire crossing the scaphoid and lunate (2). (*B*) Posttreatment PA wrist film demonstrates severe osteopenia and soft tissue swelling related to CRPS but good outcome of the distal radius fracture without indirect signs of scapholunate instability.

guidance to surgical approach of distal radius fractures or scaphoid fractures or synovectomy.[20]

Complications are rare, occurring in up to 2% of cases; however, this is probably underestimated because most of them are mild and self-limited and therefore not reported.[21,22]

Complications of arthroscopy can include the general complications of surgical procedures described in the previous section, but can also occur secondary to the traction and arm positioning used to establish arthroscopy portals or can be attributed to specific procedures. Specific complications are reviewed in further detail. The main arthroscopic portals are the dorsal 3-4 portal located between the third and fourth extensor tendon compartments 1 cm distal to the Lister tubercle. Dorsal 5-6 portal is placed between the fifth and sixth dorsal extensor compartments at the level of the radiocarpal joint. The dorsal outflow 6R portal is just radial to the extensor carpi ulnaris (ECU) tendon at the level distal to the ulnar head. Radial midcarpal portal is located 1 cm distal and 0.5 cm ulnar to the dorsal 3-4 portal.

Complications can be divided into major and minor, as well as early complications such as infections, vascular or nerve injuries, or delayed complications in the late postoperative period such as stiffness or tendinitis.

Nerve injuries can be permanent or transitory complications related to arthroscopy including nerve transection, avulsion, and secondary neuroma. There have been described lesions of the dorsal sensory branch of the ulnar nerve especially in the region of the 6R portal, therefore some surgeons recommend avoiding this portal. Injury to the distal posterior interosseous nerve is rare; however, it is possible that some of these injuries may remain underdiagnosed and a cause of chronic dorsal pain.[23,24]

Extensor tendon partial tear, tendinitis, or tenosynovitis has also been described, but most of the times they do not need further interventions.

WRIST FRACTURES
Distal Radius Fracture

Distal radius fracture is the most common injury of the wrist. This injury can be secondary to a low-energy mechanism, such as fall from standing height onto outstretched hand, but it is also associated with high-energy trauma. Stable fractures can be treated conservatively. Extra-articular unstable fractures can be treated with closed reduction and percutaneous pinning. Unstable intra-articular fractures are treated with open reduction and internal fixation (ORIF), mainly with volar locking plate that can be assisted arthroscopically.

Patients have a better prognosis with surgical treatment than conservative treatment and can restore anatomy in many cases; however, in elderly patients there is no difference in the functional outcome[25] (Figs. 4–7). Volar locking plate surgery has an overall rate of complications of 11.7%; however, a variety of rates have been reported from 6% to 26%.[26] Dorsal approach for internal fixation is limited. For open fractures or highly comminuted fractures external fixation can be used.

Instability can be assessed with radiographs, deformities such as radial inclination, dorsal angulation greater than 5°, radial shortening greater than 5 mm, and CT, which is particularly important for the evaluation of intra-articular fragments, including the number of fragments and displacement or step-off. Significant collapse of the lunate fossa, greater than 5 mm, is associated with increased risk of complications. Distal radioulnar joint (DRUJ) injury should also be evaluated. Soft tissue injuries are frequently associated with TFCC injury in 40%, scapholunate injury in 30% of the cases, and lunotriquetral injury in 15% (see Figs. 5–7).

Normal appearance
Fixation devices should not overpass the articular surface. Radial shortening should not be greater than 5 mm compared with the contralateral side, dorsal angulation should be less than 10°, and step-off should be no greater than 1 mm (see Fig. 7).

Complications
Complications of fixations are higher in severe fractures or fractures with soft tissue damage.[26]

1. Screw penetration into the radiocarpal or the DRUJ may be detected on radiographs; however, if they do not clearly show this, it can be easily seen on CT. MR can determine if there is associated cartilage injury (Fig. 8).
2. Radial shaft fractures have been reported secondary to external fixation devices at the point of the pin insertion.
3. Tendon rupture in nondisplaced fractures is most frequently related to attrition and ischemia but might be injured by long screws or dorsal plates causing injury to the extensor pollicis longus tendon (Fig. 9); conversely, flexor pollicis longus rupture is associated with distal volar plate placement on the radius, distal to the watershed line (Fig. 10).
4. Nerve injuries to the median nerve or to the radial sensory nerve can be secondary to the fracture but can also be iatrogenic.
5. Malunion and nonunion.

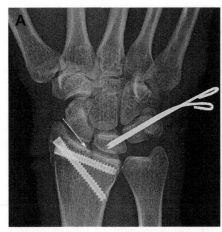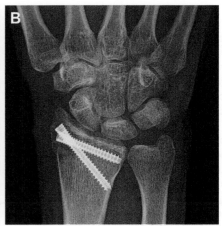

Fig. 4. Distal radius fracture treated with lateral screws. (*A*) PA wrist film shows the intra-articular fracture line (*arrow*), the lateral screws, and lunotriquetral ligament acute tear treatment with Kirschner wire. (*B*) PA wrist film demonstrates nicely the fracture healing without indirect signs of lunotriquetral instability.

- Malunion is a more prevalent complication than nonunion and occurs more frequently with casting treatment compared with fixation. However, malalignment does not always lead to unacceptable outcomes.[12]

- Restoring normal anatomy of the lunate fossa in complex surgeries requires a combination of fixation with plate and fragment-specific fixation, which might increase complications in unexperienced surgeons (see **Figs. 7** and **8**).[27]

6. Radial shortening causes secondary positive ulnar variance and overload of the ulnar side of the wrist, which with time can lead to ulnocarpal impaction syndrome (**Figs. 11** and **12**).

7. If there is a step-off greater than 1 to 2 mm, radiocarpal incongruence can lead to arthrosis, although this issue still is under controversy.

Scaphoid Fracture

Scaphoid fractures are common carpal fractures, typically occurring in young adults after a fall on an outstretched hand with the wrist in dorsiflexion. For adequate treatment, early diagnosis should be made to decrease the rate of complications. However, the diagnosis can be difficult both clinically and with early radiographs, which often leads to a delayed diagnosis and frequent complications.

Management of scaphoid fractures depends on the location of the fracture and the displacement. These fractures can be divided into nondisplaced, displaced, and proximal pole fractures. Displacement is defined as unstable if it is greater than 1 mm or 15° of lunate tilt.[28] Nondisplaced stable fractures, tubercle, or incomplete waist fractures are usually treated conservatively, using forearm cast for 8 to 12 weeks. Some stable waist fractures can also be treated with minimally invasive techniques using screw fixation to decrease recovery

Fig. 5. Distal radius fracture treated with ORIF with protrusion of the screws (*arrowheads*); note the small screw in the ulnar fovea for ulnar foveal fixation of TFCC ulnar attachment tear (*arrow*).

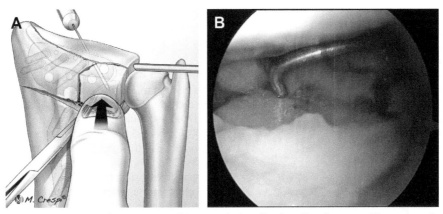

Fig. 6. (A) Arthroscopic assisted treatment of intra-articular distal radius fracture; illustration demonstrates arthroscopic treatment of complex intra-articular radial fractures, allowing normal intra-articular anatomy restoration. (B) Arthroscopic view of an intra-articular distal radius fracture. ([A] *Courtesy of* M. Crespi.)

time and earlier return to work or sports. Nondisplaced fractures should be followed up to confirm that they do not displace.[29]

Unstable fractures and proximal pole fractures are treated with reduction and internal fixation or percutaneous fixation to avoid complications such as delayed union, malunion, or nonunion.

Percutaneous technique seems to have early union, early return to functional activity, and lesser complications than open surgery. Percutaneous screw fixation is done under fluoroscopic control via palmar or dorsal approach. Dorsal approach allows placement of the screws more parallel to the long axis of the scaphoid.[30] Old untreated

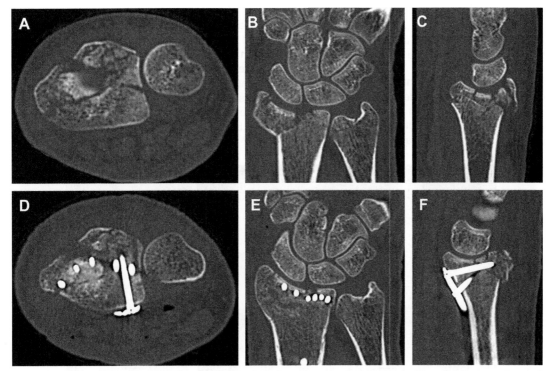

Fig. 7. (A–C) Preoperative and (D–F) postoperative imaging of a complex intra-articular radial fracture. Presurgical CT with MPR reconstructions in axial (A), coronal (B), and sagittal (C) planes show intra-articular comminuted fracture of the distal radius with significant collapse of the articular surface. Postsurgical CT with MPR in axial (D), coronal (E), and sagittal (F) planes demonstrates excellent anatomy restoration without scalloping of the articular surface.

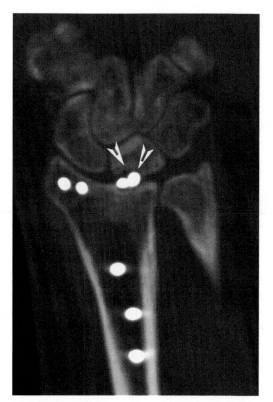

Fig. 8. Referred patient with postsurgery pain. CT with coronal MPR of a distal radius fracture treated with ORIF shows screw penetration into the radiocarpal joint compartment and protrusion into the articular side of the lunate with an osteochondral lesion (*arrowheads*).

scaphoid fractures or nonunited fractures are usually an indication for treatment.

ORIF is usually reserved for those cases with difficult position when difficult realignment is necessary or large bone graft is needed.

Eventually displaced distal fractures of the scaphoid tubercle can be treated with excision if they become symptomatic.

Assessment of healing

The healing of scaphoid fractures is influenced by the biology of fracture healing, anatomic factors, and the mechanical forces involved. The scaphoid is 80% covered by cartilage without tendinous attachments and without periosteum and therefore depends on primary direct healing and not indirect healing from callus formation. The blood supply to the scaphoid is received primarily via dorsal vessels (80%) and to a lesser extent via palmar vessels (20%) at or just distal to the waist area, and these vessels perfuse the proximal pole of the scaphoid in a retrograde manner, meaning that blood flow enters the distal portion of the scaphoid and there is no direct supply to the proximal portion of the scaphoid. Owing to the tenuous blood supply of the scaphoid, vascular compromise from fractures is often associated with the development of nonunion and avascular necrosis of the proximal pole. The attachment of the scapholunate ligament keeps the proximal pole of the scaphoid with the lunate, whereas the volar ligament and capsular attachment keep the distal pole in flexion and protonation.

Scaphoid fractures should be followed up with serial radiographs. CT with multiplanar reconstructions following the scaphoid long axis may be performed in cases in which radiographs are inconclusive. Imaging of scaphoid fracture healing is based on visualization of trabecula crossing the fracture line and sclerosis, noting that greater than 50% bridging is sufficient. MR imaging can also be used to assess healing and also to rule out

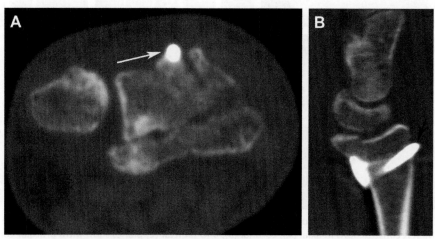

Fig. 9. (*A*) Axial and (*B*) sagittal MPR CT images display a patient with distal radial fracture treated with volar plate and screws; protrusion of one of the screws in the dorsal side at the level of Lister tubercule caused friction to the extensor pollicis longus tendon (*arrow*).

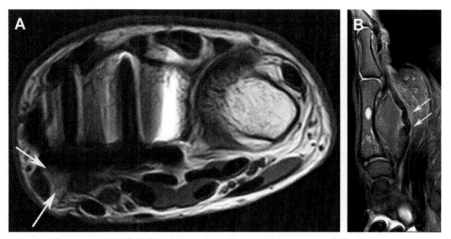

Fig. 10. Distal radial fracture treated with volar plate and secondary rupture of the flexor pollicis longus tendon. (A) Axial FSE PD MR image shows increased signal intensity in the flexor pollicis longus (*arrow*). (B) Sagittal FSE PD MR image demonstrates the retraction of the tendon, curled up into the thenar muscles (*arrow*). PD, proton density.

nonunion complications such as scaphoid proximal pole avascular necrosis.[31,32]

Acute fractures usually heal before 3 months. If there is no healing between 3 and 6 months, it is considered a delayed union, and after 6 months, it is considered a nonunion or pseudoarthrosis (**Fig. 13**).[33]

Assessment of alignment

The location of the scaphoid fracture in relation to the scapholunate ligament and the dorsal intercarpal ligament will determine the deformity. A fracture distal to the dorsal ridge of the scaphoid causes the proximal fragment to fall in extension following the lunate by the scapholunate ligament, whereas the

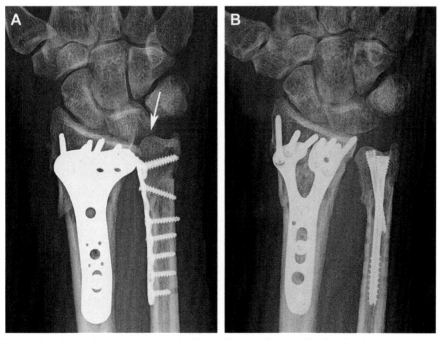

Fig. 11. (A) Frontal radiograph in a patient with ulnar side pain from a distal radial fracture treated with volar plate and secondary shortening of the radius causing positive ulnar variance (*arrow*). (B) Frontal radiograph after patient underwent a second surgery to change the volar plate of the distal radius and remove the distal ulnar plate and screw fixation of the distal ulna was performed to restore normal radiocarpal alignment.

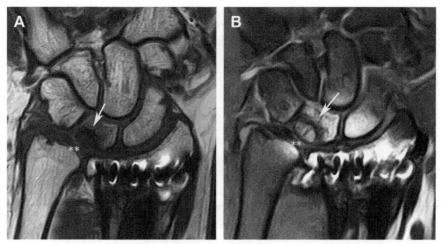

Fig. 12. (*A*) Coronal FSE T1 and (*B*) coronal FSE PD MR images of secondary ulnocarpal impaction due to shortening of a radial fracture treated with ORIF; note the central perforation of the TFCC (*asterisks*) and the osteochondral lesion on ulnar side of the lunate (*arrow*).

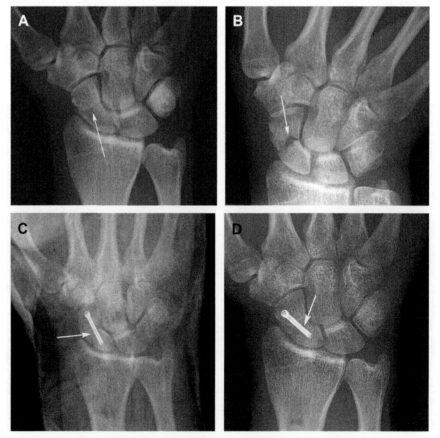

Fig. 13. Serial PA wrist radiographs of a scaphoid fracture. (*A*) Initial film shows an acute scaphoid fracture (*arrow*), which was missed at the emergency room. (*B*) Seven months later, patient came with persistent pain, and nonunion was clearly diagnosed with sclerotic margins of the fracture (*arrow*). (*C*) Patient was treated with bone graft and Herbert-type screw (*arrow*). (*D*) Healing was seen 3 months later (*arrow*).

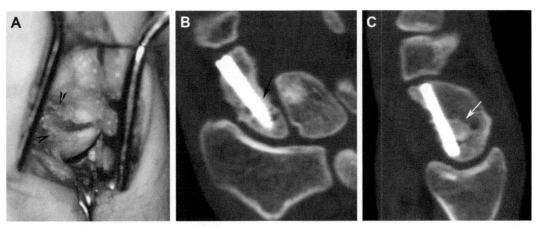

Fig. 14. Scaphoid nonunion treated with bone graft and Herbert-type of screw. (*A*) Intraoperative photograph shows a dorsal approach to the scaphoid after curettage; note the normal vascularization of both fragment edges (*arrowheads*). (*B*) CT coronal MPR shows fracture healing (*arrow*). (*C*) CT sagittal MPR shows healing of the fracture, integration of the hyperdense bone graft, and restoration of the normal shape without humpback deformity. The screw is located a bit volar avoiding interfering with the graft (*arrow*).

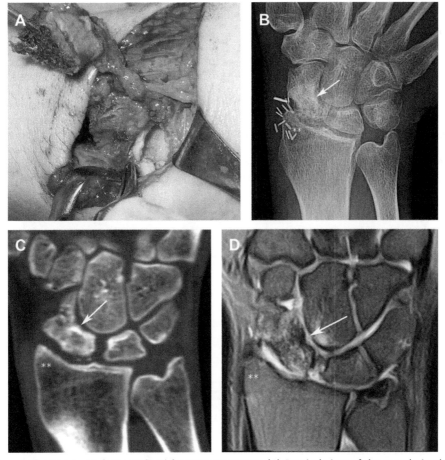

Fig. 15. Vascularized bone graft in scaphoid fracture treatment. (*A*) Surgical view of the vascularized graft procedure from the distal radius with the 1,2 intercompartmental supraretinacular artery graft. (*B*) PA wrist film. (*C*) CT coronal MPR and (*D*) coronal MR imaging FSE DP fat saturation images show postsurgical changes on the distal radius (*asterisks*) and normal healing of the scaphoid (*arrow*).

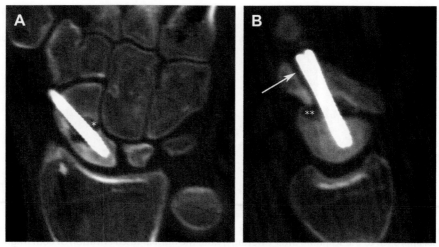

Fig. 16. Scaphoid nonunion treated with Herbert-type screw but without healing secondary to loosening of the screw. (*A*) CT coronal MPR and (*B*) CT sagittal MPR images demonstrate radiolucency surrounding the screw (*arrow*) and nonunion (*asterisks*).

distal fragment is flexed volary tethered by the scapho-trapecio-trapezoid ligament. This deformity is called humpback deformity with volar shortening and angulation of the scaphoid with the dorsal apex prominent. This deformity predisposes to nonunion, abnormal biomechanics, and progression to osteoarthritis with a predictive pattern.[33]

Complications

Nonunion and avascular necrosis: The diagnosis of nonunion is when there is absence of bone bridging after 6 months. It is important to assess the vascular state of the distal pole of the scaphoid to plan adequate treatment. Sclerosis of the proximal pole is not a reliable method to assess vascularization and MR imaging after gadolinium correlates with Green vascular grades[31,32] helping treatment planning. Bone graft and internal fixation is a good treatment option if vascularization is present in the distal pole, whereas vascularized bone graft or other techniques are necessary if no vascularization is present in the distal pole.[31,32] The most frequently used bone autograft is taken from the volar aspect of the distal radius, using the 1,2 intercompartmental supraretinacular artery vascularized bone graft (**Figs. 14** and **15**).

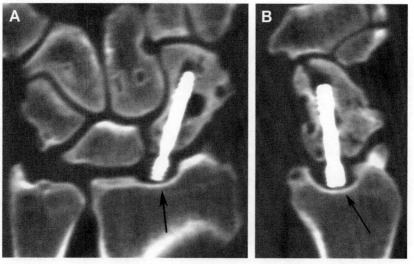

Fig. 17. Scaphoid fracture Herbert screw displacement. (*A*) CT coronal MPR and (*B*) CT sagittal MPR images demonstrate proximal displacement of the scaphoid fixation screw causing chondral lesion in the proximal radius (*arrow*).

> **Box 1**
> **Scaphoid nonunion carpal collapse classification**
>
> SNAC, scaphoid nonunion advance collapse stages
>
> Stage I artrosis in the radial side of the scaphoid
>
> Stage II in addition to stage I, arthrosis scaphocapitate and scaphohamate
>
> Stage III periscaphoid arthritis with degenerative changes hamatolunate
>
> Stage IV, carpal arthrosis

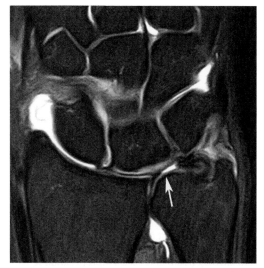

Fig. 19. Postsurgery of TFCC central debridement, coronal MR imaging PD fat-saturated MR image shows regularization of the TFC edges (*arrow*). (*From* Cerezal L, Llopis E, Canga A, Piñal FD. Postoperative Imaging of Ulnar Wrist Pain. Semin Musculoskelet Radiol. 2021 Apr;25(2):329-345 with permission.)

Screw malposition or loosening: Screws should be placed within scaphoid margins, and no radiolucency should be present within or around the screws. Displacement of a screw or pin can cause chondral lesions in the surrounding structures (**Figs. 16** and **17**).

Wrist osteoarthritis: Long-term scaphoid nonunion, with or without avascular necrosis, progresses to wrist osteoarthritis, which follows a predictive pattern starting in the radioscaphoid joint, followed with the scaphohamate joint, and finally carpal osteoarthrosis and carpal collapse. This condition is classified by the SNAC (scaphoid nonunion carpal collapse classification) (**Box 1**). If osteoarthritis develops, proximal carpectomy or partial arthrodesis of the wrist is recommended (**Fig. 18**).

TRIANGULAR FIBROCARTILAGE COMPLEX

The TFCC is a 3-dimensional structure that includes the fibrocartilage, meniscus homologue, ulnocarpal ligaments, distal radioulnar ligaments, and the subsheath of the ECU tendon. TFCC has an avascular central articular disk, but it is well vascularized in its periphery and the surrounding structures with greater healing potential. Lesions of the TFCC are closely related to the ulnar variance and should be carefully evaluated before surgical planning. Injuries have been divided by the Palmer classification into acute (type I) and degenerative (type II).[34–37]

Traumatic Acute Triangular Fibrocartilage

Type IA, traumatic TFCC tears are initially treated conservatively. If pain or instability persists, surgical treatment is advised. Central fibrocartilage type IA tears are treated with debridement of

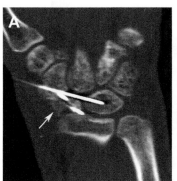
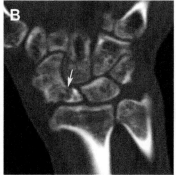
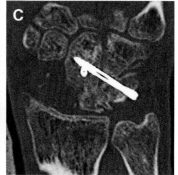

Fig. 18. Vascularized bone graft failure of a proximal pole scaphoid fracture. (*A*) CT coronal MPR following surgery showing the graft (*arrow*) and the Kirschner wires. (*B*) CT coronal MPR following wire removal demonstrates persistence of the nonunion without bone bridge within the fracture (*arrow*). (*C*) CT coronal MPR showing scaphoid resection and 4-corner partial arthrodesis, which was performed successfully.

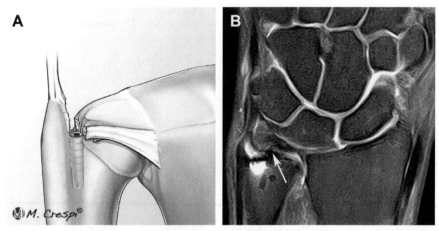

Fig. 20. Reattachment of TFCC ulnar foveal avulsion. (*A*) Illustration of the surgical procedure with fixation of the foveal attachment of the TFCC. (*B*) Coronal PD fat saturation MR image shows normal appearance postreattachment (*arrow*). (*From* Cerezal L, Llopis E, Canga A, Piñal FD. Postoperative Imaging of Ulnar Wrist Pain. Semin Musculoskelet Radiol. 2021 Apr;25(2):329-345 with permission; and (*A*) *Courtesy of M. Crespi.*)

the unstable fragments, leaving a larger central defect. In cases with neutral or positive variance, additional techniques might be needed[38,39] (**Fig. 19**).

Type IB injuries, ulnar side avulsion tears, are treated depending on the structures that are involved, the time elapsed, and the edges of the lesions, the last of which is better evaluated during arthroscopy. Capsular lesions are treated with debridement and capsular repair. Complete foveal insertion and complete ulnar tears typically require treatment to restore distal radioulnar stability through arthroscopy or mini–open procedure

inserting suture anchor in the center of the fovea. Metal artifacts and granulation tissue make it difficult to evaluate on conventional MR, thus CT or MR arthrography may help (**Fig. 20**). If positive variance is present, shortening of the distal ulnar may be recommended; however, it is not usually performed in the acute setting.[38–40]

If the injury is irreparable, tendon graft is used for reconstruction using the palmaris longus graft through tunnels in the radius and ulna to provide stability (**Fig. 21**). When cartilage lesions are present only salvage surgical procedures can be performed.[38–40]

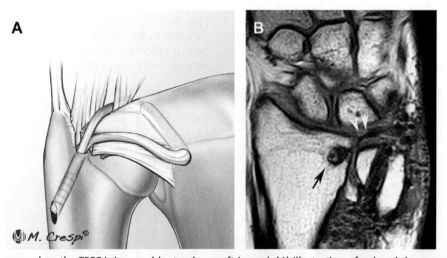

Fig. 21. In cases when the TFCC is irreparable, tendon graft is used. (*A*) Illustration of palmaris longus graft with tunnels crossing the lateral radius and ulna to provide stability. (*B*) Coronal FSE T1 MR image post–tendon graft surgery reconstruction displays the normal tunnels (*arrows*) and the graft in the ulnocarpal space (*arrowheads*). (*From* Cerezal L, Llopis E, Canga A, Piñal FD. Postoperative Imaging of Ulnar Wrist Pain. Semin Musculoskelet Radiol. 2021 Apr;25(2):329-345 with permission; and [*A*] *Courtesy of M. Crespi.*)

Ulnocarpal ligament tears (type 1C) and radial avulsion tears (type 1D) are less common. Type 1C lesions are usually repaired, whereas type 1D tears are only repaired if there is involvement of the dorsal or volar radioulnar ligament.[38–40]

Degenerative Fibrocartilage Injuries, Palmer Type 2

Degenerative TFCC tears are commonly associated with an ulnar impaction syndrome. These tears are asymptomatic in the early stages (2A), and only more advanced injuries become symptomatic, usually type 2B or 2C, and suitable for surgical treatment. In cases with neutral or positive variance additional techniques should be performed. Nowadays they are both treated with debridement and a Wafer technique through arthroscopic approach in the presence or absence of a perforation of the fibrocartilage, because it is less aggressive than open surgery. If the ulnar negative variance is lower than 3 mm, the Wafer technique is recommended, whereas if the ulnar variance is greater than 3 mm, ulnar extra-articular shortened osteotomy is recommended. The postsurgical imaging evaluation of the Wafer technique should show smooth limited ulnar head resection with regularized TFC (**Fig. 22**).[38,39]

Complications of Triangular Fibrocartilage Complex Debridement

1. Excessive debridement can result in injury of the distal radioulnar ligaments and secondary DRUJ instability.[38,39]

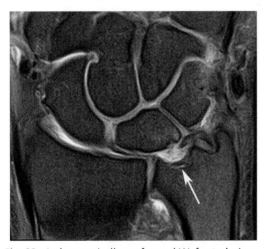

Fig. 22. Arthroscopically performed Wafer technique. Postsurgical PD fat saturation coronal MR image shows the proximal resection of the distal ulnar fovea (*arrow*) and debridement of the TFCC. (*From* Cerezal L, Llopis E, Canga A, Piñal FD. Postoperative Imaging of Ulnar Wrist Pain. Semin Musculoskelet Radiol. 2021 Apr;25(2):329-345 with permission.)

2. Scar formation with fibrosis can lead to secondary pain.[38,39]
3. Secondary positive ulnar variance can occur if shortening of the distal ulnar has not been performed leading to ulnocarpal impaction and chondral lesions in the articular side of the lunate and triquetrum.

Complications of Foveal Reattachment

Pronosupination limitation occurs if the tendon graft fixation is too tight or fibrosis. Loosening of the screws is frequently related with malposition of the screws in nonisometric fixations.[38,39]

Wafer Technique Complications

Excessive or incomplete resection is the most frequent complications of the Wafer technique. Excessive resection might lead to DRUJ instability, whereas incomplete resection might cause ulnar impaction and first row osteoarthrosis.[38,39]

WRIST INSTABILITY
Scapholunate Instability

Scapholunate instability is the most frequent pattern of wrist instability and can be acute or chronic, static or dynamic, and with or without dissociation. The scapholunate ligament is the primary stabilizer and is a C-shaped ligament, which can be divided into a dorsal site, which is the strongest; the interosseous membrane; and the volar site, which is weaker than the dorsal ligament. Scaphotrapezial ligaments, together with the extrinsic ligaments, including the radioscaphocapitate and the dorsal ligaments (dorsoradial carpal ligament and dorsal intercarpal ligament), are the secondary stabilizers. Scapholunate instability is frequently associated with distal radial fracture, especially in radial styloid fractures. Hyperextension with ulnar deviation is the main mechanism and follows a continuous pattern of ligament injuries starting with scapholunate tear followed by radiocapitate, radiotriquetral, and dorsal radiocarpal ligament injury, and ultimately the lunate follows the triquetrum in extension and dorsal intercalated segmental instability deformity occurs. Rupture of the scapholunate ligament will lead to scaphoid displacement in palmar flexion because of its oblique position and dorsal rotation around the radiocapitate ligament. The Geisseler arthroscopy classification is the most often used grading system to assess partial or total instability; however, the new Garcia-Elias different grading types can help in planning different surgical approaches. Long-term scapholunate dissociation leads to carpal osteoarthritis, scapholunate advance collapse (SLAC), which also follows a consistent pattern, including the radial styloid joint, radioscaphoid and radiolunate joints, and midcarpal joint.[41–43]

Patients with low functional demand and injuries limited to only dynamic instabilities can be treated conservatively.

Surgical techniques

Surgical approach to scapholunate ligament ruptures varies if it is an acute or a chronic lesion, acute considered within 4 hours to 6 weeks after the lesion. Acute injuries allow the reestablishment of alignment by first reduction and then fixation with a Kirschner wire. Contact of the articular surfaces with the wires should be avoided to prevent arthritis. Although many different fixation protocols have been described, there has to be a balance between stabilization and biological impairment.[41]

Acute ligament repair if diagnosed early enough can be performed either arthroscopically or with open surgery using minianchors and sutures. However, the procedure frequently requires tenodesis through the use of various tendon weaves because direct reattachment or repair of the ligament is difficult, because the ligament fragments are often retracted or short and degenerate shortly after its injury, and diagnosis is often delayed. Tenodesis can be performed with dorsal extensor carpi radialis tenodesis or Brunelli tenodesis.[42,43] Capsulodesis is recommended for augmentation together with ligament repair techniques.

The surgical treatment of chronic scapholunate dissociation depends on the state of the remaining ligament fibers, the possibility of reduction, and the degenerative status. If reduction is possible, reconstruction of the scapholunate ligament can be made using different techniques. The modified Brunelli technique uses a split of the flexor carpi radialis tendon through a tunnel in the distal pole of the scaphoid from volar to dorsal, to the lunate, and it is fixed to the ulnar side of the radius. The 3-

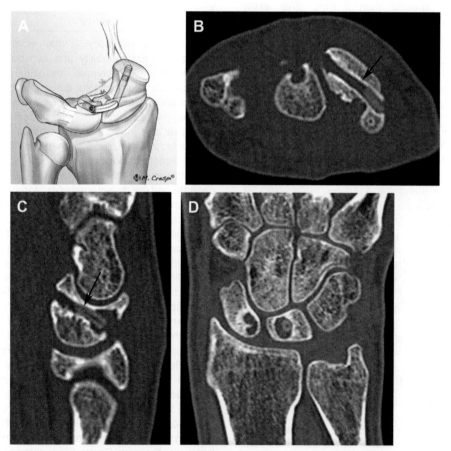

Fig. 23. Brunelli technique for treatment of scapholunate chronic rupture. (A) Illustration demonstrates surgical technique with splitting of the flexor carpi radialis tendon and the tunnels in the scaphoid and the lunate. (B) Axial CT, (C) sagittal CT MPR, and (D) coronal CT MPR images after Brunelli technique demonstrate the tunnels in the scaphoid and lunate (arrow). ([A] Courtesy of M. Crespi.)

ligament tenodesis technique is a further developed technique that improves scaphoid stabilization of the scapho-trapezio-trapezoid ligaments, and the lunate is better reduced. These techniques reduce pain, and patients have normal alignment and acceptable grip strength; however, the arc of movement is decreased (**Fig. 23**).[42,43]

Arthroscopically assisted reconstructions aim to reconstruct the dorsal and volar parts of the scapholunate ligament, which can also decrease injuries of the other ligaments.[42] Scapholunate axis method is a recently described surgical option. Dorsal Blatt capsulodesis uses the dorsal capsule as a strip to tether the distal scaphoid. Capsulodesis alone is not enough and should be combined with tenodesis. Bone alignment bone grafts have also been proposed as a technique using second or third metacarpal bone or hamate-capitate grafts; however, the consolidation of graft has been problematic, and it is no longer used.[42,43]

If scapholunate dissociation is irreducible, partial fusion is advocated, particularly with scapho-trapezoid fusion.

Surgical management of SLAC wrist is challenging, and depending on the stage of the SLAC deformity, the surgical options change. Radial styloidectomy is performed for mild cases. For more severe cases, proximal row carpectomy is usually performed for older less demanding patients and 4-corner fusion for younger, more demanding patients.

Normal imaging findings

Follow-up after surgery is done with wrist plain films; posteroanterior, lateral, ulnar, and lateral deviation views should be done early after surgery and before and after the removal of the Kirschner wires (see **Fig. 4**). Normal carpal alignment should be checked; all carpal Gilula rows should be smooth. Scapholunate distance and scapholunate angle should be compared with the presurgical radiographs and should be within the normal range angle from 30° to 60° and scapholunate distance lower than 3 mm. After the removal of the K-wires the distance and the angle increase slightly but should not be significant.

Bone tunnels can be identified on plain films and also with CT. The role of dynamic CT has not been established because of the lack of availability but can precisely demonstrate wrist stability patterns (see **Fig. 23**). If MR imaging is needed, metal reduction sequences are recommended (**Fig. 24**).

Complications

Failure in achieving stability and recurrence of instability are the more important complications and are relatively easy to diagnose. When

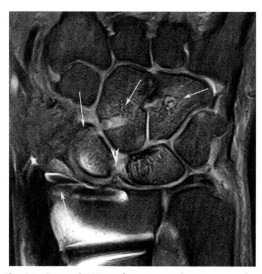

Fig. 24. Coronal FSE PD fat-saturated MR image after Brunelli surgery for scapholunate rupture. Surgical artifacts are seen next to the tunnels in the scaphoid, capitate, hamate, and proximal radius (*arrows*). Note the high signal intensity of the tendon graft in the tunnels. A residual small increase of scapholunate distance is frequently seen despite the good outcome in most of the cases (*arrowhead*).

alignment is abnormal, the carpal rows are not smooth and the scapholunate distance is greater than 3 mm or increasing with time or scapholunate angle increases or is greater than 60°. Progression of degenerative changes is seen despite treatment, but usually collapse of the wrist is slowed if no complications occur.[41–43]

Lunotriquetral Instability

Treatment of lunotriquetral instability remains controversial. In the acute setting, reduction and fixation with K-wires together with primary ligamentous repair can be tried (see **Fig. 5**). If the lesion is chronic, ligamentoplasty is less often used than partial wrist arthrodesis between the lunate and the triquetrum.

NERVE AND VASCULAR LESIONS, CARPAL TUNNEL

Carpal tunnel syndrome is the most common peripheral nerve entrapment. Treatment options are started with perineural therapeutic injections and modification of activities. Those that do not improve undergo section of the transverse ligament to release the flexor retinaculum, which can be done using US guidance, endoscopically, or with open surgery.[44,45]

Postoperative imaging can include US or MR imaging; however, US has some difficulties in the evaluation of the postsurgical retinaculum. Some investigators advocate the use of intravenous gadolinium for a better accuracy on MR imaging.[44,45]

Discontinuity and volar convexity of the transverse ligament can be seen, together with increase of the carpal tunnel size, especially at the level of the pisiform (**Fig. 25**). Increase of size or flattening of the median nerve should be evaluated with caution because this can be persistent up to 12 months despite good patient outcome.[45] Bowing of the retinaculum at the level of the inlet and the outlet of the carpal tunnel is a normal appearance after surgery. Normal decompression is considered when the carpal tunnel structures are above a line crossing at the level of the hook of the hamate to the ridge of the trapezium.[44,45]

Complications

Complications from carpal tunnel release occur in approximately 20% of the patients, and up to 10% need reexploration surgery.[45] The most frequent complication is incomplete release especially with endoscopic treatment, in which case the free margins of the transected retinaculum are not well delineated on US. With time, the sectioned carpal retinaculum can regenerate. Fibrosis and scar tissue can occur and can be depicted with MR imaging or US (**Fig. 26**). Flexor tenosynovitis can also occur. More infrequent complications are median nerve or ulnar artery laceration. Postsurgery median nerve enhancement is well correlated with recurrent carpal tunnel syndrome and might be secondary to edema and partial nerve injury.[44,45]

TRAPEZIUM METACARPAL SURGERIES

The trapezo-metacarpal joint is a common place for osteoarthritis, which can be multifactorial including ligament laxity, biomechanical properties, overuse activities, or posttraumatic injuries. Conservative treatment is the main treatment with orthosis and therapeutic joint injections. If conservative treatment fails, depending on the osteoarthritis stage, the treatment options are different. In the early stages, Eaton stage I, treatment with arthroscopic synovectomy, capsulotomy, and oblique palmar ligament reconstruction is recommended.[46]

Surgical therapies for more advanced cases have been changing in the last several years, and the goal is to decrease pain and maintain the function and strength. Trapeziectomy can be performed, and various methods have been used to fill the empty space of the resected trapezium, such as hematoma arthroplasty, tendon interposition using usually flexor carpi radialis tendon, or

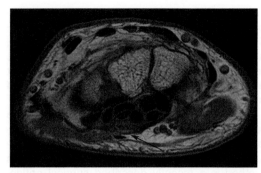

Fig. 25. Normal appearance post–carpal tunnel release; axial FSE T1 MR imaging shows normal postsurgical gap in the transverse ligament of the carpal tunnel (*arrow*).

implant placements (**Figs. 27** and **28**). There are many plasty techniques that can be performed. Ligamentoplasty reconstructing the palmar oblique ligament usually with a split of the flexor carpi radialis tendon through the base of the first metacarpal joint and the remaining tendon is used to fill the space left by the trapeziectomy. After trapeziectomy, the ulnar slip of the abductor pollicis longus tendon can be passed through a tunnel of the first and second metacarpal base and secured to the extensor carpi radialis tendon (see **Fig. 28**).[46,47]

Patients with recurrent or persistent pain after ligamentoplasty reconstructions failure, especially in high-demanding occupations, can undergo trapezio-metacarpal prosthesis (**Fig. 29**).[46,47]

TENDON RECONSTRUCTIONS

Tendon injuries of the finger are frequent in work-related injuries. These injuries are classified following the International Committee of tendon

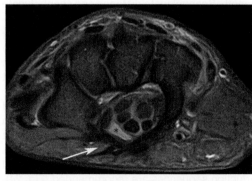

Fig. 26. Postsurgical fibrosis after carpal tunnel surgery. Axial PD fat saturation MR imaging demonstrates fibrosis with thickening and low signal intensity of the transverse ligament (*arrow*) and increased signal intensity of the median nerve (*asterisk*).

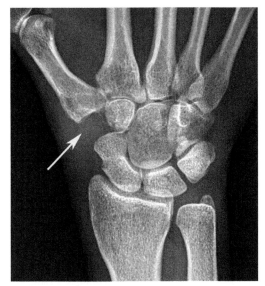

Fig. 27. Trapeziectomy was performed with hematoma arthroplasty. PA wrist radiograph displays the empty space of the trapezium resection (*arrow*).

injuries into 5 different zones, with zone I being the most frequent, affecting the flexor digitoris profundus tendon, and zone II, from the insertion of the flexor digitorum superficialis tendon to the palmar fold.[48,49]

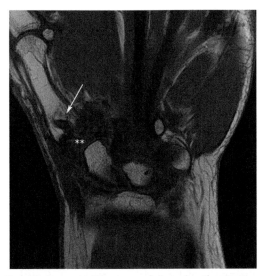

Fig. 28. Trapeziectomy was follow by the Burton-Pellegrini technique of tendon interposition and stabilization of the tendon between the first and the second metacarpals. Coronal FSE T1 MR imaging shows interposition of the tendon between the scaphoid and the first metacarpal base where the tunnel for stabilization is depicted (*arrow*). Note the hypointense signal at the resection site of the trapezium (*asterisks*).

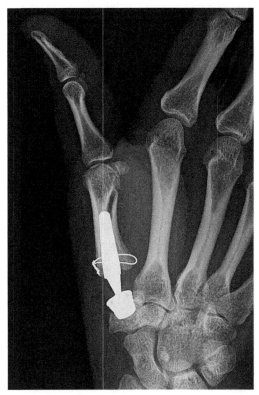

Fig. 29. PA radiograph of the thumb shows normal appearance of a trapeziometacarpal prosthesis.

There are different types of surgeries involving suture repair and plasties with grafts of the palmaris longus or tendon transfers. Tendon healing after a rupture and suture repair has an extrinsic phase in which the granulation tissue at the margin of the repair invades the rupture area and an intrinsic phase that occurs within the tendon; tendons do not regenerate; however, the granulation tissue that fills in the rupture during healing process, which takes approximately 6 weeks, makes a functional anatomically aligned tendon.

Complications of tendon reconstructions are rupture of the sutures and elongation of the tendon with some fibrous tissue or adhesions, which are difficult to diagnose on all imaging techniques. Fibrous tissue needs time to mature, and changes in its echogenicity on US or signal intensity on MR imaging can be seen with time (**Fig. 30**). Recurrent tendon ruptures following repair are seen as discontinuity on both US and MR, especially using axial planes. Peritendinous adhesions are seen as thickening of the tendon sheath and loss of the normal fat planes that surround the tendon. Laceration injuries of the tendons can also lead to injuries of nearby neurovascular structures (**Fig. 31**).[48]

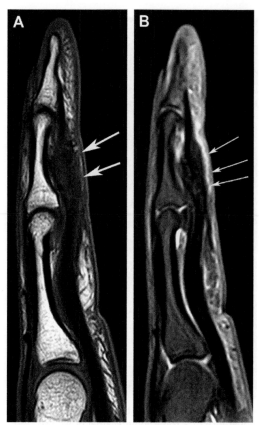

Fig. 30. Tendon reconstruction repair. (*A*) Sagittal FSE T1 and (*B*) sagittal FSE PD fat saturation MR images of a flexor tendon rupture repair in zone II, also called "no man's land," where the flexor digitorum profundus and superficialis tendons change their position. These repairs have a tendency for fibrosis in the tendon edges and within the flexor pulley system as in this case (*arrows*).

ARTHRODESIS

Arthrodesis is a well-established procedure for the treatment of osteoarthrosis from a variety of injuries and diseases such as fractures, instability, and rheumatological disorders. The goal is to reduce pain maintaining as much of the function as possible.[50,51]

Proximal row carpectomy is a motion-preserving treatment, which involves excising the scaphoid, lunate, and triquetrum bones, with the aim of creating a new articulation between the capitate bone and the distal radius.

Four-corner arthrodesis consists of the excision of the scaphoid and fusion of the capitate, hamate, lunate, and triquetrum. The fusion can be made with standard technique (screws, staples, wires) or using a circular plate and screws (**Fig. 32**). These 2 procedures, proximal row carpectomy and 4-corner arthrodesis, are effective treatments for advanced osteoarthritis secondary to SNAC and SLAC lesions with relatively low rates of complications. Complications seem to occur more frequently with circular plate 4-corner arthrodesis (**Fig. 33**).[50] The major complications are nonunion or impingement.[51]

Partial radiocarpal arthrodesis, radioscapholunate or radiolunotriquetral arthrodesis, can be performed when these joints develop pain from osteoarthritis refractory to other treatments (**Fig. 34**).

Total wrist arthrodesis involves the fusion of the radius, scaphoid, lunate, and capitate, and it is used when the lunocapitate joint has severe osteoarthritis; they can be fused with dorsal plates or pins. The purpose is to achieve fusion between the bones with bone bridges and sclerosis.

Complications

1. Loosening of the osteosynthesis, pins, or screws
2. Nonunion
3. Ruptures of tendons or tenosynovitis of the extensor tendons mainly secondary to the hardware
4. Impingement of the lunate into the dorsal radius mainly when deformities have not been corrected

ARTHROPLASTIES

Wrist arthroplasty arises as an alternative to arthrodesis, with the aim of not only relieving pain but also preserving a range of motion for daily activities.

In wrist arthroplasty, the damaged joint can be remodeled with bone resection and/or replaced with soft tissue interposition or a prosthesis.

Wrist arthroplasty has evolved substantially in the last several decades, with the improvement of implants and surgical techniques. However, the durability of prosthetic components is still limited. Therefore, the choice between arthrodesis and arthroplasty depends on the location of the disease and the existence of contraindications.

In wrist arthroplasty, like arthrodesis, there is a wide spectrum of options ranging from partial to complete arthroplasty.

The different types of resections and implant arthroplasty of the wrist are reviewed, focusing on the 2 main types of implants: total wrist arthroplasty (TWA) and DRUJ arthroplasty.

Resection Arthroplasty

Resection arthroplasty is considered as a surgical option for disease located at the DRUJ and radiocarpal joint.

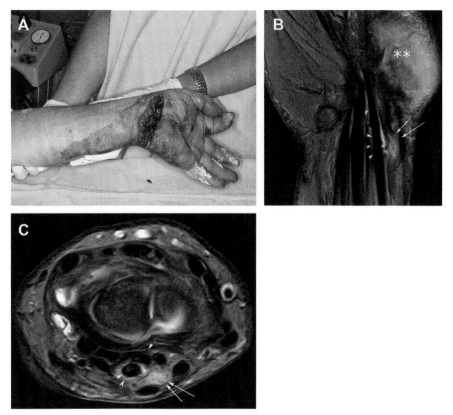

Fig. 31. Flexor tendon laceration in zone IV associated with median nerve injury. (*A*) Photograph of patient's wrist after acute laceration, which went straight to surgery without imaging. (*B*) Coronal PD fat saturation (*asterisks*) and (*C*) axial PD fat saturation MR images after surgery demonstrate continuity of the repaired tendons (*arrowheads*) and a posttraumatic neuroma of the median nerve with thickening and increased signal intensity of the nerve (*arrows*) and denervation signs in the thenar muscles with diffuse increase signal intensity.

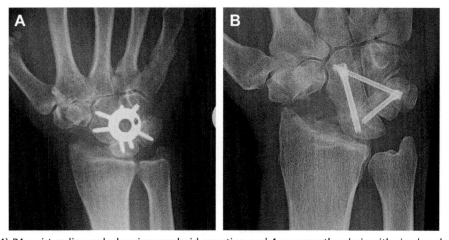

Fig. 32. (*A*) PA wrist radiograph showing scaphoid resection and 4-corner arthrodesis with circular plate. (*B*) PA wrist radiographs demonstrate scaphoid resection and 4-corner fusion with screws.

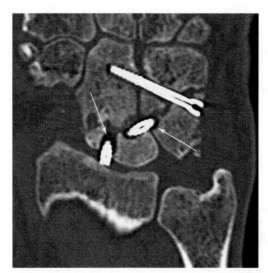

Fig. 33. Four-corner fusion failure. Coronal MPR CT shows absence of bridges between lunate, triquetrum, hamate, and capitate with radiolucency surrounding the screws (*arrows*).

The following are the classical surgical techniques for DRUJ disease:

1. The Darrach procedure is based on the resection of the distal ulna, just proximal to the sigmoid notch, with preservation of the surrounding soft tissue structures (**Fig. 35**).[52]
2. The hemiresection interposition technique involves resection of the ulnar articular head, leaving shaft and styloid relationship intact. This technique requires that the TFCC is intact or reconstructible.[53]
3. The Sauvé-Kapandji technique involves resection of a portion of the distal ulna, just proximal to the sigmoid notch, and fusion of the DRUJ, with the aim of restoring forearm rotation (**Fig. 36**).[54]

The main complication of these techniques is the instability of the distal ulna, which can lead to radioulnar impingement, and for that reason they are being replaced by implant arthroplasties.

Another potential complication of the Sauvé-Kapandji technique is reactive bone formation at the pseudoarthrosis site.[54]

Total Wrist Arthroplasty

The most common indication for TWA is advanced rheumatoid arthritis, and less frequently, for osteoarthritis and posttraumatic osteoarthritis.[55]

Since 1960, when wrist arthroplasty with silicone implants was introduced, many types of prostheses have emerged, including different materials and fixation systems, which have been refined up to the current prostheses. The most important changes include a more semiconstrained motion arc and ellipsoidal articulation,

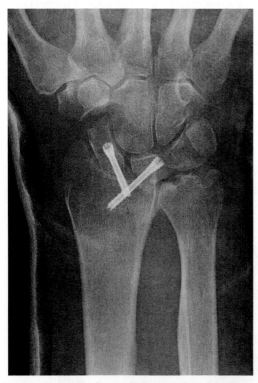

Fig. 34. PA wrist radiograph shows radioscapholunate arthrodesis with screws along the radioscapholunate joint.

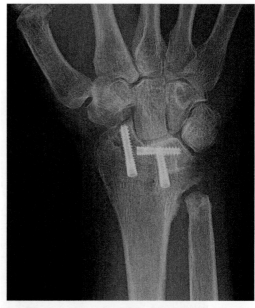

Fig. 35. PA wrist radiograph demonstrates the Darrach procedure with arthrodesis of the radius, scaphoid, and lunate and resection of the distal ulna.

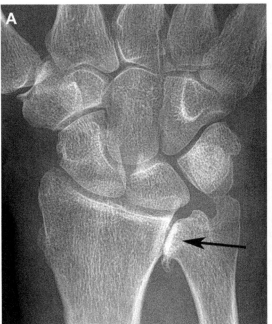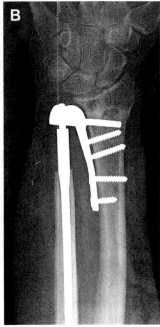

Fig. 36. (A) PA wrist radiograph in a patient with radioulnar osteoarthritis and impingement from a prominent ulnar osteophyte at the proximal facet of the lateral radial side (*arrow*). (B) Post Sauvé-Kapandji technique, showing resection of the distal ulna and posterior fixation of the distal radioulnar joint.

resulting in lower dislocation rates and less alterations to the distal component.

The requirements for a successful arthroplasty are a good bone stock and an intact extensor carpi radialis brevis and longus tendons.[56] In addition, ideal candidates are those with low demand for manual activities in their day-to-day life and who want to reduce pain without giving up wrist movement.

Normal imaging findings

At present, the most widely used prostheses are bicompartmental, formed by a radial and carpal component, made of cobalt chromium (CoCr) or titanium, with a radiolucent polyethylene insert between both components.[57]

During implantation, the proximal carpal row is resected. The distal part is fixed within the carpus by anchoring a peg to the capitate bone and 2 screws to the trapezoid and hamate bones.[58]

Over time, the carpal component favors the fusion of the carpal bones to achieve good support for anchoring the prosthesis, whereas the radial component is designed to preserve a good bone stock for possible revisions or fusions.

The concomitant management of the DRUJ in these patients depends on whether there is osteoarthritis and its severity, instability, and the patient's symptoms. At present, a prosthetic ulnar head is usually preferred instead of ulnar head resection, which

has been associated with more complications and instability.

The alignment of the prosthetic components and the preserved carpal height are 2 of the findings that should be looked for on postoperative radiographs, to confirm the correct position of the prosthesis.

Pathologic findings and complications

Despite continuous advances in TWA, instability and implant loosening are the most common TWA complications.[55,58–60]

During the first 3 years, radiographs may show thin lines of radiolucency around the radial and carpal components, which could be a normal finding in the absence of clinical symptoms[59]. However, progressive radiolucency around the stems of either the carpal or radial components should raise concern for loosening of the prosthesis.

Other possible complications are fracture, tendon laceration, DRUJ impingement or instability, screw fracture, polyethylene wear, and particle disease, subsidence, and infection.[61]

Distal Radioulnar Joint Arthroplasty

The DRUJ is critical to the function of the forearm and wrist, allowing pronosupination and load transmission, and providing stability to the wrist.

At present, arthroplasty is the treatment of choice for DRUJ pathology because resection of the ulna has been associated with long-term instability of the forearm and wrist.

Again, there are multiple implant options for DRUJ, ranging from partial ulnar head replacements to implants that replace the entirety of the DRUJ.

Ulnar head arthroplasty
The main indications of ulnar head arthroplasty are DRUJ arthrosis, both as primary and salvage treatment after failed ulnar head resections, and distal ulnar neoplasms.

Partial ulnar head arthroplasty involves resection of the ulnar head articular surface and placement of the prosthesis with minimal soft tissue disruption.[62] These prostheses preserve the ulnar styloid and the TFCC and are indicated for arthritis without instability.

Total ulnar head arthroplasty involves a complete resection of the ulnar head replacing it with an endoprostheses, composed of a stem and a head implant. Implant materials can be CoCr, pyrolytic carbon, or ceramic. Unlike partial arthroplasty, these implants require reconstruction of the soft tissue attachments and aim to treat instability in addition to pain.[63]

Common findings within the first year on postoperative radiographs are the presence of small radiolucencies adjacent to the prosthesis and remodeling of the sigmoid fossa around the metallic head. These findings should be considered pathologic if they progress over time or become symptomatic.

Potential complications include implant loosening, implant failure, infection, tendon rupture, and instability of the distal ulna.

Total distal radioulnar joint arthroplasty
Total DRUJ arthroplasty can be used for the treatment of primary DRUJ arthrosis, but it is especially useful for failed distal ulnar resections and unstable ulnar head replacements.

The Scheker prosthesis is a self-constrained device designed to treat DRUJ pathology with insufficient supporting soft tissues (**Fig. 37**).[60]

The ulnar component is an intramedullary ulnar stem and a peg that fits inside an ultra-high-molecular-weight polymer ball replacing the ulnar head. In turn, this ball sits in the hemisocket of a radial plate, which is attached to the distal radius by a peg and several cortical screws. The free movement of the peg within the ball and the ball within the socket allows full pronation and supination.[64]

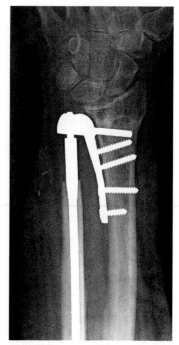

Fig. 37. PA wrist radiograph shows a Scheker prosthesis to treat DRUJ instability.

This prosthesis is contraindicated if the proximal ulnar remnant is less than 11 cm and in patients with immature skeleton or severe osteoporosis.

The DRUJ can also be replaced using nonconstrained arthroplasty, such as the sigmoid notch implant. This implant is composed of an insert that slides on a radial plate and articulates with an ulnar head component. The insert is secured with a peg and screw on the radial plate, but there are no screws linking the ulnar and sigmoid components. Therefore, malarticulation and dislocation are potential complications.

Potential complications include bone resorption around the ulnar stem or radial component, screw fracture or loosening, perihardware fracture, bearing surface wear of the polyethylene ball, soft tissue infection, ECU tenosynovitis, and heterotopic ossification.[64]

SUMMARY

General complications such as infection, CRPS, and nonunion can occur after any of the wrist and hand surgeries discussed. However, knowledge of the complexity of the different surgical techniques available in the hand and wrist is essential for posttreatment evaluation. Wrist and hand plain films together with clinical maneuvers is still the basis for posttreatment evaluation. CT with metal artifact reduction allows depiction of the healing process, location of the screw, and complications such as malposition or loosening of the screws. For the evaluation of superficial soft tissue structures, US and/or MR with metal artifact reduction techniques is the method of choice; however, careful interpretation should be made to avoid mistaking postsurgical changes from pathologic significant ones.

CLINICS CARE POINTS

- Infections are rare but mainly related to pins and hardware

- Healing assessment, healing, nonunion, and mal union, should be done with plain films and if doubts with CT using special protocols to minimize artifacts

- Posttreatment of fractures evaluation includes careful check of the location of the screws and devices to rule out complications such as articular penetration and chondral damage and tendon or nerve impingement

- Surgical approach of TFCC depends on the location of the tear and the ulnar variance. If ulnar variance is positive ulnar shortened osteotomy should be considered

- Acute tears of the intrinsic ligaments can be treated with pin or with anchors via miniopen surgery or arthroscopically, whereas chronic injuries with instability require tenodesis many times.

DISCLOSURE

The authors have nothing to disclose.

REFERENCES

1. Lipira AB, Sood RF, Tatman PD, et al. Complications Within 30 Days of Hand Surgery: An Analysis of 10,646 Patients. J Hand Surg Am 2015;40(9):1852–9.

2. Davies AM, Grainger AJ, James SJ, editors. Imaging of the hand and wrist. Springer Berlin, Heidelberg: Springer; 2013.

3. Strobel K, van der Bruggen W, Hug U, et al. SPECT/CT in Postoperative Hand and Wrist Pain. Semin Nucl Med 2018;48(5):396–409.

4. Vande Berg B, Malghem J, Maldague B, et al. Multi-detector CT imaging in the postoperative orthopedic patient with metal hardware. Eur J Radiol 2006;60(3):470–9.

5. Petscavage JM, Ha AS, Chew FS. Imaging assessment of the postoperative arthritic wrist. Radiographics 2011;31(6):1637–50.

6. Katsura M, Sato J, Akahane M, et al. Current and Novel Techniques for Metal Artifact Reduction at CT: Practical Guide for Radiologists. Radiographics 2018;38(2):450–61.

7. Wellenberg RHH, Hakvoort ET, Slump CH, et al. Metal artifact reduction techniques in musculoskeletal CT-imaging. Eur J Radiol 2018;107:60–9.

8. Johnson D, Stevens KJ, Riley G, et al. Approach to MR Imaging of the Elbow and Wrist: Technical Aspects and Innovation. Magn Reson Imaging Clin N Am 2015;23(3):355–66.

9. Olsen RV, Munk PL, Lee MJ, et al. Metal artifact reduction sequence: early clinical applications. Radiographics 2000;20(3):699–712.

10. Gupta A, Subhas N, Primak AN, et al. Metal artifact reduction: standard and advanced magnetic resonance and computed tomography techniques. Radiol Clin North Am 2015;53(3):531–47.

11. Harness NG, Inacio MC, Pfeil FF, et al. Rate of infection after carpal tunnel release surgery and effect of antibiotic prophylaxis. J Hand Surg Am 2010;35(2):189–96.

12. Chung KC, Malay S, Shauver MJ, et al, WRIST Group. Assessment of Distal Radius Fracture Complications Among Adults 60 Years or Older: A Secondary Analysis of the WRIST Randomized Clinical Trial. JAMA Netw Open 2019;2(1):e187053.

13. Patel DB, Emmanuel NB, Stevanovic MV, et al. Hand infections: anatomy, types and spread of infection, imaging findings, and treatment options. Radiographics 2014;34(7):1968–86.

14. Reuben SS. Preventing the development of complex regional pain syndrome after surgery. Anesthesiology 2004;101(5):1215–24.

15. Harden NR, Bruehl S, Perez RSGM, et al. Validation of proposed diagnostic criteria (the "Budapest Criteria") for Complex Regional Pain Syndrome. Pain 2010;150(2):268–74.

16. Marsland D, Konyves A, Cooper R, et al. Type I complex regional pain syndrome: MRI may be misleading. Inj Extra 2008;39(3):102–5.

17. Schweitzer ME, Mandel S, Schwartzman RJ, et al. Reflex sympathetic dystrophy revisited: MR imaging findings before and after infusion of contrast material. Radiology 1995;195(1):211–4.

18. Vas L, Pai R. Musculoskeletal Ultrasonography to Distinguish Muscle Changes in Complex Regional Pain Syndrome Type 1 from Those of Neuropathic Pain: An Observational Study. Pain Pract 2016;16(1):E1–13.

19. Morshed S. Current Options for Determining Fracture Union. Adv Med 2014;708574. https://doi.org/10.1155/2014/708574.

20. Beredjiklian PK, Bozentka DJ, Leung YL, et al. Complications of wrist arthroscopy. J Hand Surg Am 2004;29(3):406–11.

21. Warhold LG, Ruth RM. Complications of wrist arthroscopy and how to prevent them. Hand Clin 1995;11(1):81–9.

22. De Smet L. Pitfalls in wrist arthroscopy. Acta Orthop Belg 2002;68(4):325–9.

23. Ahsan ZS, Yao J. Complications of wrist arthroscopy. Arthroscopy 2012;28(6):855–9.

24. del Piñal F, Herrero F, Cruz-Camara A, et al. Complete avulsion of the distal posterior interosseous nerve during wrist arthroscopy: a possible cause of persistent pain after arthroscopy. J Hand Surg Am 1999;24(2):240–2.

25. Francisco del Pinal: Atlas of distal radius fractures (With e-book)Thieme Verlag, New York, Stuttgart, Delhi, Rio de Janeiro, 2018, 392 pp. 684 figs., Hardcover, ISBN: 978-1-62623-679-0.

26. Ochen Y, Peek J, van der Velde D, et al. Operative vs Nonoperative Treatment of Distal Radius Fractures in Adults: A Systematic Review and Meta-analysis. JAMA Netw Open 2020;3(4):e203497.

27. Li Y, Zhou Y, Zhang X, et al. Incidence of complications and secondary procedure following distal radius fractures treated by volar locking plate (VLP). J Orthop Surg Res 2019;14(1):295.

28. Gilley E, Puri SK, Hearns KA, et al. Importance of Computed Tomography in Determining Displacement in Scaphoid Fractures. J Wrist Surg 2018;7(1):38–42.

29. Hackney LA, Dodds SD. Assessment of scaphoid fracture healing. Curr Rev Musculoskelet Med 2011;4(1):16–22.

30. Jeon IH, Micic ID, Oh CW, et al. Percutaneous screw fixation for scaphoid fracture: a comparison between the dorsal and the volar approaches. J Hand Surg Am 2009;34(2):228–36.e1.

31. Cerezal L, Abascal F, Canga A, et al. Usefulness of gadolinium-enhanced MR imaging in the evaluation of the vascularity of scaphoid nonunions. AJR Am J Roentgenol 2000;174(1):141–9.

32. Green DP. The effect of avascular necrosis on Russe bone grafting for scaphoid nonunion. J Hand Surg Am 1985;10(5):597–605.

33. Goldfarb CA, Yin Y, Gilula LA, et al. Wrist fractures: what the clinician wants to know. Radiology 2001; 219(1):11–28.

34. Palmer AK. Triangular fibrocartilage complex lesions: a classification. J Hand Surg Am 1989;14(4):594–606.

35. Ng AWH, Tong CSL, Hung EHY, et al. Top-Ten Tips for Imaging the Triangular Fibrocartilaginous Complex. Semin Musculoskelet Radiol 2019;23(4):436–43.

36. Llopis E, Restrepo R, Kassarjian A, et al. Overuse Injuries of the Wrist. Radiol Clin North Am 2019;57(5): 957–76.

37. Cerezal L, de Dios Berná-Mestre J, Canga A, et al. MR and CT arthrography of the wrist. Semin Musculoskelet Radiol 2012;16(1):27–41. https://doi.org/10.1055/s-0032-1304299.

38. Cerezal L, Llopis E, Canga A, et al. Postoperative Imaging of Ulnar Wrist Pain. Semin Musculoskelet Radiol 2021;25(2):329–45.

39. del Piñal F. Dry arthroscopy and its applications. Hand Clin 2011;27(3):335–45.

40. Atzei A, Luchetti R. Foveal TFCC tear classification and treatment. Hand Clin 2011;27(3):263–72.

41. Jakubietz MG, Zahn R, Gruenert JG, et al. Kirschner wire fixations for scapholunate dissociation: a cadaveric, biomechanical study. J Orthop Surg (Hong Kong) 2012;20(2):224–9.

42. Corella F, Del Cerro M, Ocampos M, et al. Arthroscopic ligamentoplasty of the dorsal and volar portions of the scapholunate ligament. J Hand Surg Am 2013;38(12):2466–77.

43. Garcia-Elias M, Lluch AL, Stanley JK. Three-ligament tenodesis for the treatment of scapholunate dissociation: indications and surgical technique. J Hand Surg Am 2006;31(1):125–34.

44. Campagna R, Pessis E, Feydy A, et al. MRI assessment of recurrent carpal tunnel syndrome after open surgical release of the median nerve. AJR Am J Roentgenol 2009;193(3):644–50.

45. Ng AWH, Griffith JF, Tsai CSC, et al. MRI of the Carpal Tunnel 3 and 12 Months After Endoscopic Carpal Tunnel Release. AJR Am J Roentgenol 2021;216(2):464–70.

46. Khorashadi L, Ha AS, Chew FS. Radiologic guide to surgical treatment of first carpometacarpal joint osteoarthritis. AJR Am J Roentgenol 2012;198(5): 1152–60.

47. Munns JJ, Matthias RC, Zarezadeh A, et al. Outcomes of Revisions for Failed Trapeziometacarpal Joint Arthritis Surgery. J Hand Surg Am 2019; 44(9):798.e1–9.

48. Drapé JL, Silbermann-Hoffman O, Houvet P, et al. Complications of flexor tendon repair in the hand: MR imaging assessment. Radiology 1996;198(1):219–24.

49. Libberecht K, Lafaire C, Van Hee R. Evaluation and functional assessment of flexor tendon repair in the hand. Acta Chir Belg 2006;106(5):560–5.

50. Saltzman BM, Frank JM, Slikker W, et al. Clinical outcomes of proximal row carpectomy versus four-corner arthrodesis for post-traumatic wrist arthropathy: a systematic review. J Hand Surg Eur 2015; 40(5):450–7.

51. Daar DA, Shah A, Mirrer JT, et al. Proximal Row Carpectomy versus Four-Corner Arthrodesis for the Treatment of Scapholunate Advanced Collapse/ Scaphoid Nonunion Advanced Collapse Wrist: A Cost-Utility Analysis. Plast Reconstr Surg 2019; 143(5):1432–45.

52. Tulipan DJ, Eaton RG, Eberhart RE. The Darrach procedure defended: technique redefined and long-term follow-up. J Hand Surg Am 1991;16(3):438–44.

53. Glowacki KA. Hemiresection arthroplasty of the distal radioulnar joint. Hand Clin 2005;21(4): 591–601.

54. Slater RR Jr. The Sauvé-Kapandji procedure. J Hand Surg Am 2008;33(9):1632–8.

55. Yeoh D, Tourret L. Total wrist arthroplasty: a systematic review of the evidence from the last 5 years. J Hand Surg Eur 2015;40(5):458–68.

56. Gupta A. Total wrist arthroplasty. Am J Orthop (Belle Mead Nj) 2008;37(8 Suppl 1):12–6.

57. Srnec JJ, Wagner ER, Rizzo M. Total Wrist Arthroplasty. JBJS Rev 2018;6(6):e9.

58. Anderson MC, Adams BD. Total wrist arthroplasty. Hand Clin 2005;21(4):621–30.

59. Ferreres A, Lluch A, Del Valle M. Universal total wrist arthroplasty: midterm follow-up study. J Hand Surg Am 2011;36(6):967–73.

60. Adams BD. Complications of wrist arthroplasty. Hand Clin 2010;26(2):213–20.

61. Carlson JR, Simmons BP. Total wrist arthroplasty. J Am Acad Orthop Surg 1998;6(5):308–15.

62. Garcia-Elias M. Eclypse: partial ulnar head replacement for the isolated distal radio-ulnar joint arthrosis. Tech Hand Up Extrem Surg 2007;11(1):121–8.

63. Berger RA. Indications for ulnar head replacement. Am J Orthop (Belle Mead Nj) 2008;37(8 Suppl 1):17–20.

64. Willis AA, Berger RA, Cooney WP 3rd. Arthroplasty of the distal radioulnar joint using a new ulnar head endoprosthesis: preliminary report. J Hand Surg Am 2007;32(2):177–89.

Postoperative Hip MR Imaging

Ara Kassarjian, MD, FRCPC[a],*, Jaime Isern-Kebschull, MD, PhD[b], Xavier Tomas, MD, PhD[b]

KEYWORDS

- Hip • MR imaging • MR arthrography • Arthroscopy • Hip replacement • Complications • Labrum

KEY POINTS

- Postarthroscopy MR and MR arthrography of the hip can be challenging to interpret.
- Adhesions and capsular defects are best identified with MR arthrography.
- Detection of heterotopic ossification can be difficult on MR imaging.
- In the setting of total hip arthroplasty (THA), acetabular component positioning is one of the key factors in determining long-term clinical outcomes.
- Adverse locate tissue reactions following THA can take many forms, and a high index of suspicion and appropriate imaging protocols is recommended.

INTRODUCTION

Postoperative imaging of the hip used to be dominated by radiographs, computed tomography (CT), and occasionally nuclear medicine studies, given that most surgeries were arthroplasties or, less commonly, core decompressions. However, over the past 2 decades, hip arthroscopy has matured significantly and now represents one of the most common surgical procedures of the hip.[1] The indications and procedures performed have expanded well beyond arthroplasties and now include labral procedures (resections, repairs, and reconstructions), osteochondroplasties, acetabuloplasties, and removal of loose bodies, among others. As a result, postoperative evaluation of the hip now often includes MR imaging and MR arthrography. This article discusses normal postoperative appearances and some of the more common complications associated with hip arthroscopy and hip arthroplasty with a focus on MR imaging.

MR Imaging Following Hip Arthroscopy

Labral surgery

One of the most common current indications for hip arthroscopy is a symptomatic labral tear. Although there is controversy regarding the most appropriate treatment strategies for patients with hip pain and labral tears, hip arthroscopy is often performed to address labral pathology. As with labral tears in the shoulder, the type and extent of tear determines the optimal procedure. Possibilities include labral shaving/trimming/debridement, labral repair, and labral reconstruction. Although the details of each of these procedures is beyond the scope of this article, the postoperative appearances of the most common procedures are reviewed.

Labral shaving/trimming/debridement

With small nondisplaced labral tears and/or degenerative fraying and mild degenerative tearing of the labrum, it may not be appropriate or possible to perform a labral repair. In these cases, using an arthroscopic shaver, the irregular frayed labral margin is shaved back to a stable rim. All unstable fragments and flaps are removed while attempting to conserve the maximum amount of labral tissue possible.

Postoperatively, on MR imaging and MR arthrography, if only minimal shaving has been performed, the labrum may have a normal or near normal appearance. However, in most cases,

---

[a] Elite Sports Imaing, SL, Calle Grecia, 28224, Pozuelo de Alarcón, Spain; [b] Department of Radiology, Hospital Clínic. C. de Villarroel, 170, 08036 Barcelona, Spain
* Corresponding author.
E-mail address: kassarjian@me.com

Magn Reson Imaging Clin N Am 30 (2022) 673–688
https://doi.org/10.1016/j.mric.2022.03.003

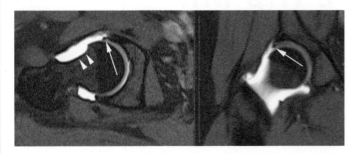

Fig. 1. Normal postoperative appearance following osteochondroplasty and labral debridement. Axial oblique and coronal T1-weighted fat-suppressed images from direct MR arthrogram demonstrate evidence of prior femoral osteochondroplasty (*arrowheads*) and a blunted anterior superior labrum following labral debridement (*arrow*).

particularly if preoperative images are available for direct comparison, the labrum will have a slightly more blunted and/or diminutive appearance (**Fig. 1**). There may be minimally increased intrinsic signal in the labrum although this is nonspecific. However, there should be no discrete fluid-filled cleft traversing the labrum itself or any evidence of labrochondral separation.[2]

Labral repair

In cases of a well-defined labral tear with associated good-quality labral substance, a labral repair can be considered; this includes both intrinsic labral tears as well as labral chondral separations. The most common form of labral repair includes suturing of the labral tear with or without associated anchors depending on the configuration location and extent of the labral tear.

Following labral repair, the findings on MR imaging can be subtle but are usually slightly more

evident than in cases of minimal labral debridement. In general, the labrum will have low signal or low to intermediate signal on all pulse sequences. Minimal susceptibility artifact may be seen in the region of the labrum itself, depending on the technique used. In addition, if anchors were used, subtle tracts may be seen along the acetabular rim at the site of anchor attachment (**Fig. 2**). On MR imaging, intermediate signal may remain along the course of the original labral tear for months; this may represent granulation tissue. However, no discrete fluid-filled cleft should be seen after successful labral repair. Similarly, if MR arthrography is performed, no gadolinium should be seen traversing the substance of the labrum or traversing the labral chondral junction following labral repair. A residual or recurrent labral tear can be diagnosed when either fluid intensity signal or gadolinium is severely traversing labral substance and/or the labral chondral junction (**Fig. 3**). In addition, attention should be paid to identify unstable labral flaps, displaced labral fragments, and displaced or malpositioned labral anchors (**Fig. 4**).[3]

Labral reconstruction

Although less commonly performed, there is a recent trend to attempt to reconstruct the labrum using autografts or allografts including the iliotibial band among other tissues. The literature regarding the normal postoperative appearance following labral reconstruction is scant. However, in general, the same principles are applied wherein no fluid intensity signal or gadolinium should be seen traversing the labrum or labral chondral junction. No unstable labral flaps or displaced labral fragments should be seen.

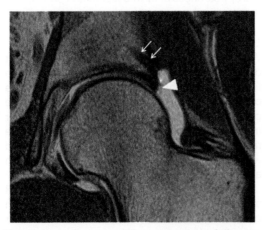

Fig. 2. Normal postoperative appearance following labral repair. Coronal T1-weighted image from direct MR arthrogram demonstrates an intact superior labrum with minimal adjacent artifact (*arrowhead*) as well as a screw tract along the superior acetabulum (*arrows*) following labral reattachment. (Reprinted with permission from R. Sutter. MRI of the Postoperative Hip in MRI of the Hip. Breitenseher Publisher. 2016.)

Osteochondroplasty

In patients with femoroacetabular impingement syndrome with CAM morphology, an osteochondroplasty (a.k.a. bumpectomy) is often performed to address the flattened or convex morphology at the femoral head neck junction; this is typically

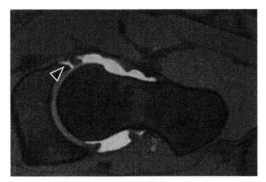

Fig. 3. Failed labral reattachment. Oblique axial T1-weighted fat-suppressed image from direct MR arthrogram demonstrates a detached anterior superior labrum (*arrowhead*) following arthroscopic labral reattachment with anchors. (Reprinted with permission from R. Sutter. MRI of the Postoperative Hip in MRI of the Hip. Breitenseher Publisher. 2016.)

performed arthroscopically using a bone burr to reestablish a concave morphology of the femoral head neck junction. After a successful osteochondroplasty, the reestablishment of a concave morphology is easily appreciated both at MR imaging and MR arthrography (**Fig. 5**).

One of the most common "complications" of osteochondroplasty is suboptimal or incomplete resection of the conflicting bump.[4] Although this has become less common, there is a significant learning curve in performing this procedure arthroscopically and for less experienced surgeons it can be challenging to assess whether adequate resection has been performed. On postoperative MR imaging and MR arthrography, regions of incomplete resection can easily be identified, particularly if radial imaging is used (**Fig. 6**).

In addition, if there is mixed type femoroacetabular impingement syndrome, acetabular rim

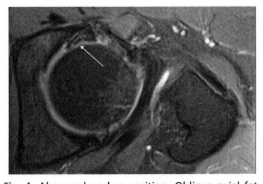

Fig. 4. Abnormal anchor position. Oblique axial fat-suppressed intermediate-weighted image demonstrates an abnormal intraarticular position of an anchor following labral reattachment (*arrow*). (*Courtesy of* V. Mascarenhas, Lisbon, Portugal.)

trimming is often performed to correct any regions of focal or global over coverage. On postoperative imaging, this can be subtle and may simply appear as a slightly attenuated acetabular rim, particularly when directly compared with preoperative images.

Cartilage Repair Procedures

Despite significant growing interest in performing cartilage repair procedures in the hip, the experience remains limited and publications remain scarce. Some of the more commonly performed procedures include microfracture and, in the setting of delaminating lesions, gluing and/or suture fixation. In general, the same concepts can be applied here as are seen in regions where cartilage repairs are more frequent such as the knee. The repaired cartilage may have increased signal on intermediate and T2-weighted sequences (**Fig. 7**). Signs of failure or complication include persistent or new fluid-filled clefts, focal cartilage defects, residual/recurrent delamination, or displaced cartilage fragments. Subchondral edema is less commonly seen following acetabular cartilage repair procedures when compared with those involving the femoral condyles or the femoral head.[5–7]

Nonspecific Postarthroscopic Complications

As with other joints, there are certain nonspecific complications that can occur following hip arthroscopy. Neurovascular injury and infections are rare but can occur as in any other joint. These will not be discussed, as the findings are similar in the hip as in other joints.

Although not very common, one of the complications occasionally seen after hip arthroscopy is a formation of adhesions. Clinically, these can present with pain/discomfort, limited range of motion, and occasionally mechanical symptoms such as locking and clicking. However, adhesions can also be seen in asymptomatic patients.[8] If no joint effusion is present, these can be difficult, if not impossible, to identify. At MR arthrography, adhesions can be seen as low-signal-intensity bands traversing portions of the hip joint, typically extending from the capsule to the femoral neck (**Fig. 8**). Smaller more focal adhesions can also be seen adjacent to the ligamentum teres. More severe adhesions can result in actual adherence of the capsule to the femoral head or neck. Of note, small thin synovial plicas that are present in most of the hips should not be confused with postoperative adhesions. The normal plica has a typical appearance and distribution in the hip joint.[9]

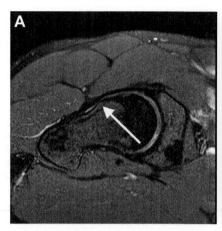
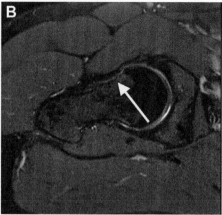

Fig. 5. Normal preosteochondroplasty and postosteochondroplasty appearance. (*A*) Oblique axial fat-suppressed intermediate-weighted image demonstrates cam morphology at the femoral head neck junction (*arrow*). (*B*) Postoperative oblique axial fat-suppressed intermediate-weighted image with subsequent reestablishment of desired concavity at the femoral head neck junction following arthroscopic osteochondroplasty (*arrow*).

There has been some interest in defining the significance of capsular defects following hip arthroscopy. The surgical community is divided regarding whether capsular closure should routinely be performed. At MR imaging, it can be challenging to identify a capsular defect unless it is quite prominent. A small amount of gadolinium present outside of the joint capsule can be seen in normal cases due to injection artifact. However, if a significant focal defect within the capsule is seen at MR arthrography, capsular deficiency or dehiscence may be present (**Fig. 9**). Despite the imaging findings, many patients with capsular defects remain asymptomatic.[8]

Heterotopic Ossification

Although heterotopic ossification is more common following open/major surgery, specifically arthroplasties, it can occasionally be seen following hip arthroscopy. The incidence is quite low and reported to occur in less than 5% of cases.[10] The most common locations for the appearance for heterotopic ossification following hip arthroscopy are along the tract of the portals or at the site of capsulotomy (**Fig. 10**).[10]

MR imaging is notoriously insensitive and often nonspecific for the detection of heterotopic ossification. Ossified bone has fatty marrow, which will have high signal on T1-weighted images and low signal on fat-suppressed T2-weighted images, therefore blending with surrounding tissues. Use of gradient echo imaging can increase the sensitivity for detection of calcification/ossification. In any case, a high index of suspicion is recommended and if any doubt exists, assessment with radiographs or CT scan can be considered to identify small regions of heterotopic ossification that may be occult on MR images (**Fig. 11**).

MR Imaging Following Hip Arthroplasty

Normal postoperative appearances

The most common indication for a total hip arthroplasty (THA) is advanced degenerative changes/osteoarthritis of the hip. Additional indications include inflammatory arthritis, osteonecrosis, and certain types of trauma. Although there are many variations of hip prostheses, one of the most common combinations is that of a cemented femoral stem and a noncemented acetabular cup.

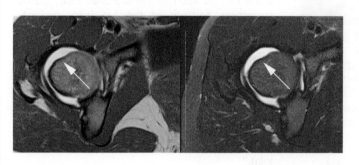

Fig. 6. Incomplete arthroscopic resection of the femoral head-neck convexity. Axial T1 and fat-suppressed T2-weighted images from direct MR arthrogram demonstrate incomplete resection of the convexity at the femoral head neck junction (*arrow*) following arthroscopic osteochondroplasty.

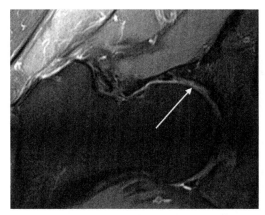

Fig. 7. Postoperative cartilage after microfracture. Fat-suppressed intermediate-weighted image from radial acquisition following arthroscopic microfracture of acetabular cartilage lesions demonstrates intact acetabular cartilage with sightly heterogeneous signal (*arrow*). No evidence of cartilage gap or fluid-filled cleft to suggest failure of the procedure. (*Courtesy of* V. Mascarenhas, Lisbon, Portugal.)

When evaluating a total hip prosthesis, the first step is to assess the proper positioning of the components; this includes ensuring that the femoral component is properly centered within the acetabular component, there is appropriate acetabular component inclination in the coronal plane (40°–50°), there is appropriate anteversion of the acetabular component in the axial plane (0°–20°, depending on anatomic and certain technical factors), and that the acetabular screws are in appropriate position. Although the position of the femoral head may be slightly inferior to the center of the acetabular cup with certain acetabular liners, a femoral head position located superiorly in the acetabular cup indicates wear of the polyethylene liner. It should be noted that a thin lucency at the metal bone interface in noncemented components as seen on radiographs is compatible with fibrous ingrowth and does not necessarily represent loosening.[11]

Improper positioning can result in discomfort and pain shortly after surgery. For example, an increased alpha angle can result in friction of the iliopsoas tendon and subsequent tendinopathy, bursitis, and tendon tears. Similarly, a malpositioned screw could affect the neurovascular bundle and result in vascular and/or neural compromise. In addition, improperly positioned components are at risk for rapid wear and failure (**Fig. 12**).

Positioning of the acetabular component is critical, especially in metal-on-metal implants, as it seems to be one of the key determinants of clinical outcomes at 10 years following THA.[12]

Aseptic mechanical loosening

The most frequent complications following THA include aseptic mechanical loosening (AML), a septic prosthesis, and a granulomatous pseudotumor reaction. These 3 conditions seem to occur in different time frames, with AML occurring at an average of 39 months following surgery, infection occurring at an average of 55 months following surgery, and granulomatous pseudotumor reaction occurring at an average of 126 months following surgery.[13] On radiographs, AML is characterized by radiolucency greater than 2 mm at the prosthesis-bone interface; this represents a periprosthetic membrane, which is characterized histologically by a lack of fibroblasts and inflammatory cells. In the case of a cemented prosthesis, fragmentation of the cement can be seen. Although these lucencies can be quite difficult to detect at MR imaging due to artifact from inhomogeneities in the local magnetic field, advanced metal artifact reduction sequences may occasionally sufficiently reduce artifact to demonstrate these findings of AML. In such cases, the lucency seen on radiographs is typically seen as regions of periprosthetic T2 hyperintensity. Although the term "aseptic" indicates lack of infection, oftentimes what is clinically and preoperatively thought to represent aseptic loosening is

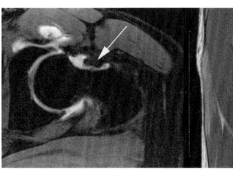
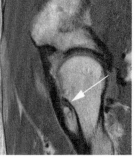

Fig. 8. Postoperative intraarticular adhesions. Oblique axial fat-suppressed T1-weighted image and sagittal proton density–weighted image demonstrate adhesions extending from the capsule to the femoral neck (*arrows*) following arthroscopic osteochondroplasty.

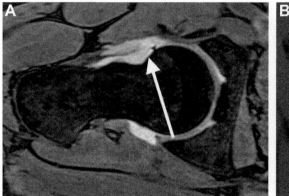
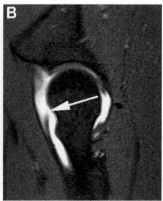

Fig. 9. Postoperative capsular defect. Oblique axial fat-suppressed T1-weighted VIBE (volumetric interpolated breath hold examination) image (*A*) and sagittal fat-suppressed T1-weighted image (*B*) from direct MR arthrogram demonstrate a large capsular defect (*arrow*) anteriorly following arthroscopic osteochondroplasty.

shown to represent septic mechanical loosening when sonification cultures are performed; this was seen to be the case in greater than 50% of prosthesis in one study, particularly in those patients with severe osteolysis.[14]

Granulomatous Pseudotumor or Adverse Local Tissue Reactions

There is extensive variability in the terminology used to describe reactions surrounding prostheses, which include granulomatous pseudotumor,[13,15] pseudotumors,[16] adverse local tissue reaction (ALTR),[17,18] adverse reaction to metal debris,[19] aseptic lymphocytic vasculitis–associated lesions due to a delayed type IV hypersensitivity,[20] metallosis,[21,22] trunnionosis,[23]

and so forth. There is a general lack of consensus regarding which terminology to use with significant overlap between the terms (**Table 1**).[23] Although the term "pseudotumor" traditionally has been described in the context of metal-on-metal total hip arthroplasties,[24] it has also been detected in other types of arthroplasties including nonmetal on metal, metal on polyethylene, ceramic on polyethylene, and ceramic on metal prostheses.[25–27]

What all of these entities usually have in common is the absence of malignancy or infection although those 2 entities can rarely coexist. For the purposes of this section, the authors use the term "adverse local tissue reaction" (ALTR) to include all adverse reactions/responses including wear-related reactions and biological reactions.

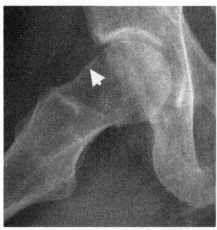
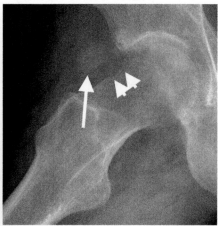

Fig. 10. Postoperative heterotopic ossification. Preoperative and postoperative frog lateral radiographs of the hip demonstrate convexity at the femoral head neck junction (*arrowhead*), which was subsequently resected arthroscopically via osteochondroplasty. Postoperative radiograph demonstrates the osteochondroplasty (*double arrowhead*) as well as the formation of a small region of heterotopic ossification along the superolateral aspect of the hip (*arrow*). (*Courtesy of* E. Llopis. Valencia, Spain.)

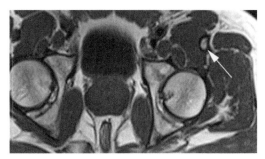

Fig. 11. Postoperative heterotopic ossification. Axial T1-weighted image demonstrates a small focus of heterotopic ossification anterior to the hip joint (*arrow*) with internal high signal from fatty marrow and peripheral ring of low signal from the cortical-type calcification.

ALTR in the setting of metallosis represents a well-organized connective tissue predominantly composed of a foreign body reaction to metal debris (a.k.a. metal reactivity) with macrophages/ histiocytic giant cells, which may then undergo apoptosis with resultant tissue necrosis (**Fig. 13**). Alternatively, a complex immune reaction may occur, which involves lymphocytes and a type IV delayed hypersensitivity reaction (a.k.a. metal sensitivity).[28,29]

In cases of ALTR, one can find extensive synovitis with soft tissue periprosthetic masses, tissue necrosis, and bursal hypertrophy.[30–32] If there is associated extensive metal wear, metal ions from cobalt-based alloys can be released, resulting in both local and systemic sequela, with the former sometimes referred to as arthroprosthetic cobaltism. Subsequent cobalt toxicity may result in hematological, neurologic, cardiac, and endocrine consequences, which, in rare cases, can be fatal.[33–36]

The presence of periprosthetic collections, whether fluidlike, mixed, or solid, is compatible with synovitis. These collections were classified by Hauptfleisch and colleagues into 3 types. Type 1 collections consist of thin-walled cystic lesions that

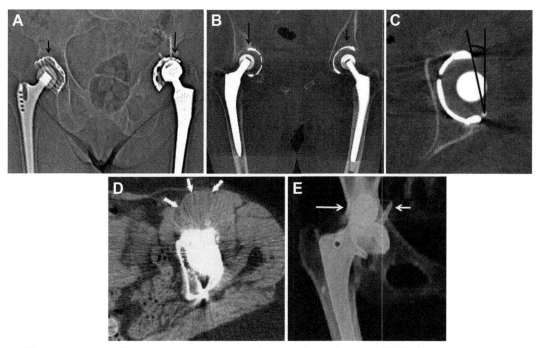

Fig. 12. Analysis of prosthetic component position of a total hip arthroplasty (THA). (*A*) Scout anteroposterior localizer radiograph shows that femoral head component must be centered within the acetabular component (*short arrow*). An eccentric position is pathologic (*long arrow*) and indicates polyethylene liner wear. (*B*) Coronal CT image shows that acetabular component inclination in the coronal plane should be between 40° and 50° (*short arrow*). Right THA shows a greater, abnormal inclination angle of around 90° (*long arrow*). (*C*) Axial CT image shows that appropriate anteversion of acetabular component in the axial plane should be between 0° and 20° ("alpha angle"). (*D*) Axial CT image shows that iliopsoas impingement usually occurs when the alpha angle of acetabular component overhangs the bone structure chronically irritating the iliopsoas tendon and producing an iliopsoas bursitis (*arrows*). (*E*) Coronal volume–rendered 3-dimensional CT image demonstrates acetabular screw (*short arrow*) markedly exceeding the cortical bone and inappropriately nearing the anatomic area of the iliopsoas muscle and the iliac vessels. Also notice the cranial dislocation of the prosthetic femoral head (*long arrow*).

Table 1
Overlapping terminology used in the literature to describe the presence of periprosthetic soft tissue lesions

Term	Definition
Pseudotumor	Describes the clinical and radiological presentation of an aseptic periprosthetic soft tissue (solid or cystic) mass
Granulomatous pseudotumor or foreign body reaction	Describes the presence of histiocytes and giant cells in the histopathological specimen forming periprosthetic osteolysis with expansile periosteal reaction[5]
Adverse local tissue reaction (ALTR)[a]	Describes all periprosthetic adverse reactions whether attributable to wear or not[8]
Adverse reaction to metal debris (ARMD)	Describes all adverse periprosthetic reactions attributable to metal alloy wear
Metallosis	Describes local deposition of metal wear debris with resultant gray/black discoloration of the periprosthetic soft tissues[12]
Aseptic lymphocytic vasculitis–associated lesions (ALVAL)	Describes the histologic sequelae of adverse periprosthetic reactions particularly related to metal ion release (rather than particle wear)
Trunnionosis	Metal wear and/or corrosion at a tapered modular interface with concomitant cobalt ion release, most commonly at the head-neck junction in THA[13]
Arthroprosthetic cobaltism	Soft tissue reaction generating a catastrophic wear–related failure of THA components and systemic toxicity described exclusively with cobalt-based alloys[13]

[a] ALTR includes all adverse responses resulting from biological and wear-related causes and could be the most appropriate, inclusive term.

Adapted from Shulman RM, Zywiel MG, Gandhi R, et al. Trunnionosis: the latest culprit in adverse reactions to metal debris following hip arthroplasty. Skeletal Radiol. 2015 Mar;44(3):433-440.

communicate with the joint. Type 2 collections consist of thick-walled cystic lesions, whereas type 3 collections are more solid lesions and may be pseudoencapsulated or decompressed into surrounding bursae such as the iliopsoas or trochanteric bursa. The latter are more commonly found posterior to the joint and seem to be associated with more severe symptoms and higher revision rates.[37] Other classifications for periprosthetic collections also exist. One of these is the Anderson criteria for metal-on-metal total hip arthroplasties, which categorize periprosthetic soft tissue masses and ranges from grade A (normal or acceptable) to grade C3 (severe). These criteria include changes in the surrounding tendons, bone marrow, and bone cortices. Of note, the grade B category includes infections.[38] At MR imaging, osteolysis due to bone resorption can be seen and is a hallmark of immune reactions with elevated osteoclastic activity. Isern-Kebschull and colleagues published that periprosthetic osteolysis with expansile

periosteal reaction was significantly higher in the ALTR group (71.9%) compared with aseptic mechanical loosening (10.3%) and infection (13.6%).[13] The synovitis may invade the surrounding bone marrow, thereby replacing the normal higher signal of intramedullary fat with the low to intermediate signal of T1-weighted images[17] (**Fig. 14**). Rarely, other findings such as an iliopsoas mass mimicking a psoas abscess[39] or a "cementoma" (**Fig. 15**) can be seen.

Periprosthetic Fluid Collections and Infection

Numerous studies have described periprosthetic soft-tissue alterations such as edema, fluid collections, and infections.[13,40,41] Initially, these findings were seen on ultrasound[42] and CT.[13,41] However, MR imaging with metal artifact reduction sequences has become very sensitive for the detection of periprosthetic collections and other complications.[43]

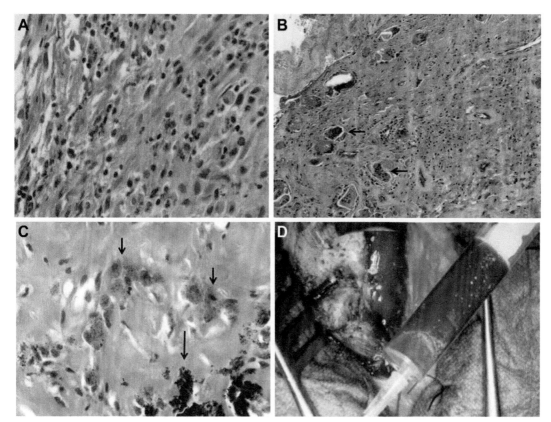

Fig. 13. Histology of infection and adverse local tissue reaction (ALTR). (*A*) A 40-year-old male patient with a right THA because of femoral head necrosis. Light-microscopic view of biopsy of periprosthetic tissue with a magnification of x20 shows a typical picture of an acute infection with several polymorphonuclear leukocytes (>20). (*B*) A 61-year-old female patient with a right THA. Light-microscopic view of the biopsy of periprosthetic tissue with a magnification of x10. Note presence of histiocytes and giant cells (*arrows*) that indicate ALTR. (*C*) A 37-year-old female patient with a right THA because of severe rheumatoid arthritis. Light-microscopic view of biopsy of the periprosthetic tissue with a magnification of x40. Macrophages with cytoplasm containing pigmented grains (short *arrows*) and metal wear debris (long *arrow*) indicating ALTR with metallosis. (*D*) A 62-year-old man with a left THA. Surgical image showing a large volume of black fluid surrounding the periprosthetic soft tissues, indicating ALTR with metallosis.

Another sign that has been related to infections following hip arthroplasty is the presence of ipsilateral iliac chain adenopathy, which can be visualized by CT or MR imaging.[13,41,43,44]

It is critical that the MR sequences are tailored to the specific clinical context, as the presence of periprosthetic collections can also be a finding associated with other conditions such as biomechanical alteration (eg, in the form of iliopsoas bursitis)[45] or foreign body reactions (eg, ceramic-on-polyethylene and metal-on-metal resurfacing arthroplasties).[46]

The pattern of the fluid in periprosthetic collections seen on MR imaging has proved to be useful in elucidating a specific diagnosis.[47] The lamellar pattern (layering) of a thickened hyperintense synovium suggests an infected hip arthroplasty,

as has also been reported in cases of knee prostheses.[47,48] Likewise, the presence of debris is frequently visualized in these cases.

These collections can be associated with edematous changes of the periarticular soft tissues, abscesses, or even sinus tracts including some that may extend to the skin surface. Although rarely visualized (or very subtle) on MR imaging, the presence of gas in these collections suggests a septic complication (**Figs. 16** and **17**).

The recognition of osteolysis around the components of the prosthesis can be seen by MR imaging, especially if it is an aggressive pattern of bone loss.[47] However, a recent study has shown that the presence of early signs such as periosteal reaction by MR imaging is typically related to infection.[43]

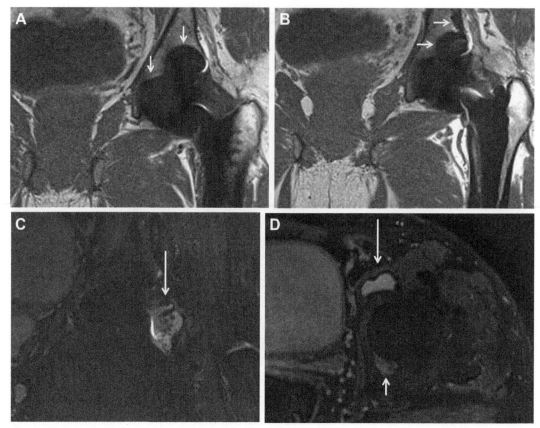

Fig. 14. Adverse local tissue reaction (ALTR) in a left THA. Coronal T1 (*A, B*), Coronal STIR (*C*), and axial STIR (*D*) MR images demonstrate areas of osseous resorption replacing the intramedullary fat compatible with osteolysis surrounding the acetabular component (*A, B, D; short arrows*). Pseudocapsulated area containing fluid signal intensity with solid debris, suggesting mixed synovitis (*C; long arrow*). Fluid signal intensity (fluid synovitis) in the iliopsoas bursa (*D; long arrow*).

Tendon Tears and Muscle Atrophy

Although most of the literature has focused on the infectious and abnormal local tissue reactions to total hip arthroplasties, other periprosthetic pathologies are also important to consider. Chang and colleagues demonstrated that patient pain was more associated with gluteal tendon tears (gluteus medius and minimus) and bone marrow edema surrounding the femoral component prosthesis as opposed to the presence or size of pseudotumors.[49] Another study demonstrated that fatty atrophy of the gluteus medius as demonstrated on MR imaging was more common in patients with limping and trochanteric pain when compared with asymptomatic patients.[50,51] As such, further attention and investigation is recommended into the presence and significance of

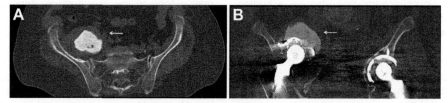

Fig. 15. 75-year-old man with bilateral THA. (*A*) Axial and (*B*) coronal CT images show a significant superomedial protrusion of the right prosthetic acetabular component, with migration of the cement into the pelvis invading the iliopsoas muscle and forming a pseudomass (*arrows*). The native acetabulum shows severe osteolysis and expansive periosteal displacement, suggesting an ALTR. Compare with the properly positioned left THA.

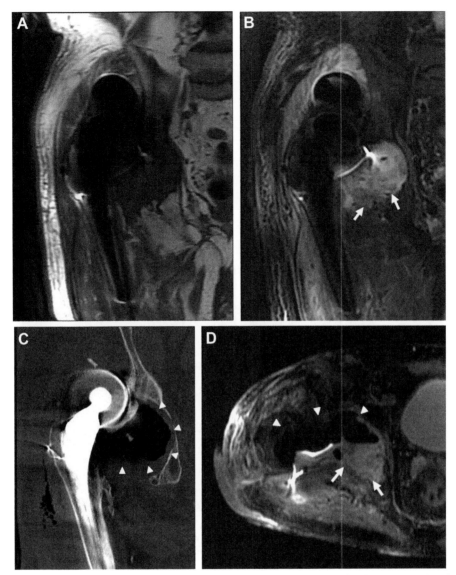

Fig. 16. Complete dislocation of an infected hip prosthesis. Coronal T1-weighted (*A*) and coronal and axial STIR (*B, D*) MR images show displacement of the prosthetic components toward the gluteal muscles, associated with edematous changes in the adjacent soft tissues and a voluminous fluid collection with thickened synovium in a lamellar pattern (*arrows* in *B, D*) and air-fluid level (*arrowheads* in *D*). Coronal reconstruction from a CT scan (*C*) confirms the dislocation of the prosthesis as well as the presence of gas (*arrowheads*) in the collection seen on MR imaging.

abductor tendon pathology and marrow edema in patients after THA.

As an example, Ibrahim and colleagues demonstrated that in a group of more than 100 patients, there was a higher incidence of gluteus medius tendon degeneration in patients following revision hip arthroplasty than those with primary osteoarthritis and controls with femoral neck fractures.[52] Additional recent studies have suggested that a direct lateral approach as opposed to the posterior or anterior approach results in more gluteus medius

tendon degeneration and fatty atrophy. However, despite another study showing that a direct anterior approach resulted in less atrophy of hip musculature, there were no significant differences in patient-related outcome scores 1 year following THA.[52–56] As opposed to the findings with the gluteus medius muscle and tendon, fatty atrophy of the gluteus minimus is quite common following THA and does not seem to correlate with trochanteric pain syndromes.[57] Given the aforementioned, a radiologist should be aware of the surgical

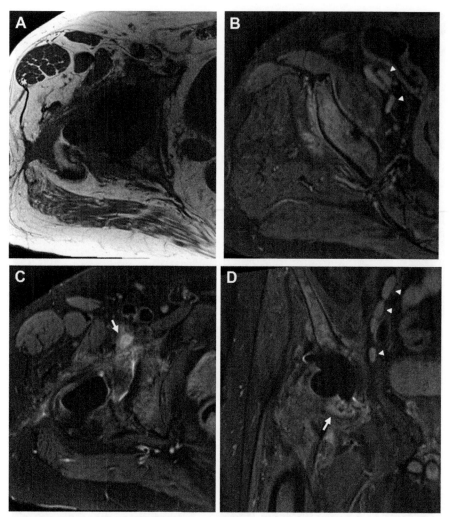

Fig. 17. Infected total hip prosthesis. Axial T1 (A), axial STIR (B, C), and coronal STIR (D) MR images show edematous changes surrounding the prosthesis in the form of fluid with changes of synovitis (*arrows* in C, D). Prominent lymph nodes are present along the iliac chain (*arrowheads B, D*).

approach used and should look specifically for pathology involving the gluteal muscles and tendons, specifically the gluteus medius, even in cases when the arthroplasty seems to be in proper position/alignment (**Fig. 18**).[49,52] Another potential postoperative complication following THA is impingement of the iliopsoas tendon with subsequent tendinopathy, bursitis, and rarely tendon tears; this can occur when there is improper positioning of the acetabular component in the setting of an oversized acetabular component.[58–60]

Periprosthetic Osseous Stress Reaction and Fractures

The occurrence of periprosthetic fractures is relatively frequent (around 20%), typically seen in association with the femoral component and generally caused by osseous resorption due to micromotion stress.[47] Radiographs are the initial technique of choice to diagnose fractures.[61] CT is reserved for cases where there is a high clinical suspicion for a fracture but normal-appearing radiographs and in cases where surgical planning is required.[62]

When a fracture is not evident on radiographs or CT, particularly in the setting of significant demineralization, MR is useful, as it can detect subtle signs of stress reactions such as localized marrow edema, endosteal edema, and thickening of the cortex (initially without the presence of a fracture line).[47,63,64] This finding is common but often asymptomatic on short-term follow-up.[65] The identification of a linear component on MR helps differentiate a stress fracture from a stress reaction.[47,66,67] It is important to emphasize that the

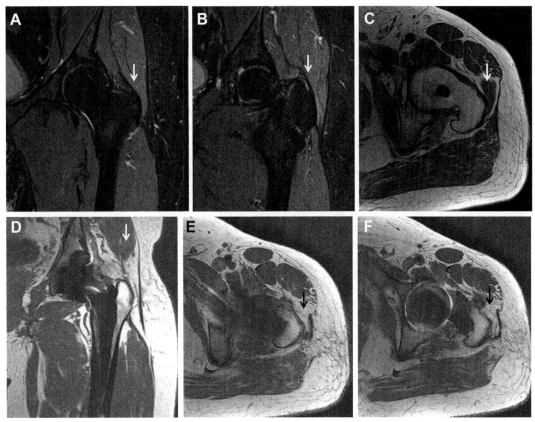

Fig. 18. Tendinopathies in the postoperative hip. Coronal STIR-weighted (*A, B*) and axial T1-weighted (*C*) MR images show homogeneous, hypointense intact gluteus minimus and gluteus medium tendons at anterior and lateral facets of greater trochanter (*arrows*). In another patient status post-THA with a direct lateral surgical approach, coronal (*D*) and axial T1-weighted MR images (*E, F*) demonstrate gluteus tendon tear and fatty atrophy (*arrows*).

presence of hyperintense marrow signal alteration on all pulse sequences can be considered an artifact,[40] but if it is only observed in fluid-sensitive sequences in the form of marrow edema surrounding the femoral component, it is associated with pain.

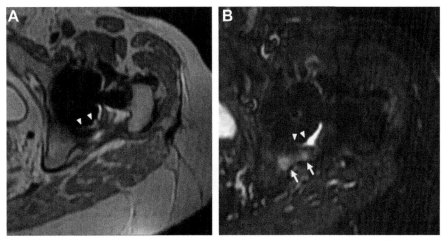

Fig. 19. Periprosthetic stress reaction of the acetabulum. (*A*) Axial T2 TSE MR image shows a thick layer of increased signal intensity (*arrowheads*) at the acetabular implant-bone interface that suggests bone resorption along the posterior wall. (*B*) Axial STIR MR image shows a bone marrow edema pattern underlying the cortex, indicating an associated stress reaction (*arrows*).

Demonstration of edema adjacent to prosthetic components may also indicate a stress reaction related to loosening (**Fig. 19**). The presence of a hyperintense band at the bone-metal interface with a thickness greater than 2 mm suggests loosening of the prosthesis.[47]

SUMMARY

MR imaging of the postoperative hip can be challenging. Following hip arthroscopy, depending on the clinical indication, high-resolution MR or direct MR arthrography may be indicated. Following THA, although the initial imaging modalities are radiography and CT, MR imaging has been taking on an increasing role, particularly due to advances of metal artifact reduction sequences. In both setting, it is critical to know the type of surgery performed as well as the clinical indications for the examination to properly interpret the imaging findings.

CLINICS CARE POINTS

- Following hip arthroscopy, knowledge of the surgical procedure is imperative to determine whether the MR findings represent expected postoperative change versus complications.

- Despite clinical and imaging findings consistent with aseptic mechanical loosening following THA, greater than 50% of prosthesis, especially those with severe osteolysis, may demonstrate evidence of infection on sonification cultures

---

REFERENCES

1. Kassarjian A. Hip hype: FAI Syndrome, Amara's Law, and the Hype cycle. Semin Musculoskelet Radiol 2019;23(3):252–6.

2. Blankenbaker DG, De Smet AA, Keene JS. MR arthrographic appearance of the postoperative acetabular labrum in patients with suspected recurrent labral tears. AJR Am J Roentgenol 2011;197(6): W1118–22.

3. Foreman SC, Zhang AL, Neumann J, et al. Postoperative MRI findings and associated pain changes after arthroscopic surgery for femoroacetabular impingement. AJR Am J Roentgenol 2020;214(1):177–84.

4. Meier MK, Lerch TD, Steppacher SD, et al. High prevalence of hip lesions secondary to arthroscopic over- or undercorrection of femoroacetabular impingement in patients with postoperative pain. Eur

Radiol 2021. https://doi.org/10.1007/s00330-021-08398-4.

5. Kaya M, Hirose T, Yamashita T. Bridging suture repair for acetabular chondral carpet delamination. Arthrosc Tech 2015;4(4):e345–8.

6. Tzaveas AP, Villar RN. Arthroscopic repair of acetabular chondral delamination with fibrin adhesive. Hip Int 2010;20(1):115–9.

7. Bretschneider H, Trattnig S, Landgraeber S, et al. Arthroscopic matrix-associated, injectable autologous chondrocyte transplantation of the hip: significant improvement in patient-related outcome and good transplant quality in MRI assessment. Knee Surg Sports Traumatol Arthrosc 2020;28(4): 1317–24.

8. Kim CO, Dietrich TJ, Zingg PO, et al. Arthroscopic hip surgery: frequency of postoperative MR arthrographic findings in asymptomatic and symptomatic patients. Radiology 2017;283(3):779–88.

9. Bencardino JT, Kassarjian A, Vieira RL, et al. Synovial plicae of the hip: evaluation using MR arthrography in patients with hip pain. Skeletal Radiol 2011; 40(4):415–21.

10. Zheng L, Hwang JM, Hwang DS, et al. Incidence and location of heterotopic ossification following hip arthroscopy. BMC Musculoskelet Disord 2020; 21(1):132.

11. Miller TT. Imaging of hip arthroplasty. Eur J Radiol 2012;81(12):3802–12.

12. Amstutz HC, Le Duff MJ, Johnson AJ. Socket position determines hip resurfacing 10-year survivorship. Clin Orthop Relat Res 2012;470:3127–33.

13. Isern-Kebschull J, Tomas X, García-Díez AI, et al. Value of multidetector computed tomography for the differentiation of delayed aseptic and septic complications after total hip arthroplasty. Skeletal Radiol 2020;49(6):893–902.

14. Sierra JM, García S, Martínez-Pastor JC, et al. Relationship between the degree of osteolysis and cultures obtained by sonication of the prostheses in patients with aseptic loosening of a hip or knee arthroplasty. Arch Orthop Trauma Surg 2011;131(10): 1357–61.

15. Tomas X, Bori G, Garcia S, et al. Accuracy of CT-guided joint aspiration in patients with suspected infection status post-total hip arthroplasty. Skeletal Radiol 2011;40(1):57–64.

16. Pandit H, Glyn-Jones S, McLardy-Smith P, et al. Pseudotumours associated with metal-on-metal hip resurfacings. J Bone Joint Surg Br 2008;90:847–51.

17. Nawabi DH, Gold S, Lyman S, et al. MRI predicts ALVAL and tissue damage in metal-on-metal hip arthroplasty. Clin Orthop Relat Res 2014;472(2): 471–81.

18. Amstutz HC, Le Duff MJ, Campbell PA, et al. Complications after metal-on-metal hip resurfacing arthroplasty. Orthop Clin North Am 2011;42:207–30, viii.

19. Langton DJ, Joyce TJ, Jameson SS, et al. Adverse re- action to metal debris following hip resurfacing: the influence of component type, orien- tation and volumetric wear. J Bone Joint Surg Br 2011;93:164–71.

20. Willert HG, Buchhorn GH, Fayyazi A, et al. Metal-on-metal bearings and hyper- sensitivity in patients with artificial hip joints: a clinical and histomorphological study. J Bone Joint Surg Am 2005;87:28–36.

21. Ollivere B, Darrah C, Barker T, et al. Early clinical failure of the Birmingham metal-on-metal hip resurfacing is associated with metallosis and soft-tissue necrosis. J Bone Joint Surg Br 2009;91:1025–30.

22. Cipriano CA, Issack PS, Beksac B, et al. Metallosis after metal-on-polyethylene total hip arthroplasty. Am J Orthop 2008;37(2):E18–25.

23. Shulman RM, Zywiel MG, Gandhi R, et al. Trunnionosis: the latest culprit in adverse reactions to metal debris following hip arthroplasty. Skeletal Radiol 2015;44(3):433–40.

24. Grammatopolous G, Pandit H, Kwon YM, et al. Hip resurfacings revised for inflammatory pseudotumour have a poor outcome. J Bone Joint Surg (Br) 2009; 91(8):1019–24.

25. Cooper HJ, Della Valle CJ, Berger RA, et al. Corrosion at the head-neck taper as a cause for adverse local tissue reactions after total hip arthroplasty. J Bone Joint Surg Am 2012;94(18):1655–61.

26. Bisseling P, Tan T, Lu Z, et al. The absence of a metal-on-metal bearing does not preclude the formation of a destruc- tive pseudotumor in the hip-a case report. Acta Orthop 2013;84(4):437–41.

27. Koper MC, Mathijssen NMC, van Ravenswaay Claasen HH, et al. Pseudotumor after bilateral ceramic- on-metal total hip arthroplasty: a case report. J Bone Joint Surg 2014;4(1):1–6.

28. Schmalzried TP. Metal-metal bearing surfaces in hip arthroplasty. Orthopedics 2009;32. https://doi.org/10.3928/01477447-20090728-06.

29. Gill IP, Webb J, Sloan K, et al. Corrosion at the neck-stem junction as a cause of metal ion release and pseudotumour formation. J Bone Joint Surg (Br) 2012;94(7):895–900.

30. Gil-Albarova J, Laclériga A, Barrios C, et al. Lymphocyte response to polymethylmethacrylate in loose total hip prostheses. J Bone Joint Surg Br 1992;74(6):825–30.

31. Potnis PA, Dutta DK, Wood SC. Toll-like receptor 4 signaling path- way mediates proinflammatory immune response to cobalt-alloy particles. Cell Immunol 2013;282(1):53–65.

32. Jacobs JJ, Campbell PA, T Konttinen Y. How has the biologic reaction to wear particles changed with newer bearing surfaces? J Am Acad Orthop Surg 2008;16(Suppl 1):549–55.

33. Wassef AJ, Schmalzried TP. Femoral taperosis: an accident waiting to happen? Bone Joint J 2013;95-B(11 Suppl A):3–6.

34. Mao X, Wong AA, Crawford RW. Cobalt toxicity-an emerging clinical problem in patients with metal-on-metal hip prostheses? Med J Aust 2011; 194(12):649–51.

35. Tower SS. Arthroprosthetic cobaltism associated with metal on metal hip implants. BMJ 2012;344: e430.

36. Zywiel MG, Brandt JM, Overgaard CB, et al. Fatal cardiomyopathy after revision total hip replacement for fracture of a ceramic liner. Bone Joint J 2013; 95-B(1).

37. Hauptfleisch J, Pandit H, Grammatopoulos G, et al. A MRI classification of periprosthetic soft tissue masses (pseudotumours) associated with metal-on-metal resurfacing hip arthroplasty. Skelet Radiol 2012;41(2):149–55.

38. Anderson H, Toms AP, Cahir JG, et al. Grading the se- verity of soft tissue changes associated with metal-on-metal hip replacements: reliability of an MR grading system. Skeletal Radiol 2011;40(3): 303–7.

39. Abdul N, Fountain J. Stockley I infection versus ALVAL: acute presentation with abdominal pain. BMJ Case Rep 2013;2013. bcr2013009976.

40. Cyteval C, Hamm V, Sarrabere MP, et al. Painful infection at the site of hip prosthesis: CT imaging. Radiology 2002;224(2):477–83.

41. Isern-Kebschull J, Tomas X, García-Díez AI, et al. Accuracy of computed tomography-guided joint aspiration and computed tomography findings for prediction of infected hip prosthesis. J Arthroplasty 2019;34(8):1776–82.

42. Sdao S, Orlandi D, Aliprandi A, et al. The role of ultrasonography intheassessment of peri-prosthetic hip complications. J Ultrasound 2014;18(3): 245–50.

43. Galley J, Sutter R, Stern C, et al. Diagnosis of periprosthetic hip joint infection using MRI with metal artifact reduction at 1.5 T. Radiology 2020;296(1): 98–108.

44. Albano D, Messina C, Zagra L, et al. Failed total hip arthroplasty: diagnostic performance of conventional MRI features and locoregional lymphadenopathy to identify infected implants. J Magn Reson Imaging 2021;53(1):201–10.

45. Hessmann MH, Hübschle L, Tannast M, et al. Irritation der Iliopsoassehne nach totalendoprothetischem Hüftgelenkersatz [Irritation of the iliopsoas tendon after total hip arthroplasty]. Orthopade 2007;36(8):746–51. German.

46. Bisseling P, de Wit BW, Hol AM, et al. Similar incidence of periprosthetic fluid collections after ceramic-on-polyethylene total hip arthroplasties and metal-on-metal resurfacing arthroplasties: results of a screening metal artefact reduction sequence-MRI study. Bone Joint J 2015;97-B(9): 1175–82.

47. Fritz J, Lurie B, Miller TT, et al. MR imaging of hip arthroplasty implants. Radiographics 2014;34(4): E106–32.

48. Plodkowski AJ, Hayter CL, Miller TT, et al. Lamellated hyperintense synovitis: potential MR imaging sign of an infected knee ar- throplasty. Radiology 2013;266(1):256–60.

49. Chang EY, McAnally JL, Van Horne JR, et al. Metal-on-metal total hip arthroplasty: do symptoms correlate with MR imaging findings? Radiology 2012; 265(3):848–57.

50. Pfirrmann CW, Notzli HP, Dora C, et al. Abductor tendons and muscles assessed at MR imaging after total hip arthroplasty in asymptomatic and symptomatic patients. Radiology 2005;235(3): 969–76. https://doi.org/10.1148/radiol.2353040403. Available at.

51. Hoffmann A, Pfirrmann CW. The hip abductors at MR imaging. Eur J Radiol 2012;81(12):3755–62. https:// doi.org/10.1016/j.ejrad.2010.03.002. Available at.

52. Ibrahim M, Hedlundh U, Sernert N, et al. Histological and ultrastructural degenerative findings in the gluteus medius tendon after hip arthroplasty. J Orthop Surg Res 2021;16:339. https://doi.org/10. 1186/s13018-021-02434-1. Available at.

53. Pai VS. A modified direct lateral approach in total hip arthroplasty. J Orthop Surg (Hong Kong) 2002;10: 35–9.

54. Masonis JL, Bourne RB. Surgical approach, abductor function, and total hip arthroplasty dislocation. Clin Orthop Relat Res 2002;405:46–53.

55. Kwon MS, Kuskowski M, Mulhall KJ, et al. Does surgical approach affect total hip arthroplasty dislocation rates? Clin Orthop Relat Res 2006;447:34–8.

56. Enocson A, Hedbeck CJ, Tidermark J, et al. Dislocation of total hip replacement in patients with fractures of the femoral neck. Acta Orthop 2009;80(2):184–9.

57. Wendt RE 3rd, Wilcott MR 3rd, Nitz W, et al. MR imaging of susceptibility-induced magnetic field inhomogene- ities. Radiology 1988;168:837–41.

58. Lachiewicz PF, Kauk JR. Anterior iliopsoas impingement and tendinitis after total hip arthroplasty. J Am Acad Orthop Surg 2009;17:337–44.

59. Piggott RP, Doody O, Quinlan JF. Iliopsoas tendon rupture: a new differential for atraumatic groin pain post-total hip arthroplasty. BMJ Case Rep 2015; 2015. bcr2014208518.

60. Maheshwari AV, Malhotra R, Kumar D, et al. Rupture of the ilio-psoas tendon after a total hip arthroplasty: an unusual cause of radio-lucency of the lesser trochanter simulating a malignancy. J Orthop Surg Res 2010;5:6.

61. Vanrusselt J, Vansevenant M, Vanderschueren G, et al. Postoperative radiograph of the hip arthroplasty: what the radiologist should know. Insights Imaging 2015;6:591–600. https://doi.org/10.1007/ s13244-015-0438-5. Available at.

62. Roth TD, Maertz NA, Parr JA, et al. CT of the hip prosthesis: appearance of components, fixation, and complications. Radiographics 2012;32(4): 1089–107.

63. Gill SK, Smith J, Fox R, et al. Investigation of occult hip fractures: the use of CT and MRI. ScientificWorldJournal 2013;2013:830319.

64. Hargunani R, Madani H, Khoo M, et al. Imaging of the painful hip arthroplasty. Can Assoc Radiol J 2016;67(4):345–55.

65. Cooper HJ, Ranawat AS, Potter HG, et al. Early reactive synovitis and osteolysis after total hip arthroplasty. Clin Orthop Relat Res 2010;468(12):3278–85.

66. Walde TA, Weiland DE, Leung SB, et al. Comparison of CT, MRI, and radiographs in assessing pelvic osteolysis: a cadaveric study. Clin Orthop Relat Res 2005;437:138–44.

67. Nachtrab O, Cassar-Pullicino VN, Lalam R, et al. Role of MRI in hip fractures, including stress fractures, occult fractures, avulsion fractures. Eur J Radiol 2012;81(12):3813–23.

Postoperative MR Imaging of the Pubic Symphysis and Athletic Pubalgia

Riti M. Kanesa-thasan, MD[a], Adam C. Zoga, MD, MBA[b],*,
William C. Meyers, MD, MBA[c], Johannes B. Roedl, MD, PhD[d]

KEYWORDS

• Athletic pubalgia • Postoperative findings • MR imaging • Pelvic floor repair

KEY POINTS

- MR imaging findings in patients with prior surgery for athletic pubalgia do not mimic those in the nonoperative patient; thus it is important for radiologists to differentiate healing and expected findings from new and unexpected lesions.
- Preoperative secondary clefts are typically present postoperatively; however, a new contralateral secondary cleft after ipsilateral repair should raise suspicion for new injury.
- Edema at the adductor longus myotendinous junction is a common MR imaging finding after core muscle surgery and can be considered an expected postoperative finding.
- Evaluation for internal hip derangement should be included in the evaluation of groin pain after surgery and may be further evaluated with MR arthrography, if indicated.

INTRODUCTION

Athletic pubalgia, also referenced in the literature as "core muscle injury," "inguinal disruption," "sports hernia," or "sportman's hernia," refers to groin-pain centered about and near the pubic symphysis exacerbated by activity and specific ranges of motion. Both MR imaging and surgical lesions generally involve the rectus abdominis muscle, the adductor longus origin, the pubic tubercle, and often the pubic symphysis itself. Physical examination typically demonstrates pain with palpation of the inguinal region just above the inguinal ligament and near the pubic tubercle, or superficial inguinal ring without a true hernia, with or without decreased internal and external rotation of the hip. Pain at the pubic tubercle or crest is often exacerbated by resisted sit up.[1] Diagnostic criteria established by the 2014 British Hernia Society meeting are based on the presence of 3 of the following: pinpoint tenderness over the pubic tubercle at the conjoint tendon insertion, palpable tenderness over the deep inguinal ring, pain and/or dilation of the external ring without obvious hernia, pain at the adductor longus tendon origin, or dull, diffuse groin pain often radiating to the perineum and inner thigh or across the midline.[1,2] (The "conjoint tendon" refers to the aponeurosis of the lower rectus abdominis and the adductor origin spanning the anteroinferior aspect of the pubic bone just lateral to midline.) The 2015 Doha Agreement meeting divided groin pain into 3 categories: "defined clinical entities for groin pain (adductor-related, iliopsoas-related, inguinal-related, or pubic-related), hip-related groin pain, or other causes of groin pain in athletes."[3]

DISCUSSION

Normal Anatomy and Preoperative Findings

The musculoskeletal core can be loosely interpreted to include all muscle and tendon

[a] Department of Radiology, Division of Musculoskeletal Imaging, University of Pennsylvania, 3737 Market Street, Mailbox #4, Philadelphia, PA 19072, USA; [b] Department of Radiology, Thomas Jefferson University Hospitals, 132 South 10th Street, Suite 1096, Philadelphia, PA 19107, USA; [c] Vincera Institute, Sidney Kimmel Medical Collegs at Jefferson, 1200 Constitution Avenue #110, Philadelphia, PA 19112, USA; [d] Department of Radiology, Thomas Jefferson University Hospitals, 132 South 10th Street, Philadelphia, PA 19107, USA
* Corresponding author.
E-mail address: adam.zoga@jefferson.edu

Magn Reson Imaging Clin N Am 30 (2022) 689–702
https://doi.org/10.1016/j.mric.2022.04.002
1064-9689/22/© 2022 Elsevier Inc. All rights reserved.

attachments on the pelvis, proximal femora, lumbar spine, and lower thoracic cage, but the clinical syndrome of athletic pubalgia, also termed "core muscle injury," almost always focuses on the pubic symphysis joint and its regional muscle, tendon, and ligamentous attachments. The normal pubic symphysis is a stable joint with a central fibrocartilaginous disc and articular cartilage stabilized by a group of ligaments, most notably the arcuate ligament extending bilaterally along the anteroinferior joint and lateral along a jagged ridge on the anteroinferior pubic bone, or the pubic tubercles. The lower rectus abdominis muscles from above and the common adductor origins from below blend with the arcuate ligament along its pubic tubercle attachment, forming a thick, broad, fibrocartilaginous plate (or aponeurosis) bilaterally that is considered the primary stabilizer of the musculoskeletal core and the location of most core muscle injuries leading to the clinical scenario of athletic pubalgia. The lateral margin of this fibrocartilaginous pubic plate forms the posteromedial reinforcement of the superficial inguinal ring. Deficiencies of the plate frequently lead to a patulous superficial ring and can subsequently generate a physical presentation confusing for inguinal hernia.[4–6]

The pubic plate (or rectus abdominis aponeurosis or conjoined pubic attachment) and its anatomic relationship with the superficial ring is most often the focus of operative intervention for athletic pubalgia lesions. Various patterns of pubic plate injury are documented in imaging literature. Some lesions involve an elongated detachment of the plate from the pubic bone, centered at the pubic tubercle, often with accompanying detachment of the pubic periosteum. Other lesions show a clear transverse breech of the plate, which can occur at its medial margin anterior to the symphysis or more laterally anterior to the pubic tubercle. More severe lesions include complete rupture of the pubic plate with avulsion of the combined adductor origin and retraction of the adductor tendons into the proximal thigh, with or without abruption and retraction of the rectus abdominis muscle cephalad. Chronic athletic pubalgia lesions often show deficiency of the pubic plate on imaging, with asymmetric atrophy and a subsequent patulous superficial inguinal ring.

Instability of the pubic symphysis itself can also be a source of pain in athletic pubalgia and core muscle injury; this can manifest on imaging with reciprocal or asymmetric subchondral bone marrow edema and/or osseous productive change, a scenario termed "osteitis pubis." This instability is often considered a result of pubic plate deficiency or detachment but can also occur after traumatic ligamentous injury from high-velocity trauma or pregnancy and childbirth. Imaging findings of superior and secondary clefts described in athletic pubalgia can be considered indicators of pubic symphysis instability.[7] These clefts were described as lateral or inferolateral extensions of contrast with pubic symphysis injection correlating with the situs of symptoms. However, they can often be seen on fluid-sensitive MR imaging sequences and are important imaging observations in the preoperative athletic pubalgia patient. MR imaging protocols and imaging findings in athletic pubalgia and core muscle injury have been well described, including osteitis pubis, superior and secondary clefts, disruption or deficiencies of the pubic plate, and adductor tendon or muscle strains.[8–10]

Imaging Technique/Protocols

MR imaging with a dedicated athletic pubalgia protocol has been established as the imaging standard in the workup of athletic pubalgia or core muscle injury.[4,11] When imaging is warranted after percutaneous or surgical intervention, the same MR imaging protocol can be useful to assess for recurrent injury or new core muscle lesions that may prolong or prohibit full recovery. A dedicated noncontract athletic pubalgia MR imaging protocol optimizes evaluation of the pubic symphysis and musculoskeletal core muscle attachments compared with a standard pelvis protocol. The noncontrast athletic pubalgia protocol is acquired in 4 anatomic planes using a phased array torso receiver coil placed anteriorly on the supine patient, centered on the pubic symphysis. Large field-of-view axial (T2-weighted fat-suppressed fast spin echo [FSE] sequence) and coronal (T1-weighted FSE sequence and short inversion time inversion recovery sequence) imaging is obtained from the level of the umbilicus to the proximal third of the thighs, extending from skin to skin in the anteroposterior and transverse planes.[12] Small field-of-view sagittal (proton density–weighted fat-suppressed FSE sequence) and axial oblique (proton density–weighted fat-suppressed FSE sequence and proton density FSE nonfat-suppressed sequence) imaging is then acquired, with oblique planes angled along the arcuate line of the pelvis or the anterior cortex of the iliac bone from a sagittal localizer.[12] These smaller field-of-view sagittal and axial oblique acquisitions optimize evaluation of the anatomy at the aponeuroses of the rectus abdominis and adductor origins at the pubic tubercle.[12] In the postoperative setting, imaging at 3 T or 1.5 T with strong gradient strength and a high-quality

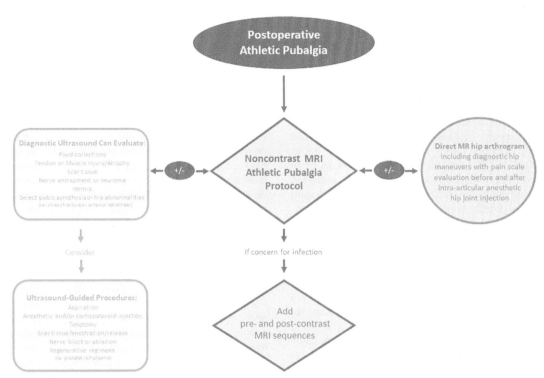

Fig. 1. Recommended imaging algorithm for patients with new, persistent, or recurrent athletic pubalgia symptoms after percutaneous or surgical intervention.

receiver coil (16 channels or higher) is optimal, as strong signal and contrast can help distinguish healing granulation tissue from recurrent/persistent fluid gaps between structures or true superior and secondary clefts from expected postoperative findings.[13]

In our experience, administration of intravenous gadolinium-based contrast agents adds little to the assessment of mechanical sources of postoperative athletic pubalgia, whereas deviation from a preoperative protocol may limit direct comparison to preoperative imaging.[13] In addition, enhancing granulation tissue in the operative bed can be very difficult to distinguish from early perioperative soft tissue infection, with note that the standard noncontrast protocol should still demonstrate potential infectious complications including osteomyelitis and abscess. Additional imaging after administration of intravenous contrast can always be added later when warranted in difficult scenarios for the imager.[13] For these reasons, the standard postoperative protocol is performed without contrast and with an identical protocol to the standard preoperative athletic pubalgia/core muscle injury MR imagings.

A detailed clinical and therapeutic history is essential for the imager to optimally interpret the postoperative MR imaging. We strongly advocate for the use of a patient questionnaire specific to core muscle injury, as well as review of clinical presentation and therapeutic history. Our recommended questionnaire includes a diagram for patients to mark sites of symptoms; pain scale region to list activities related to symptoms; and areas for chronology of symptoms, rehab programs, and interventions.

Adjunct imaging studies and procedures can be performed for additional evaluation, diagnosis, and/or treatment (**Fig. 1**). For example, MR arthrography of the hip joint is valuable in the evaluation for concurrent internal hip derangement. Ultrasound can evaluate for scar tissue, nerve entrapment/neuroma, or hernia. Ultrasound-guided diagnostic and/or therapeutic procedures frequently add value, noting that the chosen imaging modality may vary based on specific clinical scenarios and physician preference.

Operative Techniques

Both surgical and percutaneous treatments are frequently performed for athletic pubalgia, either in the acute setting for severe lesions or with more chronic lesions refractory to treatment with rehabilitation.[1] Many operative techniques have been described with varying levels of impact on outcomes. Both open and laparoscopic procedures are common, with or without mesh placement, adductor tenotomy/release, or neurectomy. To date, some of the strongest reported outcomes have been with open core muscle injury repair.[1,8,14–17]

Open surgical repair for inguinal-related groin pain has been performed using varying techniques that involve different layers of the abdominal wall, including, but not limited to, the modified Bassini, Muschaweck, Shouldice, Meyers anterior pelvic floor, Gilmore, and Lichtenstein repair techniques.[14,18,19] Poor and colleagues use an open pelvic floor approach targeted toward restoring normal anatomy and balance between opposing muscle groups across the pubic bone, with reinforcement of the aponeurotic pubic plate attachment to the pubic tubercle just lateral to the midline symphysis.[20] Sheen and colleagues describe an open suture repair targeted toward strengthening the posterior inguinal wall, involving continuous suture from the medial toward the deep inguinal ring to create a free fascial lip, reversal of the suture at the pubic bone (including the free lip brought to the inguinal ligament), lateralization of the rectus abdominis muscle with sutures, preservation of the cremaster muscle if possible, and external fascia and subcuticular suture closure.[21] Choi and colleagues describe an open suture repair focused on both repairing the rectus abdominus and stabilizing the conjoined tendon/rectus abdominus interface while reinforcing the inguinal canal's posterior wall.[22] Their technique involves roughening the pubic tubercle with electrocautery to create an inflammatory surface, with or without adductor longus tendon release/lengthening or injection with steroid or platelet-rich plasma (PRP).[22] Some repairs, including the Lichtenstein procedure, include mesh reinforcement.[18,19,22] Dehydrated placental allograft placement at the site of adductor tenotomy has also been described as a means to decrease scar formation.[23] Inguinal neurectomy or nerve division is sometimes performed with open operative repair, noting that nerve decompression can also be performed through more minimally invasive methods such as radiofrequency denervation or local injection.[1,19,24] Hip arthroscopy may also be combined with core muscle repair to address associated hip pathology, such as femoroacetabular or psoas impingement.[25]

Laparoscopic techniques are also frequently used, including transabdominal preperitoneal repair (TAPP) and total extraperitoneal repair, both of which predominantly use mesh placement.[18,21,24,26] Adductor tenotomy/release has been performed in isolation or in conjunction with mesh repair. Meshes can have various weights and are typically placed behind the injured groin area, with lightweight meshes reportedly demonstrating various advantages.[24] Meshes can be made from various synthetic material (such as polypropylene or polyester).[21,24] The use of bioactive prosthetic materials (such as mesh made from porcine intestine) has been reported, in addition to placement of hybrid mesh material consisting of a mix of polypropylene and bioactive prosthetic materials.[27,28] Mesh placement can vary from either no fixation to fixation of the mesh with either tacks, glue, or staples.[24] Variations of these techniques have also been reported, such as the "Manchester Groin Repair," a modification of the laparoscopic totally extraperitoneal repair with increased dissection within the pre-peritoneal plane, placement of a larger mesh, and fixation of the mesh with fibrin sealant.[29,30]

Percutaneous Interventions

Percutaneous interventions have also shown some success in the treatment of athletic pubalgia and core muscle injury. Techniques including trigger point injections, targeted steroid injections, dry needle tenotomy, and regenerative regimens (such as PRP or stem cells) have shown promise with ultrasound, fluoroscopic, or computed tomography guidance (**Fig. 2**). In the posttreatment setting, it is vital for the imager to understand what interventions were performed and in what proximity to the MR imaging.[31,32]

Postoperative Imaging Findings

Multiple factors can cause groin pain after surgical treatment of athletic pubalgia, including new injury, recurrent or residual symptoms from an incompletely effective repair, concomitant core muscle injuries, referred sources of pain from the hip or spine, complications of intervention, or unrelated traumatic insults (such as pregnancy and childbirth).[13] Although strict data were not available, Meyers and colleagues reported that 4.6% of 5218 surgical patients had previously undergone unsuccessful prior traditional hernia repair.[33] Piozzi and colleagues reported an inguinal disruption recurrence rate of 2.5% on 13-year follow-up after laparoscopic TAPP repair.[26] Clinically, Meyers and colleagues reported that repeat surgery after prior repair was most frequently performed for contralateral symptoms after unilateral surgery, with less than 1% incidence of repeat injuries occurring ipsilateral to site of prior repair or with history of bilateral repair.[13,33] MR imaging is not a standard, scheduled examination after surgery for athletic pubalgia. Many patients respond well to surgery or percutaneous intervention and subsequently no further imaging is indicated. MR

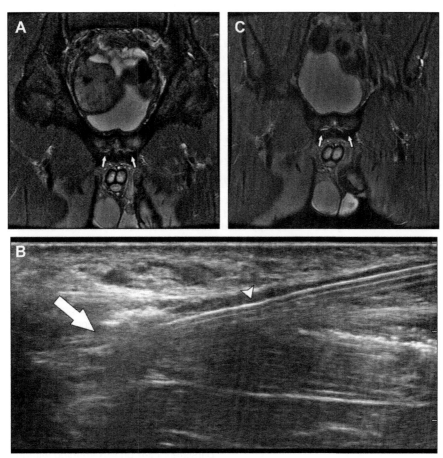

Fig. 2. Football player with a bilateral core muscle injury: axial oblique proton density fat-suppressed MR image showing bone marrow edema spanning the pubic tubercles and disruption of the pubic plates (*arrows*) (*A*), a longitudinal image from ultrasound-guided dry needle tenotomy therapy with needle (*arrowhead*) at the site of injury (*arrow*) (*B*), and a similar axial oblique MR image 8 months after tenotomy showing improvement of the bone marrow edema and granulation tissue formation at the site of injury (*arrows*) (*C*).

imaging is indicated after intervention for athletic pubalgia in the following scenarios:

- When there is an unexpected recurrence of symptoms
- When there is a significant new injury either at the site of treatment or at a new location
- When there is failure to respond or return to the expected level of activity
- When there is clinical concern for an adverse outcome such as infection or repair failure

Given the complex anatomy and myriad of potential interventions, MR imaging interpretation in the setting of postoperative athletic pubalgia can be daunting. Postoperative MR imaging findings are not always predictive of clinical outcomes, and the imager's role is to distinguish expected findings from those that are likely to be clinically significant.[34] For example, Knapik and colleagues found that 53% of National Football League

players who underwent MR imaging after prior surgical repair for athletic pubalgia demonstrated positive imaging findings, without significant difference in performance compared with those without surgery.[34,35] Athletes with a history of surgical repair within 1 year of imaging showed higher odds of having positive imaging findings reported.[35] Granulation tissue at sites of repair must be differentiated from new or recurrent tears, and some athletic pubalgia MR imaging findings will never return to normal on postoperative imaging studies. Distinguishing expected postoperative MR imaging findings and healing lesions from new injuries and sources of persistent or recurrent pain is the primary role of MR imaging in the postintervention setting and will add value to treatment planning for the managing clinical team.[13]

Access to preoperative imaging, surgical history, and detailed knowledge of injury history and current clinical presentation is essential when

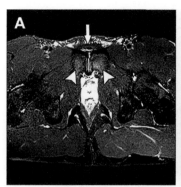 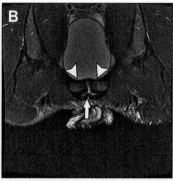 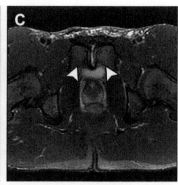

Fig. 3. Initial axial T2-weighted fast-spin echo (FSE) fat-suppressed image (*A*) from an NFL running back with groin pain demonstrates osteitis pubis (*arrowheads*) and bilateral secondary clefts (*arrow*). Axial oblique proton density (*B*) and axial T2 (*C*)-weighted FSE fat-suppressed sequences obtained 1 year after bilateral core muscle repair demonstrate resolution of bone marrow edema (*arrowheads*) and asymptomatic residual secondary clefts not meeting fluid signal intensity, typical for expected granulation tissue at the site of prior injury.

interpreting MR imaging for the postoperative athletic pubalgia patient. Diligent use of a musculoskeletal patient history questionnaire directed to athletic pubalgia and core muscle injury at the time of imaging is an essential step in the operation, as blind interpretation of postoperative MR imaging is very likely to lead to misidentification of lesions.[12] We will detail our experience in interpreting MR imaging examinations in the setting of persistent or recurrent groin pain or delayed return to expected activity after intervention for athletic pubalgia and core muscle injury.

Osteitis pubis

Osteitis pubis typically improves in a majority (75%) of postoperative MR imagings after surgical repair, likely reflecting better stabilization of the pubic symphysis as a joint.[13,36] In particular, bone marrow edema about the pubic symphysis should decrease within 6 weeks of surgery, although osseous productive change is likely to be a permanent finding on imaging. Interval worsening of bone marrow edema across the pubic symphysis on postoperative imaging should thus be noted, as findings could correlate with progressive instability, increased stress across the joint, overaggressive rehabilitation, premature return to play, or possibly repair failure.[13] Eventually, after months or years, bone marrow edema at the pubic symphysis can completely resolve after successful intervention for athletic pubalgia (**Fig. 3**), but in athletes, some degree of subchondral bone marrow edema at the pubic symphysis generally persists throughout the playing career.

Secondary and superior clefts

T2-weighted hyperintense clefts at the site of prior injury are an expected postoperative MR imaging finding. Secondary clefts on postoperative MR

imaging have been reported in approximately 68% of patients, highlighting the importance of distinguishing healing and granulation tissue from true fluid clefts concerning new injury.[13] Secondary clefts should slowly decrease in size and T2 hyperintensity over time, and a persistent secondary cleft at MR imaging but relative decreased T2 hyperintensity when compared with the preoperative MR imaging can be considered a sign of healing (**Fig. 4**). In fact, in the immediate postoperative period (0–6 weeks), clefts at the site of initial injury often meet fluid signal, despite an intact repair. A persistent cleft on MR imaging without significant distraction of soft tissue structures after core muscle surgery should NOT be considered an indicator of repair failure.

New contralateral secondary or superior clefts, however, can be an indicator of new injury (**Fig. 5**).[13] Meyers and colleagues reported that additional surgery was most frequently performed for contralateral symptoms in patients with ipsilateral repair, and a new contralateral secondary cleft was a common finding at MR imaging (**Fig. 6**). Repeat ipsilateral injury/surgery is relatively rare (although possible), despite the persistence of ipsilateral secondary cleft on MR imaging.[33] From our experience, new contralateral secondary clefts often extend lateral to the external margin of the pubic plate and the superficial inguinal ring. In contrast, preoperative midline defects and secondary clefts ipsilateral to the site of unilateral or bilateral surgical repair are expected MR imaging findings postoperatively (see **Fig. 3**). Rarely, a more extensive secondary cleft or enlarging fluid signal gap could suggest the ipsilateral propagation of soft tissue injury or recurrent/new tear, but this finding should be correlated with the clinical scenario of a significant new injury (see **Fig. 5**).[13]

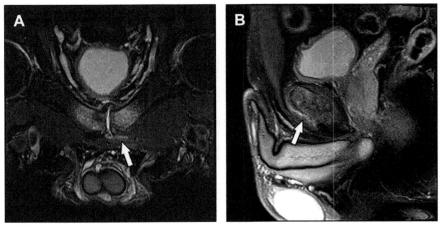

Fig. 4. Axial oblique (*A*) and sagittal (*B*) proton density–weighted FSE fat-suppressed images from an athletic pubalgia MR imaging protocol acquired 3 months after left-sided core muscle repair show an MR secondary cleft
not meeting fluid signal (*arrows*), typical for expected granulation tissue at the site of injury in the postoperative
healing phase.

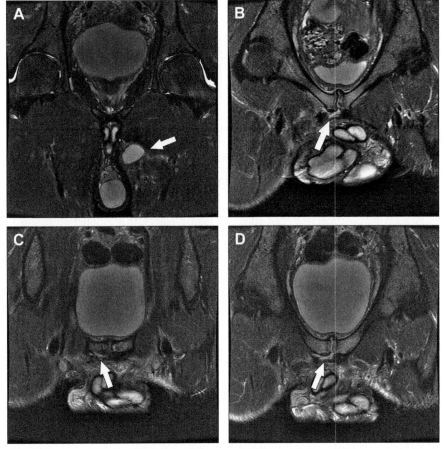

Fig. 5. Axial oblique proton density–weighted FSE fat-suppressed images from different postoperative patients.
Image A demonstrates a postoperative adductor hematoma (*arrow*). Image B obtained from a patient with new
right-sided injury/pain 15 months after left core muscle repair demonstrates corresponding abnormal new secondary cleft contralateral to the site of prior repair with associated osteitis pubis (*arrow*). Images C and D obtained from a patient with right-sided injury/pain 5 months after right core muscle repair demonstrates
reinjury with secondary cleft and associated osteitis pubis (*arrows*).

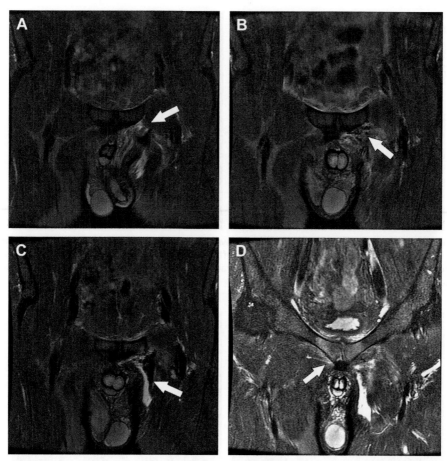

Fig. 6. Axial oblique proton density–weighted FSE fat-suppressed images from a professional baseball player obtained initially (*A*), 3 weeks postoperatively (*B*), 7 weeks postoperatively (*C*), and 12 postoperatively due to right-sided pain during rehab (*D*). Image A demonstrates left core muscle injury with retraction of the combined adductor group (*arrow*). Image B demonstrates expected postoperative granulation tissue and susceptibility artifact after left core muscle repair (*arrow*). Image C demonstrates new hematoma ipsilateral to the side of prior repair (*arrow*). Image D demonstrates new right-sided core muscle injury with associated worsening osteitis pubis (*arrow*). The player subsequently underwent a second surgery for right-sided core muscle repair.

Pubic plate

As the fibrocartilaginous pubic plate is the most common site for incipient athletic pubalgia lesions, the plate should show improvement when compared with preoperative imaging (**Fig. 7**). Elongated regions of detachment should show approximation to the pubic bone and T2 hyperintense granulation tissue, not meeting the signal of fluid (**Fig. 8**). Gaps between the plate and retracted adductor tendons should be decreased, and focal breeches in the plate should show intermediate signal that indicates involuting granulation tissue. Most surgical techniques do not involve the medial margin of the pubic plate. Thus a stable, persistent midline lesion can be considered an expected postoperative finding if the more lateral aspect of any plate lesion seems improved. Suture artifact at the lateral margin of the plate near the

superficial inguinal ring is an expected finding with many repairs. In the setting of prior percutaneous interventions, intermediate signal granulation tissue at sites of prior plate detachment or tear and greater approximation of the plate to the pubic tubercle when compared with preoperative MR imaging are reassuring findings.

Rectus abdominis

The postoperative appearance of the rectus abdominis is variable, particularly its morphology. There should be good tissue approximation between the lower rectus abdominis muscle and the pubic bone at the site of any fluid-filled gap on preoperative imaging. If suture was primary source of repair, although midline defects are difficult to evaluate by MR, an intact hypointense suture line extending from the lateral edge of the

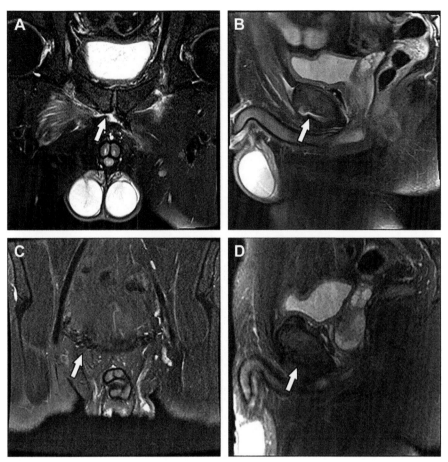

Fig. 7. Axial oblique (*A*) and sagittal (*B*) proton density–weighted FSE fat-suppressed images from an NFL lineman after a game show a confluent bilateral pubic plate disruption (*arrows*) extending from the right lateral plate into the left proximal adductor longus. Similar images (*C*, *D*) with an identical athletic pubalgia MR imaging protocol obtained 12 months later show bilateral core muscle repairs and resolution of the fluid signal and clefts (*arrows*) at the sites of injury, expected postoperative MR imaging findings.

lower rectus abdominis to its attachment at the external oblique aponeurosis is expected (**Fig. 9**). Edema in the lower rectus abdominis muscle can be expected through the initial postoperative period, and strains can occur during postoperative rehabilitation despite an intact repair. Preoperative morphologic atrophy of the rectus abdominis muscle will remain postoperatively. New atrophy, particularly at the lateral edge of the rectus abdominis, can be associated with ipsilateral pain despite an intact repair and should thus be reported, although the finding is nonspecific in the surgical literature. Note that intrinsic fatty atrophy could theoretically represent an expected postoperative finding after nerve division or neurectomy; however, there is no specific literature to support or refute this possibility or its clinical significance.

Adductor longus

Assessment of the postoperative adductor tendons at the pubic symphysis is inherently dependent on review of the degree of preoperative injury and understanding of the interventional/ operative technique. Many operative techniques involve debridement or release of the proximal adductors, and this must be taken into account. Adductors that were abnormal at preoperative MR imaging will not look normal postoperatively.

In the setting of prior avulsion of the common adductor stump, the conjoined adductor origin should be reapproximated to the pubic plate, without a visible stump or large fluid gap on MR imaging, but the imager should expect T2 hyperintense signal throughout the region, with decreasing hyperintensity throughout the postsurgical interval. Eventually, the adductor tendons will regain normal signal, but the adductor longus will always remain enlarged and fibrotic. Even with lower grade athletic pubalgia lesions, the proximal adductor longus biomechanical axis is generally shortened and tightened after repair, and low-

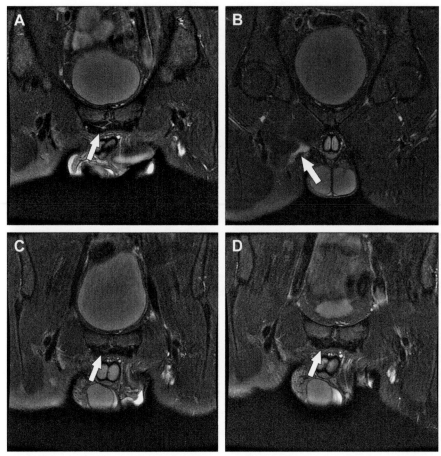

Fig. 8. Sequential axial oblique proton density–weighted FSE fat-suppressed images from an athletic pubalgia MR imaging protocol (*A*, *B*) show intrasubstance tearing of the right pubic plate (*A*) and partial avulsion of the right adductor longus (*B*). Like acquisitions from 7 months (*C*) and 18 months (*D*) after core muscle repair and subsequent percutaneous tenotomy show progressive healing of the pubic plate defect (*arrows*).

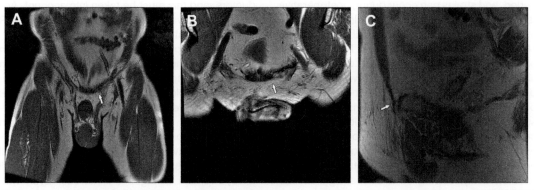

Fig. 9. A coronal large field-of-view T1-weighted FSE image (*A*), an axial oblique proton density–weighted FSE image (*B*), and a sagittal proton density FSE image (*C*) show a typical left-sided core muscle repair with reinforcement of the external oblique aponeurosis and the lateral edge of the pubic plate attachment to the pubic tubercle (*arrows*), expected MR imaging findings after core muscle repair.

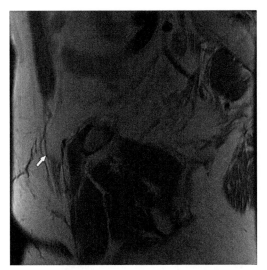

Fig. 10. A sagittal proton density–weighted nonfat-suppressed FSE image in a patient with recurrent pain after ipsilateral core muscle repair shows a fat containing indirect inguinal hernia (*arrow*), new after a core muscle repair.

grade myotendinous strains are an expected finding during the rehabilitation phase. Myotendinous edema with a grade 1 strain pattern can be considered an expected MR imaging finding after almost intervention for athletic pubalgia lesions; this should not be overinterpreted as a repair failure.[13]

Peritendinous edema, slightly hypointense relative to fluid can also reflect healing and granulation tissue, and care should be taken to distinguish this finding from true fluid gaps.[13] Occasionally, complete tendon release has been noted where the surgically transected tendon is expected and allowed to retract, and interpretation of expected healing versus recurrent injury is nearly impossible. Intrinsic fatty atrophy of the adductor longus muscles can also be considered an expected finding for several years after an adductor release or debridement. Even after percutaneous tenotomy, adductor tendons can be expected to show enlargement and regions of T2 hyperintensity with other regions of hypointensity on all MR imaging sequences, but there should be no complete disruption or fluid gaps.

New or persistent adductor pathology was also noted as the second most common reason for reoperation by Meyers and colleagues, with the lesions treated with adductor release, but a common source of pain was reported to be entrapment of adductor muscle fibers within a disrupted epimysium.[33] Myotendinous junction strains ipsilateral to the side of repair were the dominant finding in approximately 38% of postoperative MR imagings; however bilateral strains are also possible.[13,37] The strains are typically located at the proximal adductor longus myotendinous junction, approximately 8 to 12 cm distal to the common adductor tendon origin. Myotendinous strains can be graded based on presence of peritendinous edema (grade 1), partial tear (grade 2), or complete disruption (grade 3).

Other adductor tendons are often involved in athletic pubalgia lesions, and imagers should attempt to detail morphologic or signal abnormalities in the smaller adductor brevis, more posterior adductor magnus, and even the gracilis and obturator externus.

Hip flexors

Occasionally, psoas muscle release is performed as a part of athletic pubalgia repair techniques. Once released, the psoas muscle remains atrophied with loss of bulk and intrinsic fatty signal indefinitely. These findings at MR imaging should be reported, but are not unexpected. Iliopsoas tendons should remain intact, and fluid in the iliopsoas bursa is not an expected finding after psoas release. Rectus femoris tendons and muscles are generally not involved in surgical treatment of athletic pubalgia lesions, and any rectus femoris pathology should be reported.

Mesh repair

Evaluation for the presence and location of mesh is important on postoperative MR imaging. Because lesions located inferior to the lower edge of the mesh can be frequently encountered in patients with refractory pain after prior mesh repair, it is important to evaluate the caudal attachment of the rectus abdominis, origin of the adductor tendon, and rectus abdominis/adductor aponeurosis.[13,33] Borders of the mesh should also be evaluated for focal soft tissue edema; T1 hypointense signal, which can indicate scarring/fibrosis; lobular areas of hypointense fat, which can indicate fat necrosis; and/or nerve entrapment.[13] Scar tissue can be a source of neuralgia in the region and may be treated percutaneously if indicated. Fatty atrophy, specifically along the caudal and lateral aspect of the rectus abdominus attachment, can also occur after traditional herniorrhaphy and correlate with localized pain.[13] Although uncommon, true hernias through or around the mesh are possible.[13] In our experience, assessment of mesh is best achieved with T1-weighted nonfat-suppressed imaging of the lower abdomen in sagittal and coronal planes.

Differential considerations

Other pathologies may cause groin pain in the postoperative setting and should be included in the

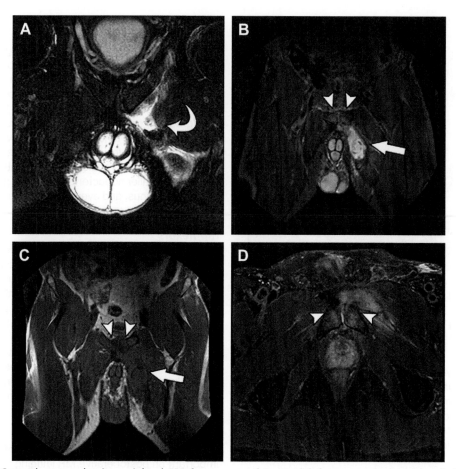

Fig. 11. Coronal proton density–weighted FSE fat-suppressed image (*A*) from a professional baseball pitcher shows a large core muscle injury on the left with retraction of the combined adductor group (*curved arrow*). Large field-of-view STIR (*B*) and T1-weighted FSE (*C*) images 3 weeks postrepair show a complex, tense collection in the adductor bed with a pigtail catheter (*arrows*). Image B and an axial T2-weighted FSE fat-suppressed sequence from the same study (*D*) demonstrate a symphysial joint effusion and new T2 hyperintensity at the pubic symphysis [with associated T1 signal hypointensity on image (*C*)], indicating a postoperative septic pubic symphysis joint and osteomyelitis (*arrowheads*).

postoperative MR search pattern. These pathologies can include inguinal hernia (**Fig. 10**), hematoma (see **Fig. 5**), infection (**Fig. 11**), hip pathology, nerve compression, lumbar disc disease, strains of the hip flexors, bursitis, osseous stress injury/fracture, soft tissue tumors, or other pelvic floor, urogenital, or intraabdominal findings.[1,13]

Postoperative collection, such as seroma or hematoma, can be a source of pain in the more immediate postoperative setting (see **Fig. 5**). Rarely, the collection can extend into the inguinal canal and be associated with severe pain. Meyers and colleagues reported that 0.3% of patients had hematomas requiring reoperation. In our experience, most symptomatic hematomas can be managed with percutaneous decompression, with or without continued catheter decompression, depending on size and discomfort level. Any aspirated fluid should

be sampled for laboratory analysis. Infection is a rare complication but can present with enlarging, complex collections, and even occasionally MR imaging findings typical for osteomyelitis at the pubic symphysis (see **Fig. 11**). Remember, T2 hyperintense signal at the symphysis should DECREASE after surgery, and increased T2 hyperintensity of bone with T1-weighted bone marrow replacement should be reported as concerning for osteomyelitis. Clinically, Meyers and colleagues reported a wound infection rate of 0.4%, noting that all wound infections in the cohort were superficial in location, but if clinical and/or imaging findings raise concern for postoperative infection, additional MR imaging sequences after administration of intravenous contrast can be useful.

Internal derangements of the hip, such as femoroacetabular impingement, articular chondrosis, or acetabular labrum tear, are common sources of groin pain that can mimic athletic pubalgia lesions. Although hip lesions in the prearthritic patient warrant dedicated imaging of the hip, pathology can often be identified with an athletic pubalgia MR imaging protocol; these should be reported, both on preoperative and postoperative MR examinations, and dedicated hip imaging can be recommended as appropriate. Identifying the true cause of groin pain in the presence of both hip and pubic symphysis pathology can be difficult on physical examination. MR arthrography of the hip joint, including evaluation of hip pain with hip maneuvers before and after intraarticular anesthetic instillation, is often a valuable imaging examination in this setting.

SUMMARY

MR imaging of the postoperative patient with recurrent or persistent athletic pubalgia can be daunting for the imager but can also be valuable to the clinical management team in the setting of unexpected pain or delay in recovery. Imagers should make every effort to study the clinical and interventional history, and comparison with preoperative imaging is essential. MR imaging findings concerning for infection, new injury, contralateral injury without overcalling repair failure, and concomitant sources of symptoms (including hip pathology) should be reported when present.

CLINICS CARE POINTS

- In the recent perioperative setting, T2 hyperintense secondary clefts at the site of surgery are expected and should not be overinterpreted as recurrent injury or repair failure.
- Adductor tendons often show abnormal signal and morphology for years after surgery, and grade 1 myotendinous strains of the adductor longus can be an expected MR imaging finding during postoperative rehabilitation.
- Imagers should note the presence of mesh or suture material.
- In general, pubic plate structures should show anatomic reapproximation, but extensive granulation tissue in the proximal adductor region is common with intact repairs.

- Osteitis pubis should improve in the postoperative patient.
- Small fluid collections are expected after repair of severe lesions, but they should resolve in the perioperative period without evidence for loculation or tensity at MR imaging.

DISCLOSURE

The authors have nothing to disclose.

REFERENCES

1. Hopkins JN, Brown W, Lee CA. Sports hernia: definition, evaluation, and treatment. JBJS Rev 2017;5(9): e6.
2. Sheen AJ, Stephenson BM, Lloyd DM, et al. Treatment of the sportsman's groin": British Hernia Society's 2014 position statement based on the Manchester Consensus Conference. Br J Sports Med 2014;48(14):1079–87.
3. Weir A, Brukner P, Delahunt E, et al. Doha agreement meeting on terminology and definitions in groin pain in athletes. Br J Sports Med 2015;49(12): 768–74.
4. Omar IM, Zoga AC, Kavanagh EC, et al. Athletic pubalgia and "sports hernia": optimal MR imaging technique and findings. Radiographics 2008;28(5): 1415–38.
5. Brittenden J, Robinson P. Imaging of pelvic injuries in athletes. Br J Radiol 2005;78(929):457–68.
6. Robinson P, Bhat V, English B. Imaging in the assessment and management of athletic pubalgia. Semin Musculoskelet Radiol 2011;15(1):14–26.
7. Murphy G, Foran P, Murphy D, et al. Superior cleft sign" as a marker of rectus abdominus/adductor longus tear in patients with suspected sportsman's hernia. Skeletal Radiol 2013;42(6):819–25.
8. Meyers WC, Foley DP, Garrett WE, et al. Management of severe lower abdominal or inguinal pain in high-performance athletes. PAIN (Performing Athletes with Abdominal or Inguinal Neuromuscular Pain Study Group). Am J Sports Med 2000;28(1): 2–8.
9. O'Connell MJ, Powell T, McCaffrey NM, et al. Symphyseal cleft injection in the diagnosis and treatment of osteitis pubis in athletes. AJR Am J Roentgenol 2002;179(4):955–9.
10. Brennan D, O'Connell MJ, Ryan M, et al. Secondary cleft sign as a marker of injury in athletes with groin pain: MR image appearance and interpretation. Radiology 2005;235(1):162–7.
11. Zoga AC, Kavanagh EC, Omar IM, et al. Athletic pubalgia and the "sports hernia": MR imaging findings. Radiology 2008;247(3):797–807.

12. Mizrahi DJ, Poor AE, Meyers WC, et al. Imaging of the pelvis and lower extremity: demystifying uncommon sources of pelvic pain. Radiol Clin North Am 2018;56(6):983–95.

13. Zoga AC, Meyers WC. Magnetic resonance imaging for pain after surgical treatment for athletic pubalgia and the "sports hernia. Semin Musculoskelet Radiol 2011;15(4):372–82.

14. Kraeutler MJ, Mei-Dan O, Belk JW, et al. A systematic review shows high variation in terminology, surgical techniques, preoperative diagnostic measures, and geographic differences in the treatment of athletic pubalgia/sports hernia/core muscle injury/inguinal disruption. Arthrosc The J Arthroscopic Relat Surg 2021;37(7):2377–90.e2.

15. Di Marzo F. Sports Hernia: a comparison of the different surgical techniques. In: Zini R, Volpi P, Bisciotti GN, editors. Groin pain syndrome: a multidisciplinary guide to diagnosis and treatment. Springer International Publishing; 2017. p. 109–15.

16. Zuckerbraun BS, Cyr AR, Mauro CS. Groin Pain Syndrome Known as Sports Hernia: A Review. JAMA Surg 2020;155(4):340–8.

17. Larson CM. Sports hernia/athletic pubalgia: evaluation and management. Sports Health 2014;6(2):139–44.

18. Otten R, Vuckovic Z, Weir A, et al. Rehabilitation and return to play following surgery for inguinal-related groin pain. Oper Tech Sports Med 2017;25(3):172–80.

19. Paksoy M, Sekmen Ü. Sportsman hernia; the review of current diagnosis and treatment modalities. Ulus Cerrahi Derg 2015;32(2):122–9.

20. Poor AE, Warren AT, Roedl JB, et al. Diagnosis and Management of Core Muscle Injuries. Oper Tech Orthopaedics 2019;29(4):100738.

21. Sheen AJ, Montgomery A, Simon T, et al. Randomized clinical trial of open suture repair versus totally extraperitoneal repair for treatment of sportsman's hernia. Br J Surg 2019;106(7):837–44.

22. Choi HR, Elattar O, Dills VD, et al. Return to Play After Sports Hernia Surgery. Clin Sports Med 2016;35(4):621–36.

23. Roach RP, Clay TB, Emblom BA. Pelvis and hip injuries/core injuries in football. In: Farmer KW, editor. Football injuries: a clinical guide to in-season management. Springer International Publishing; 2021. p. 169–89.

24. Paajanen H, Montgomery A, Simon T, et al. Systematic review: laparoscopic treatment of long-standing groin pain in athletes. Br J Sports Med 2015;49(12):814–8.

25. Poor AE, Roedl JB, Zoga AC, et al. Core muscle injuries in athletes. Curr Sports Med Rep 2018;17(2):54–8.

26. Piozzi GN, Cirelli R, Salati I, et al. Laparoscopic approach to inguinal disruption in athletes: a retrospective 13-year analysis of 198 patients in a single-surgeon setting. Sports Med Open 2019;5:25.

27. Edelman DS. Hybrid mesh for sports hernia repair. Mini-invasive Surg 2017;1:31–4.

28. The SAGES Manual of Groin Pain. SAGES. Available at: https://www.sages.org/publications/sages-manuals/sages-manual-groin-pain/. Accessed December 22, 2021.

29. Pilkington JJ, Obeidallah MR, Zahid MS, et al. Outcome of the "manchester groin repair" (laparoscopic totally extraperitoneal approach with fibrin sealant mesh fixation) in 434 consecutive inguinal hernia repairs. Front Surg 2018;5:53.

30. Pilkington JJ, Obeidallah R, Baltatzis M, et al. Totally extraperitoneal repair for the 'sportsman's groin' via 'the Manchester Groin Repair': a comparison of elite versus amateur athletes. Surg Endosc 2021;35(8):4371–9.

31. McCarthy E, Hegazi TM, Zoga AC, et al. Ultrasound-guided interventions for core and hip injuries in athletes. Radiol Clin North Am 2016;54(5):875–92.

32. Poor AE, Warren A, Zoga AC, et al. Ultrasound-guided procedures allow delay of definitive treatment for core muscle injuries. Med Sci Sports Exerc 2022;54(2):206–10.

33. Meyers WC, McKechnie A, Philippon MJ, et al. Experience with "sports hernia" spanning two decades. Ann Surg 2008;248(4):656–65.

34. Meyers WC. Editorial Commentary: Core Muscle Injuries or Athletic Pubalgia-Finally the Real Sausage, Not Just the Same Ole Baloney. Arthroscopy 2017;33(5):1050–2.

35. Knapik DM, Gebhart JJ, Nho SJ, et al. Prevalence of surgical repair for athletic pubalgia and impact on performance in football athletes participating in the National Football League Combine. Arthroscopy 2017;33(5):1044–9.

36. Kunduracioglu B, Yilmaz C, Yorubulut M, et al. Magnetic resonance findings of osteitis pubis. J Magn Reson Imaging 2007;25(3):535–9.

37. Zajick DC, Zoga AC, Omar IM, et al. Spectrum of MRI findings in clinical athletic pubalgia. Semin Musculoskelet Radiol 2008;12(1):3–12.

Postoperative Magnetic Resonance Imaging of the Knee Ligaments

Saeed Dianat, MD, Jenny T. Bencardino, MD*

KEYWORDS

- ACL • Anterior cruciate ligament • PCL • Posterior cruciate ligament • Autograft • Reconstruction
- Revision

KEY POINTS

- Magnetic resonance imaging (MRI) is a noninvasive preferred method to evaluate the reconstructed ligaments of the knee.
- ACL reconstruction is a common procedure in patients with ligamentous injuries and radiologists need to be familiar with the surgical procedures as well as new imaging techniques to accurately interpret the postoperative images.
- Expected postoperative signal changes and evolution over time need to be considered in the graft evaluation.
- The anatomic positioning of the osseous tunnels is important to restore the isometric function of the ligament throughout the entire range of motion.
- Multiligamentous knee injuries (MLKI) are infrequent, with relatively complex postoperative changes following reconstruction, and careful interpretation of the postoperative magnetic resonance imaging (MRI) in correlation with the detailed surgical report is required.

INTRODUCTION

Anterior cruciate ligament (ACL) tears are common orthopedic injuries with approximately 200,000 cases per year in the United States. Approximately 100,000 to 150,000 of these patients undergo ligamentous reconstruction. The prevalence of ACL reconstruction showed a significant increase between 1994 and 2006 particularly in the younger than 20-year age category as these patients are now more active in high-level athletics for a longer time.[1]

The ACL is one of the most frequently torn ligaments of the knee.[2] The main goal of ACL reconstruction is to restore the biomechanical stability of the knee joint and reduce secondary injury to the articular cartilage and menisci. It has been postulated that ACL reconstruction may prevent the development of posttraumatic osteoarthritis; however, long-term studies have reported that about 50% of patients develop osteoarthritis after ACL reconstruction within 12 to 14 years.[3,4] Elevated inflammatory markers in the knee joint following ACL injury can contribute to the development of osteoarthritis, which cannot be reversed by ACL reconstruction. Advanced imaging of the knee joint, particularly of the articular cartilage, after ACL reconstruction is helpful for early identification of chondral abnormalities that may require treatment to delay symptomatic osteoarthritis and need for joint replacement.[5]

A meta-analysis study reported ACL graft rupture of about 6.2% (0%–13.4%) and clinical failure of about 10.3% (1.9%–25.6%) at longer than 10-years clinical follow-up.[6] Early graft failures within the first 6 months are often secondary to technical problems, failure of graft incorporation or errors in rehabilitation. However, late graft

Division of Musculoskeletal Radiology, Department of Radiology, Penn Medicine, University of Pennsylvania, 3737 Market Street, Philadelphia, PA 19104, USA
* Corresponding author.
E-mail address: Jenny.Bencardino@pennmedicine.upenn.edu

Magn Reson Imaging Clin N Am 30 (2022) 703–722
https://doi.org/10.1016/j.mric.2022.02.002
1064-9689/22/

failure occurring more than 1 year after surgery are likely related to new injuries resulting in graft tear.[7,8] Other complications include graft roof impingement, postoperative graft stiffness, tunnel widening due to cyst formation, iliotibial band friction syndrome, hardware failure, and infection.[8,9]

Revised ACL reconstruction surgery has a slightly lower 1-year clinical success outcome and higher rate of cartilage injuries when compared with primary ACL reconstruction. Posterolateral (PL) corner injury at the time of ACL revision and use of allograft is associated with relatively poorer patient-reported outcome.[10] Another systematic review demonstrates that 0% to 25% of revision ACL grafts may re-rupture which likely underestimates the real failure rate if objective clinical criteria are also included.[11]

Knee dislocation is a rare injury that commonly results in tears of the cruciate and collateral ligaments, and joint capsule. In addition, there can be associated vascular and nerve injuries that need to be addressed. Nonoperative treatment with immobilization has been historically used in patients with multi-ligament injury of the knee. However, studies have shown the benefit of surgical stabilization of multi-ligament injuries and there has been a shift in the management of those cases over time.[12]

Great advances in surgical techniques for the reconstruction of the injured ligaments of the knee have been made. Postoperative MR imaging of the knee ligaments is increasingly used in clinical practice to evaluate the status of the repaired or reconstructed ligaments and to rule out any evidence of new internal joint derangement that may require additional procedures. Radiologists need to be familiar with the various surgical techniques of ligament reconstruction, expected postoperative appearance, and imaging manifestations of failed reconstructed ligaments and associated complications.

Review of the operative report is very helpful to identify the used surgical technique and correlate with the imaging findings. The time interval between the surgery and imaging is another important piece of information to consider for the interpretation of the postoperative MR imaging. Serial imaging should also be compared for the evolution of postoperative signal and morphologic alterations.

ANTERIOR CRUCIATE LIGAMENT
Normal Anterior Cruciate Ligament Reconstruction and Morphologic Changes

There are different types of grafts and techniques available for ACL reconstruction.

Bone–patellar tendon–bone and hamstring autografts are the 2 most commonly used methods for ACL reconstruction. Bone–patellar tendon–bone (BPTB) graft is harvested from the middle third of the patellar tendon with bone plugs attached to each end and is considered the reference standard given the inherent strength and stiffness of the graft (**Fig. 1**). However, anterior knee pain and patellar tendon dysfunction are not infrequent after this type of reconstruction.[8] Another common graft is quadrupled hamstring

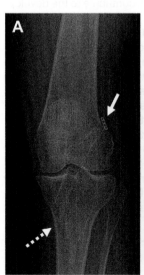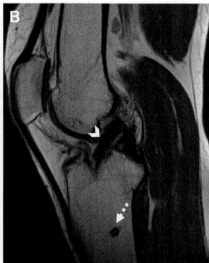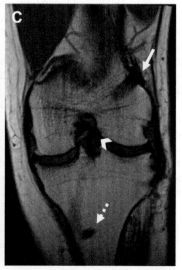

Fig. 1. 30-year-old woman with normal intact ACL reconstruction using bone-patellar tendon-bone graft (*arrowhead*) fixated by femoral endobutton (*arrow*) and tibial bioabsorbable screw (dashed *arrow*) demonstrated on frontal radiograph (*A*), Sagittal PD-weighted (*B*), and Coronal T1-weighted images (*C*).

autograft from the semitendinosus tendon, the gracilis tendon, or both which are folded and braided together (**Fig. 2**). This graft type has low morbidity related to the donor site.[13,14] Both grafts are viable options for ACL reconstruction. In a meta-analysis, the hamstring autograft failed at a higher rate than BPTB in a short-to mid-term follow-up with a generally low rate of failure in both groups.[15] However, an earlier meta-analysis showed lower postoperative complications of hamstring compared with BPTB autografts but reported a slight benefit of using BPTB in rotation stability and return to higher levels of activity.[16] Additional randomized controlled trials are needed to compare the outcome of reconstruction using different grafts based on clear and specified criteria and outcome measures. Allografts and synthetic grafts have also been used.[17,18] In some cases, extra-articular augmentation of the ACL reconstruction using iliotibial band autograft for the reconstruction of the anterolateral ligament is performed (**Fig. 3**).

Single Versus Double-Bundle Anterior Cruciate Ligament

The primary role of ACL is resisting against anterior tibial translation which is achieved by the anteromedial (AM) bundle as it tightens with knee flexion. On the other hand, the PL bundle is tight in knee extension and results in anterolateral rotational stability. Single-bundle ACL reconstruction has been the standard surgical option over the past years.[19] However, it has been postulated that the standard single-bundle reconstruction technique is less efficient in tibial rotational stability and

may contribute to arthrofibrosis or degenerative changes.[19,20] A recent meta-analysis demonstrated that while normal knee kinematics can be restored by both techniques, the double-bundle ACL reconstruction technique is associated with better restoration of anteroposterior stability. However, it is unclear which technique results in better rotational stability.[19]

Double-bundle ACL reconstruction techniques incorporate 2 femoral and 2 tibial tunnels and are associated with relatively similar complications and magnetic resonance imaging (MRI) findings of the graft.[21] The expected postoperative appearance of the double-bundle grafts on the PD-weighted images includes increased signal intensity at 6 months which is decreased at 12 months after surgery.[22,23] It has been reported that the PL graft is increased in signal intensity compared with AM graft on T2-weighted images at 12 months after surgery using hamstring grafts which may indicate the different roles of these bundles in knee stability.[24] It has been reported that the increased T1-and T2-weighted signal intensity of the single-bundle graft is reflected by the ligamentization period during 3 to 24 months after operation.[25,26]

Graft Fixation Devices

ACL graft fixation devices include interference screws, endobuttons, screw-washer constructs, and staples. Interference screws and endobuttons are the more commonly used fixation devices (**Fig. 4**)

Biodegradable interference screws have a few advantages over metallic screws such as better postoperative assessment by MR imaging given

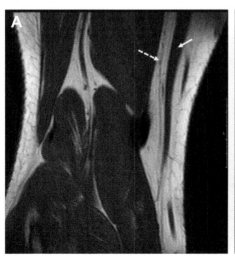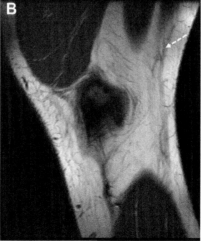

Fig. 2. Postoperative coronal (*A*) and Sagittal T1-weighted (*B*) images of semitendinosus and gracillis tendon harvesting for ACL reconstruction in a 16-year-old man with ACL tear due to football injury. Sartorius (*A, arrow*), area of gracillis (*A and B, dashed arrow*) which is harvested for ACL reconstruction.

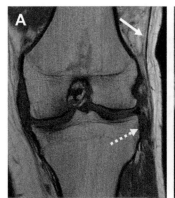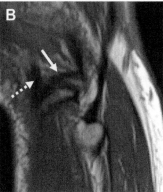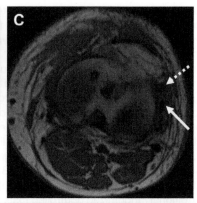

Fig. 3. A 21-year-old semi-professional man football athlete 2 weeks after surgery presenting with concern for infection. Preoperative midcoronal T1-weight image (*A*) shows intact iliotibial band (*arrow*), and tear of tibial stump of anterolateral ligament (dashed *arrow*). Postoperative sagittal T1-weighted image demonstrates extra-articular stabilization of ACL reconstruction using iliotibial band autograft (*B, C,* dashed *arrow*) for the reconstruction of anterolateral ligament (*B, C, arrow*).

the relatively absent artifact, no adverse effect on the bone marrow signal intensity, and no long-term interference with the surrounding tissues. Several disadvantages of the biodegradable screws include a slow rate of graft remodeling/ligamentization, incomplete ossification and tunnel widening, higher risk of fracture with rapid loss of the screw strength, inadequate stiffness and higher rate of breakage, inflammation, or foreign body reactions resulting in osteolysis or cyst formation.[27]

Tunnel Position and Technique

Knowledge of the anatomic position of the native ACL bundles is important to achieve isometric placement of the ACL graft. Isometry of the ACL graft refers to consistent length and tension of the graft during the entire range of motion of the knee joint.[8] The isometric ACL graft minimizes graft-tunnel motion, promotes graft healing into the bone, avoids graft loosening or tear, and potential tunnel enlargement.[28]

As discussed in the previous section, the native ACL consists of 2 bundles; AM and PL bundles which are called based on their attachment to the tibial footprint (**Fig. 5**). Coronal oblique planes in the long axis of the ACL bundles are prescribed from the intercondylar notch roof or Blumensaat line and seem helpful to identify the individual bundles and evaluate for injuries.[21,29,30] The coronal and sagittal elevation angles of the native ACL are reported in the range of 66° to 74°[31-34] and 43° to 59°,[31,34,35] respectively.[36]

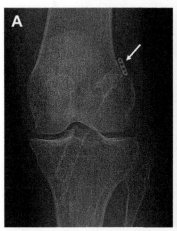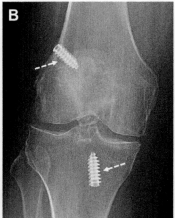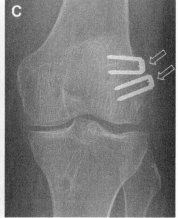

Fig. 4. ACL graft fixation devices on frontal radiographs. (*A*) Tibial fixation using bioabsorbable screw and femoral fixation using endobutton (*arrow*). (*B*) Femoral and tibial metallic screw fixation (dashed *arrows*). (*C*) Femoral fixation with metallic staples (block *arrows*) and tibial fixation using bioabsorbable screw.

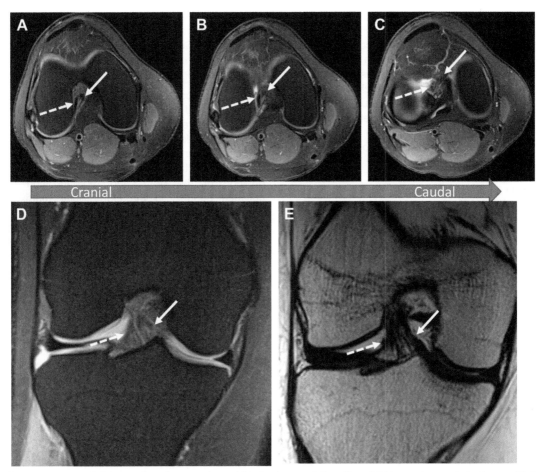

Fig. 5. Anteromedial (*arrows*) and posterolateral (dashed *arrows*) bundles of ACL are demonstrated on multiple axial PD fat-saturated images (*A–C*), Coronal PD fat-saturated images (*D*), and coronal oblique reconstructed T2 3D SPACE (*E*) of a 19-year-old man.

Forsythe and colleagues[37] have reported the anatomic positions of the AM and PL bundles of the ACL; the tibial positions of the AM and PL bundles were reported at 25 ± 2.8% and 46.4 ± 3.7% in the anterior–posterior direction and 50.5 ± 4.2% and 52.4 ± 2.5% in the medial–lateral direction, respectively. The femoral positions of the AM and PL bundles were, respectively, reported at 21.7 ± 2.5% and 35.1 ± 3.5% along a line parallel to Blumensaat line and 33.2 ± 5.6% and 55.3 ± 5.3% along a line perpendicular to Blumensaat line.

The clock-face approach is a simple method for the evaluation of the femoral tunnel position on frontal radiographs. In the right knee, the femoral tunnel for AM bundle and PL bundle reconstruction is located at approximately 10 to 11 o'clock and 9 to 10 o'clock positions, respectively. The symmetric clock-face positions are considered for the left knee.[21]

The correct positioning of the femoral and tibial tunnels for ACL reconstruction remains challenging and nonanatomical graft placement may result in failure of about 88% of cases.[38] Higher sagittal elevation angle and deviation angle in the transverse plane may result in nonanatomical graft orientation and failure. Posteromedial placement of the tibial and anterior placement of the femoral tunnels relative to the native ACL bundles can result in tunnel malposition and graft failure.[36] The femoral tunnel should be placed as far posteriorly as possible without disrupting the posterior femoral cortex with a remaining 1–2-mm-thick cortical rim.[8] During the surgery, anterior notchplasty may be performed if roof impingement is present with knee extension. With notchplasty, a few millimeters of bone are removed from the anterolateral aspect of the intercondylar roof.[8,39] The graft length and tension are increased with knee extension if the femoral tunnel is placed too high and increased with knee flexion if the femoral tunnel is placed too far anteriorly (**Fig. 6**).

The transtibial approach is the commonly used technique for ACL reconstruction in which femoral tunnel is drilled through a tibial tunnel placed in the posterior half of the tibial attachment of the ACL.[40,41] This technique may result in improper positioning of the femoral tunnel in the high femoral notch, often at the edge or outside of the anatomic femoral ACL footprint, producing a vertically oriented graft in sagittal and coronal planes.[40,42]

While a vertically oriented ACL graft may resist anterior tibial translation, it may not resist against a combination of anterior tibial translation and internal rotation in pivot-shift phenomenon.[43–45] The 2-incision technique is an alternative technique for independent drilling of the femoral tunnel using an AM portal.[38,46]

In a cadaveric study, the use of preprocedural 3D MR imaging to roadmap the femoral and tibial footprints of the native ACL showed no significant help in the anatomic placement of the tunnels when compared with standard technique without roadmap of ACL footprints.[47]

Graft Healing

The healing process of intra-articular portion of the graft is referred to "ligamentization" with 3 stages described as "early," "remodeling," and "maturation" in chronologic order. The biologic processes that occur during ligamentization include neovascularization of the graft, fibroblastic cellular repopulation of the graft, and reorganization of collagen bundles in the extracellular matrix.[48] The timing of graft ligamentization varies among reports. Rougraff and colleagues[49,50] demonstrated that the timing for remodeling of the BPTB autografts include neovascularization at 3 weeks, focal areas of acellularity at 8 weeks, degeneration at 6 to 10 months, with resolution at 1 to 3 years postoperatively. More recent studies by Sanchez and colleagues[51] showed ligamentization achieved at around 2 years after

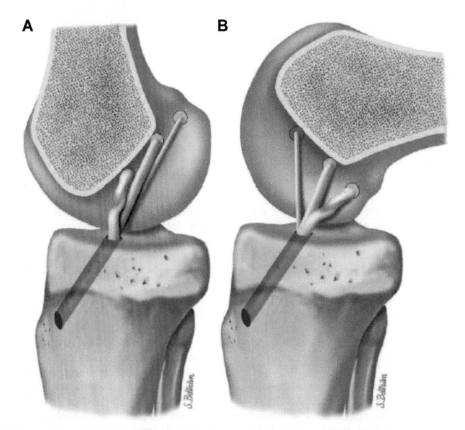

Fig. 6. Effects of femoral tunnel placement on graft length and tension. Diagrams of the knee in extension (*A*) and flexion (*B*) show anterior (*red circle*), isometric (*green circle*), and over-the-top (blue circle) positions of the femoral tunnel site in ACL reconstruction. (NEEDS REPRINT PERMISSION REQUEST FROM Bencardino JT, Beltran J, Feldman MI, Rose DJ. MR imaging of complications of anterior cruciate ligament graft reconstruction. Radiographics. 2009 Nov;29(7):2115–26. https://doi.org/10.1148/rg.297095036. PMID: 19926766.)

surgery at which time no further changes are identified in the graft.

Tunnel expansion is associated with poor incorporation of the graft, particularly in cases using cortical suspension devices and may result in the suboptimal function of the graft.[52] Using 3D MR imaging of the ACL graft in patients who underwent ACL reconstruction using hamstring tendon autograft and femoral cortical suspension device, it has been demonstrated that the expansion of the femoral tunnel involves the portion of the tunnel containing the graft, particularly at the anteroinferior wall of the femoral tunnel. Femoral tunnel expansion occurs early postreconstruction at 6 months and reduces by 24 months after reconstruction. While femoral tunnel expansion has been correlated with less favorable graft maturation, similar clinical outcomes in patients with and without femoral tunnel expansion have been demonstrated.[53]

Signal changes: ACL graft signal change is a 3-stage process based on timing after surgery. Early postoperative images demonstrate the low signal intensity of the graft on all pulse sequences. The signal is increased during the remodeling period (4–8 months after surgery) when the graft undergoes revascularization and resynovialization. In most cases, graft hypointensity on all pulse sequences should return after about 1 to 2 years.[21] Therefore, MR findings should be interpreted alongside clinical presentation. Radiologists need to be familiar with the expected postoperative signal intensity evolution and graft healing/maturation process.

Graft Maturation

Graft type, graft source (autograft vs allograft), and time after reconstruction are independent predictive variables for the normalization of the graft MR imaging signal. A systematic review demonstrates that the predicted normalized MR imaging signal intensity of the graft significantly decreases for hamstring autografts while increases for bone-patellar tendon-bone (BPTB) allografts between 6 and 12 months after surgery. By 12 months after surgery, the predicted normalized MR imaging signal intensity of BPTB autograft is significantly greater than hamstring graft and hamstring graft with minimal debridement/remnant preservation surgical technique.[54]

Revision

Revised ACL graft reconstruction has been associated with inferior clinical outcomes and approximately 3 to 4 times higher rate of failure as compared with primary ACL reconstruction.[55]

The prevalence of chondral injuries is higher in patients with revised ACL reconstruction. The presence of PL corner injury and allograft utilization are predictive factors for inferior patient-reported clinical outcomes.[10]

Anterior Cruciate Ligament Reconstruction in Adolescents

The incidence rate of pediatric ACL injuries is approximately 1 in 10,000 children.[56] This represents about 3% of pediatric knee injuries.[57] Due to the presence of open growth plates and potential growth disturbance with procedures affecting the growth plate, the best treatment of pediatric ACL injuries remain controversial.[58]

Complete transphyseal ACL reconstruction is a modified version of adult ACL reconstruction with the tunnels crossing both the femoral and the tibial physeal plates using smaller drill holes to minimize the risk of growth plate disturbance. This technique was reported as a viable option in adolescent patients after an average of 3 years which were followed up with good functional outcome and good return to physical activity without leg length discrepancy or angular deformity.[58]

Postoperative Findings/Complications

The main complications of ACL reconstruction include graft tear, graft roof impingement, arthrofibrosis, tunnel cyst formation, and hardware failure and dislodgment.

Graft Tear

Acute ACL graft tears are usually the result of major trauma. Chronic ACL graft tears are typically partial and due to graft roof impingement with repetitive friction and secondary attrition of the graft which is described in further detail in the roof impingement section.

Partial graft tear is most reliably identified on MR imaging as focal thinning of the graft due to fiber discontinuity.[59] Increased signal on PD- and T2-weighted images can also be associated with partial graft tear but when present in isolation is not a reliable MR imaging indicator of partial tear.[26,60] This underscores the necessity for radiologists to be familiar with the expected maturation and ligamentization period when there is expected increased T2 signal intensity within the graft, which is discussed in the previous section.

Complete graft tear can have different MR imaging appearances depending on whether it is acute or chronic. Acute complete graft tears typically demonstrate MR imaging findings similar to native ACL tears such as graft swelling, complete discontinuity of the fibers, laxity, retraction of the graft stump, and reciprocating bone marrow impaction injuries due to the underlying pivot shift biomechanics (**Fig. 7**). Chronic complete graft tears usually demonstrate graft attenuation and resorption, abnormal orientation, scarring in the intercondylar notch, signs of graft laxity such as buckling of PCL and anterior tibial translation (**Fig. 8**). Comparison with previous MR imaging studies is very helpful.

In a study by Kiekara and colleagues, double-bundle ACL grafts were evaluated with MR imaging at 2 years after surgery to assess the MR imaging findings following the ligamentization period. Disruption of the AM graft was noted in 3% of patients, while 6% of patients had a disrupted PL graft, and 3% of patients had disruption of both grafts. Compared with the original values, the decrease in mean graft thickness of the PL bundle graft was greater than that of AM bundle graft (18% vs 9%). The signal intensity was increased in 17% of AM grafts and in 61% of PL grafts on all pulse sequences.[23]

Graft fiber discontinuity is the most reliable MR imaging finding of surgically proven full-thickness graft tear (sensitivity 72% and specificity 100%).[59] Other primary findings of graft tear such as graft thinning or attenuation, signal intensity changes, and deranged orientation do not improve accuracy for the detection of full-thickness graft tear.

The most frequently noted pattern (35%) of double-bundle ACL graft failure among patients

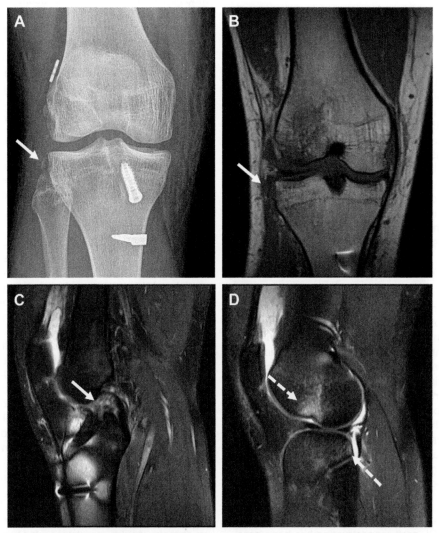

Fig. 7. 18-year-old woman soccer athlete with torn hamstring ACL graft in the right knee after soccer injury. AP radiograph (*A*) and corresponding coronal T1-weighted image (*B*) demonstrate Segond fracture (*arrow*). Sagittal PD-weighted fat sat images demonstrate torn ACL graft (*C, arrow*) and reciprocal bone contusions due to pivot-shift injury (*D,* dashed *arrows*).

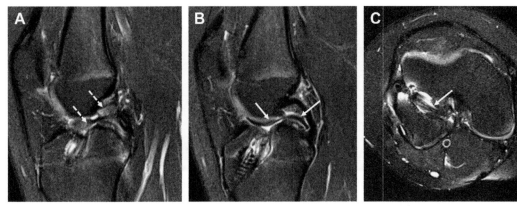

Fig. 8. Chronic complete tear of ACL graft in a 14-year-old woman with soccer-related injury 2 years prior presenting with pain. Sagittal T2-weighted fat-saturated images (*A, B*) at the level of intercondylar notch demonstrate completely torn ACL graft with absence of fibers (*A, dashed arrows*) causing significant 12 mm anterior tibial translation (not shown). Associated bucket handle tear of medial meniscus (*B, arrow*). Axial T2 fat sat (*C, arrow*) demonstrates the femoral tunnel of the torn ACL graft which was normally positioned.

presenting for revision surgery has been reported as mid-substance tear of the AM graft and mid-substance tear of PL graft, while the PL graft has been intact in 19% of cases.[61]

The clinical significance of persistent intrasubstance T2 hyperintensity of the ACL graft beyond the maturation period remains controversial. Small areas of increased signal intensity (less than 25% of the maximal cross-sectional area of the graft) on PD- and T2-weighted images were reported in a long-term study (4–12 years) after ACL reconstruction; however, there was no definite correlation with clinical findings of instability or subjective functional limitations.[60] The clinical significance of signal changes affecting double-bundle reconstruction has not been elucidated.

Correlation of increased signal intensity of the graft on T2-weighted images 1 year after surgery with laxity using functional testing has been reported.[24] In a recent study, the association between double-bundle graft signal intensity at 1-year postoperative MR imaging, tibial tunnel positioning, and the clinical outcomes was demonstrated. Tunnel malpositioning, another reason for reconstruction failure, correlated with increased intrasubstance graft signal, focal arthrofibrosis (cyclops lesion), and graft tear with residual instability (**Figs. 9 and 10**).[62]

Anterior Knee Laxity

Anterior knee laxity is a complication of ACL reconstruction that is attributed to postoperative posterior joint capsule thickening. Anterior

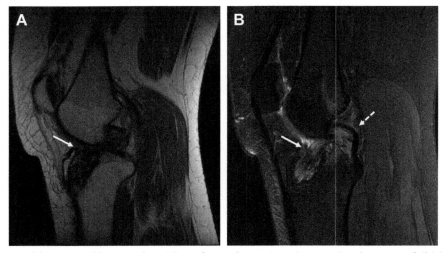

Fig. 9. 28-year-old woman with a complete ACL graft tear due to excessive anterior placement of tibial tunnel on Sagittal PD-weighted (*A, arrow*) and Sagittal T2 FS (*B, arrow*). Associated bowing of PCL (*B, dashed arrow*).

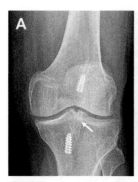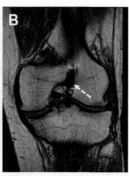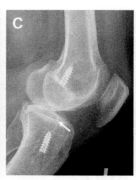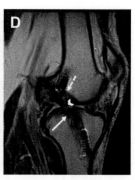

Fig. 10. 45-year-old man with ACL graft tear (*D, arrowhead*) due to excessive vertical placement of tibial tunnel (*A, C, D, arrow*) and femoral tunnel (*B, D,* dashed *arrow*) on frontal and lateral radiographs (*A,C*) and Coronal T1-weighted (*B*) and Sagittal T2-weighted (*D*) images.

translation of the tibia more than 7 mm on MR imaging in the presence of an intact ACL graft is highly specific when compared with mechanical arthrometric tests.[63] Clinical examination is more sensitive for the evaluation of anterior knee laxity. Therefore, MR imaging findings should be interpreted as an adjunct to clinical examination.

Graft Impingement

There are 3 different types of graft impingement including anterior notch roof impingement, posterior impingement with PCL, and lateral notch roof impingement (**Fig. 11**).[64] Anterior roof notch impingement is usually caused by excessive anterior positioning of the AM tibial tunnel which results in loss of terminal extension. The relationship of the graft with the intercondylar roof is best evaluated in the sagittal plane.[21] The risk of anterior notch roof impingement depends on the size of the tibial ACL footprint, the tibial tunnel diameter, and the drill-guide angle of the tibial tunnel.[62,65] Lateral notch roof impingement with the intercondylar notch is caused by a narrow intercondylar notch and a too laterally placed tibial tunnel. Posterior impingement with PCL occurs when the tibial tunnel is too medial and vertical, causing contact between the graft and PCL during flexion.[64]

Arthrofibrosis

Excessive postoperative scar formation results in painful, restricted range of motion with extension deficit, snapping, and effusion. There are diffuse and focal types of arthrofibrosis. Diffuse arthrofibrosis is joint capsule thickening causing stiffness and can be treated with physical therapy and sometimes arthrolysis.[64] Focal arthrofibrosis, the so-called cyclops lesion, seems as focal nodular scarring with intermediate signal on T2-weighted images just anterior to the distal aspect of the

ACL graft near the tibial attachment and is arthroscopically treated.[21] Cyclops lesions are identified in up to 25% of cases after ACL reconstruction, usually develop within the first 6 months after surgery and do not significantly change over a period of 2 years.[66]

Partially torn ACL graft fibers may lie in the anterior intercondylar notch which is called "Pseudocyclops lesion."[67]

Septic Arthritis

Septic arthritis is a rare complication with a risk of less than 0.5% after ACL reconstruction. In the presence of clinical suspicion for infection, MR imaging findings of joint effusion, synovial proliferation, soft tissue edema, and abscess are supportive of a septic arthritis diagnosis (**Fig. 12**).[68]

Fixation Device Failure

The complications associated with failure of the fixation devices include fragmentation, loosening, displacement, and dislodgment.[21] These are usually early complications related to surgical technique or trauma. The subcutaneous prominence of the fixation devices may become symptomatic requiring removal of the device. On the other hand, the partially dislodged or fragmented cross-pin fixation of the hamstring graft may potentially cause iliotibial band friction syndrome or tearing.[8,69] Loosening of the interference screws might be due to mechanical loosening or infectious etiology. The bioabsorbable screws may cause foreign-body granuloma formation and result in widening of the tunnels.

Tunnel Cyst Formation

Cystic degeneration of the graft or ganglion cyst formation is a rare complication that can cause

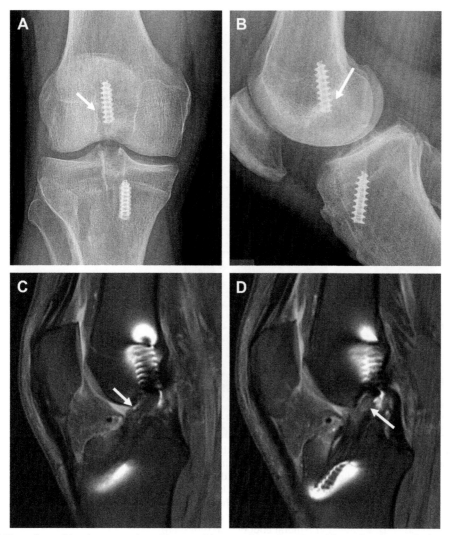

Fig. 11. ACL graft roof impingement in a 48-year-old man with pain. AP and lateral radiographs (*A, B*) demonstrate excessive vertical placement of femoral tunnel in both coronal (*A, arrow*) and sagittal planes (*B, arrow*). Sagittal PD-weighted fat-saturated images demonstrate slight laxity of the graft with increased signal (*C, D, arrows*).

pain and limitation of motion, although it is not generally associated with graft failure. The individual graft fibers are intact on MR imaging and are splayed around the cystic lesion.[21] This is a relatively late complication, which occurs more frequently following reconstruction using hamstring tendons and endobutton fixation. Cystic changes in the graft are associated with the widening of the tunnel on the radiograph. Cysts may extend distally into the tibial tunnel aperture and may result in pretibial subcutaneous edema. A small amount of fluid in the tunnels during the first 18 months postoperative period is considered normal especially in the tibial tunnel after hamstring graft reconstruction. Even though there is no objective definition for tibial tunnel widening

in the literature, the presence of a subjectively widened tunnel helps to differentiate tunnel cyst formation from normal postoperative fluid in the tunnels.[64] However, tibial tunnel enlargement has been reported to frequently occur within the first 6 months after surgery and is continued until 12 months after reconstruction. Afterward, most authors report only minimal changes in tibial tunnel size for up to 2 years after reconstruction.[70,71]

The average proximal tibial tunnel diameter of cases using bone-patellar tendon-bone graft has been reported as 12 ± 1.9 mm postoperatively and 14 ± 2.2 mm (mean ± standard deviation) at 3 months.[72] Although tibial tunnel widening is not correlated with graft failure, additional bone grafting might be needed in revision ACL

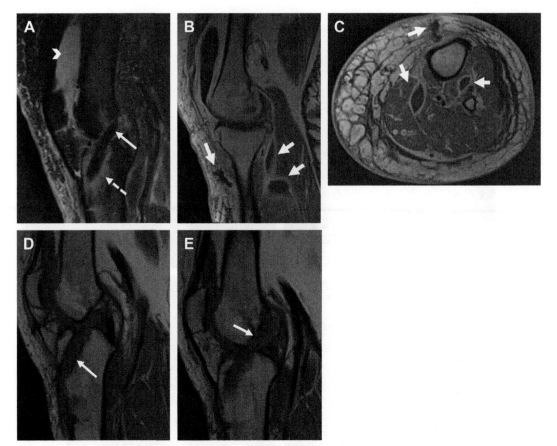

Fig. 12. 38-year-old woman presenting with pain 1 month after revision ACL reconstruction complicated by infection and multiple intramuscular abscesses. Sagittal STIR image shows intact ACL graft (*A, arrow*) associated with bone marrow edema surrounding the tibial tunnel (*A, dashed arrow*) and large joint effusion (*A, arrowhead*). Sagittal (*B*) and axial (*C*) postcontrast T1-weight WARP images demonstrate multiple intramuscular and subcutaneous abscesses (*B, C, arrows*). Next day arthroscopy showed infection, and septic arthritis. Patient underwent incision and debridement of the tibial incision, and removal of the ACL graft (*E, arrow*) and fixation hardware including tibial screw (*D, arrow*), and femoral endodutton (not seen).

reconstruction. Differential diagnosis of the tibial tunnel widening includes foreign-body granuloma formation, infection, and tibial screw extrusion.[73] Unlike graft rupture, the graft fibers remain intact and only splayed with ganglion cyst.[9]

Pretibial cyst is identified in 2.2% of cases. The incomplete graft incorporation in the tibial tunnel and subsequent tissue necrosis may allow the passage of the joint fluid through the tibial tunnel to the pretibial soft tissue and cystic formation.[74]

Multiligamentous Reconstruction

Multiligamentous knee injuries (MLKI) are relatively uncommon injuries with approximately 0.02% to 0.20% incidence among the orthopedic injuries.[75] These are defined as injuries to at least two of the cruciate and collateral ligaments, commonly associated with knee dislocation.[76] There is approximately 18% risk of vascular injury and up to 40%

risk of common peroneal nerve injury associated with knee dislocation and MLKI.[77,78] Furthermore, there is a risk of missing the injuries due to spontaneous reduction following the injury. Both low-energy trauma particularly in obese patients as well as high-energy trauma may result in knee dislocation and MLKI.[76] While the immediate management of these injuries is focused on the treatment of the associated vascular and nerve injuries, the timing and decision to perform single-session versus staged surgical repair or reconstruction of the ligaments remain controversial (**Figs. 13** and **14**). It is important to note that synovial proliferation and synovitis are often in the early postoperative period after MLKI and can be considered within the spectrum of expected postoperative changes (**Fig 15**).

The staged repair or reconstruction of the ligaments includes acute repair or reconstruction of the extra-articular structures (medial and lateral

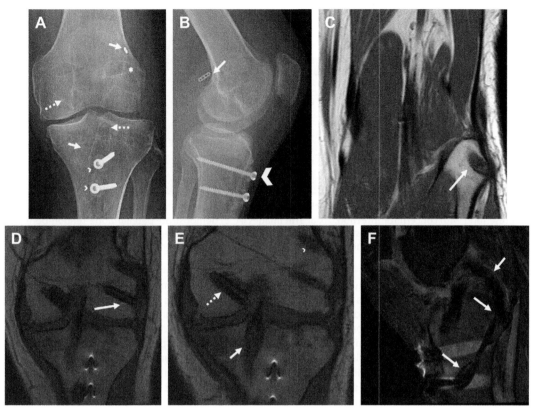

Fig. 13. Postsurgical changes of multiligamentous reconstruction in a 24-year-old man. AP and lateral radiographs (*A, B*) demonstrate postsurgical changes in fixation/reconstruction of FCL (*A, asterisk*), ACL (*A, B arrow*), and PCL (*A,* dashed *arrow*), and tibial tuberosity fracture fixation (*A, B, arrowhead*). Coronal T1-weighted image (*C*) shows fibular fixation of FCL (*C, arrow*). Coronal T1-weighted image (*D*) shows popliteus tendon fixation (*D, arrow*). Coronal T1-weighted image (*E*) demonstrates fixation/reconstruction changes of ACL (*E, arrow*), PCL (*E,* dashed *arrow*), and FCL (*E, arrowhead*). Sagittal PD-weight fat-saturated image (*F*) demonstrates PCL fixation (*F, arrows*).

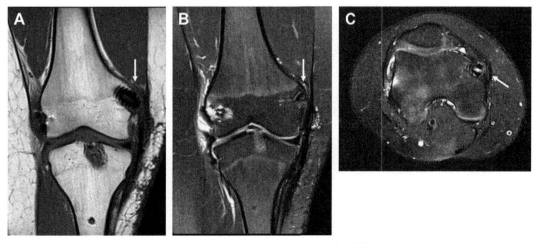

Fig. 14. 14-year-old woman with soccer-related injury 2 years prior and multiligamentous reconstruction presenting with pain. Patient had a chronic tear of ACL graft (shown in previous Fig. 8). Coronal T1-weight (*A*) and T2-weighted fat-saturated images (*B*) demonstrate intact MCL fixation to the medial femoral condyle (*A, B, arrow*). Axial T2-weighted fat-saturated image (*C*) similarly shows intact MCL fixation (*C, arrow*).

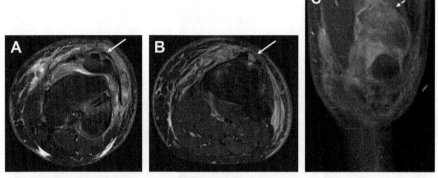

Fig. 15. 21-year-old semi-professional man football athlete 2 weeks after multiligamentous reconstruction of the knee presenting with concern for infection. Axial STIR images (*A, B*) demonstrate patellar bone-tendon-bone harvesting site (*A, B, arrows*). Coronal post-contrast T1 fat-saturated image (*C*) demonstrates synovial enhancement (*C, dashed arrow*) in keeping with synovitis and early postoperative changes.

structures) with a 6 to 8 weeks delayed the reconstruction of the cruciate ligaments following the complete restoration of range of motion.[76,79]

Graft choice for ligament reconstruction includes BPTB autograft or allograft, quadriceps tendon autograft, hamstring (gracilis and semitendinosus) tendon autograft, Achilles tendon allograft, Tibialis anterior allograft, and synthetic grafts such as Ligament Augmentation and Reconstruction System. The graft selection depends on the number of injured ligaments requiring reconstruction, graft availability, surgeon preference and the surgical technique.[76]

The most commonly injured posteromedial corner structure is the posterior oblique ligament, which is the primary stabilizer for the internal rotation of the tibia during the knee flexion and is injured in 99% of patients with AM rotatory instability.[80,81] This ligament can be repaired or reconstructed in the acute setting after injury and medial collateral ligament repair or reconstruction.[81]

The avulsion of the fibular collateral ligament from femoral and fibular attachments can be repaired in the acute setting but the midsubstance tears need to be reconstructed (**Figs. 16 and 17**). The fibular sling reconstruction of PL

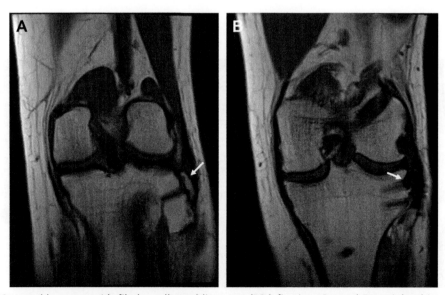

Fig. 16. 30-year-old woman with fibular collateral ligament (FCL) fixation. Coronal T1-weighted images (*A, B*) demonstrate a chronically avulsed fragment of fibular head (*A, arrow*) which presumably prompted the surgeon to fixate the FCL graft to the lateral tibial condyle due to deficient attachment site of FCL in the fibula. The FCL fixation screws in the tibia are shown (*B, arrow*).

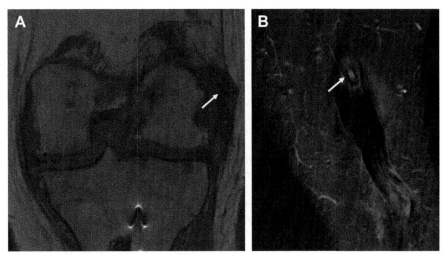

Fig. 17. 24-year-old man with the history of multiligamentous reconstruction presenting with pain. Coronal T1-weighted (*A*) and Sagittal PD-weighted fat-saturated images demonstrate dislodged screw at the proximal/femoral aspect of FCL fixation (*A, B, arrow*).

corner injury can be anatomic with a single femoral tunnel or nonanatomic with 2 femoral tunnels.[82]

Posterior Cruciate Ligament

The injury to the posterior cruciate ligament (PCL) commonly occurs in the setting of severe trauma and joint dislocation in which there are additional concurrent injuries to the supportive ligaments and tendons (**Fig. 18**).

Complete ligamentization of the PCL graft may take up to 24 months. Graft failure and impingement are the main complications of PCL reconstruction.[83] Tunnel malpositioning is contributing to about one-third of the graft failures through graft laxity and/or impingement.[83,84] Tunnel centers are commonly assessed by CT. Femoral tunnel placement is assessed using a grid and the position is assessed in 2 directions, shallow-deep and high-low.[83,85] It has been reported that the anterolateral bundle of the PCL typically lies approximately 40% in the shallow-deep and approximately 14.5% in the high-low direction in the femoral footprint, whereas the

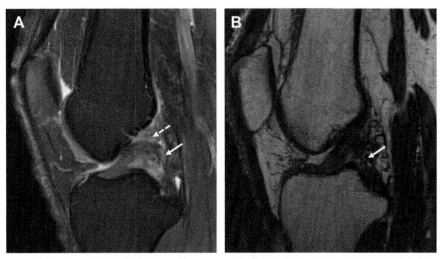

Fig. 18. 42-year-old male undergoing MR imaging 1 month after twisting injury while at heavy labor and construction work. Sagittal PD-weighted fat-saturated image shows disrupted PCL at the midportion (*A, arrow*) and thickened proximal portion of PCL with intermediate signal (*A, dashed arrow*) in keeping with tear at the midportion and high-grade sprain at the femoral portion. 3D isotropic reconstructed Sagittal T2-weighted image demonstrates disrupted PCL at the mid-portion (*B, arrow*).

posteromedial bundle lies at 56% and 36.5% in the shallow-deep and high-low directions, respectively.[84] The tibial insertion is placed in the posterior 48% of the area between tibial intercondylar fossa and posterior cortex.[86]

MR imaging is a noninvasive method for the evaluation of grafts. Given the oblique and curvilinear appearance of the native PCL and graft, acquiring additional images in the oblique coronal plane (PCL view) may improve diagnostic performance.[87] Of course, acquisition of PCL view images in addition to standard protocol requires extra-scanning time. Therefore, 3D isotropic T2-weighted MR imaging with thin slices and no gap provide an opportunity to reconstruct the images in any plane such as PCL view. PCL view potentially provides more accurate evaluation given better visualization of the entire width of the graft and decreases the volume averaging as compared with sagittal images.[87,88] In addition, it was reported that there is no significant difference in the diagnostic performance of the PCL view using 3D or 2D images either solitary or in the combination of orthogonal images to identify PCL graft complications.[87]

Double-bundle PCL reconstruction using the ligament advanced reinforcement system (LARS), a synthetic ligament composed of polyethylene terephthalate, has been an alternative option to the standard PCL reconstruction technique using autograft or allograft. The interpretation of signal of the artificial ligaments on MR imaging is difficult and differs from autograft or allograft in which grafts demonstrate low signal in the first 2 years after reconstruction.[83,89] Fibrous tissue ingrowth into the artificial ligament results in intermediate signal on MR imaging in cases without LARS rupture. In addition, LARS maintains a relaxed PCL morphology after reconstruction which promotes healing.[90] It has been reported that the LARS thickness after fibrous tissue ingrowth is moderately and inversely correlated with the instability of the knee. This study defined knee stability as side-to-side difference (SSD) $\leq$ 3 mm and instability as SSD greater than 3 mm and showed that the optimal cutoff point of LARS midsubstance thickness in the receiver operating characteristic (ROC) curve analysis was 14.3 mm or greater to achieve knee stability.[89]

SUMMARY

MR imaging is an accurate noninvasive method for the evaluation of knee ligament repair and reconstruction. Postoperative signal changes of the graft and expected evolving signal changes need to be considered in the interpretation of the postoperative imaging studies. Anatomic positioning of the grafts enables the restoration of the maximal biomechanical properties of the ligament repair. Imaging assessment of the graft includes the evaluation of the graft integrity, signal changes, abnormal configuration caused by roof impingement, arthrofibrosis, abnormal placement and cystic changes of the tunnels, healing status of the tunnel, and general postoperative complications such as infection or hardware-related failure.

CLINICS CARE POINTS

- When evaluating the postoperative MR imaging of the knee after ligamentous reconstruction, look for graft discontinuity, signal changes, and hardware failure.
- The time interval between the postoperative MR imaging and surgery is crucial in the interpretation of the signal changes that may otherwise lead to misdiagnosis.
- Comparison of the postoperative MR imaging with prior images is important.
- Postoperative MR imaging findings should be interpreted with caution and in correlation with clinical findings and implications.

DISCLOSURE

The authors have nothing to disclose.

REFERENCES

1. Mall NA, Chalmers PN, Moric M, et al. Incidence and trends of anterior cruciate ligament reconstruction in the United States. Am J Sports Med 2014;42(10): 2363–70.
2. Giaconi JC, Allen CR, Steinbach LS. Anterior cruciate ligament graft reconstruction: clinical, technical, and imaging overview. Top Magn Reson Imaging 2009;20(3):129–50.
3. Lohmander LS, Ostenberg A, Englund M, et al. High prevalence of knee osteoarthritis, pain, and functional limitations in female soccer players twelve years after anterior cruciate ligament injury. Arthritis Rheum 2004;50(10):3145–52.
4. Barenius B, Ponzer S, Shalabi A, et al. Increased risk of osteoarthritis after anterior cruciate ligament reconstruction: a 14-year follow-up study of a randomized controlled trial. Am J Sports Med 2014; 42(5):1049–57.
5. Cheung EC, DiLallo M, Feeley BT, et al. Osteoarthritis and ACL reconstruction-myths and risks. Curr Rev Musculoskelet Med 2020;13(1):115–22.

6. Crawford SN, Waterman BR, Lubowitz JH. Long-term failure of anterior cruciate ligament reconstruction. Arthroscopy 2013;29(9):1566–71.

7. Lind M, Menhert F, Pedersen AB. The first results from the Danish ACL reconstruction registry: epidemiologic and 2 year follow-up results from 5,818 knee ligament reconstructions. Knee Surg Sports Traumatol Arthrosc 2009;17(2):117–24.

8. Bencardino JT, Beltran J, Feldman MI, et al. MR imaging of complications of anterior cruciate ligament graft reconstruction. Radiographics 2009;29(7):2115–26.

9. Papakonstantinou O, Chung CB, Chanchairujira K, et al. Complications of anterior cruciate ligament reconstruction: MR imaging. Eur Radiol 2003;13(5):1106–17.

10. Svantesson E, Hamrin Senorski E, Kristiansson F, et al. Comparison of concomitant injuries and patient-reported outcome in patients that have undergone both primary and revision ACL reconstruction-a national registry study. J Orthop Surg Res 2020;15(1):9.

11. Grassi A, Kim C, Marcheggiani Muccioli GM, et al. What is the mid-term failure rate of revision acl reconstruction? A systematic review. Clin Orthop Relat Res 2017;475(10):2484–99.

12. Skendzel JG, Sekiya JK, Wojtys EM. Diagnosis and management of the multiligament-injured knee. J Orthop Sports Phys Ther 2012;42(3):234–42.

13. Rispoli DM, Sanders TG, Miller MD, et al. Magnetic resonance imaging at different time periods following hamstring harvest for anterior cruciate ligament reconstruction. Arthroscopy 2001;17(1):2–8.

14. Aglietti P, Buzzi R, Zaccherotti G, et al. Patellar tendon versus doubled semitendinosus and gracilis tendons for anterior cruciate ligament reconstruction. Am J Sports Med 1994;22(2):211–7 [discussion: 217-8].

15. Samuelsen BT, Webster KE, Johnson NR, et al. Hamstring Autograft versus Patellar Tendon Autograft for ACL Reconstruction: Is There a Difference in Graft Failure Rate? A Meta-analysis of 47,613 Patients. Clin Orthop Relat Res 2017;475(10):2459–68.

16. Xie X, Liu X, Chen Z, et al. A meta-analysis of bone-patellar tendon-bone autograft versus four-strand hamstring tendon autograft for anterior cruciate ligament reconstruction. Knee 2015;22(2):100–10.

17. Goetz G, de Villiers C, Sadoghi P, et al. Allograft for anterior cruciate ligament reconstruction (ACLR): a systematic review and meta-analysis of long-term comparative effectiveness and safety. results of a health technology assessment. Arthrosc Sports Med Rehabil 2020;2(6):e873–91.

18. Dhammi IK, Rehan Ul H, Kumar S. Graft choices for anterior cruciate ligament reconstruction. Indian J Orthop 2015;49(2):127–8.

19. Oh JY, Kim KT, Park YJ, et al. Biomechanical comparison of single-bundle versus double-bundle anterior cruciate ligament reconstruction: a meta-analysis. Knee Surg Relat Res 2020;32(1):14.

20. Chouliaras V, Ristanis S, Moraiti C, et al. Effectiveness of reconstruction of the anterior cruciate ligament with quadrupled hamstrings and bone-patellar tendon-bone autografts: an in vivo study comparing tibial internal-external rotation. Am J Sports Med 2007;35(2):189–96.

21. Casagranda BU, Maxwell NJ, Kavanagh EC, et al. Normal appearance and complications of double-bundle and selective-bundle anterior cruciate ligament reconstructions using optimal MRI techniques. AJR Am J Roentgenol 2009;192(5):1407–15.

22. Poellinger A, Scheffler S, Hamm B, et al. Magnetic resonance imaging of double-bundle anterior cruciate ligament reconstruction. Skeletal Radiol 2009;38(4):309–15.

23. Kiekara T, Järvelä T, Huhtala H, et al. MRI of double-bundle ACL reconstruction: evaluation of graft findings. Skeletal Radiol 2012;41(7):835–42.

24. Sonoda M, Morikawa T, Tsuchiya K, et al. Correlation between knee laxity and graft appearance on magnetic resonance imaging after double-bundle hamstring graft anterior cruciate ligament reconstruction. Am J Sports Med 2007;35(6):936–42.

25. Vogl TJ, Schmitt J, Lubrich J, et al. Reconstructed anterior cruciate ligaments using patellar tendon ligament grafts: diagnostic value of contrast-enhanced MRI in a 2-year follow-up regimen. Eur Radiol 2001;11(8):1450–6.

26. Howell SM, Clark JA, Blasier RD. Serial magnetic resonance imaging of hamstring anterior cruciate ligament autografts during the first year of implantation. A preliminary study. Am J Sports Med 1991;19(1):42–7.

27. Ramos DM, Dhandapani R, Subramanian A, et al. Clinical complications of biodegradable screws for ligament injuries. Mater Sci Eng C Mater Biol Appl 2020;109:110423.

28. Wan F, Chen T, Ge Y, et al. Effect of nearly isometric ACL reconstruction on graft-tunnel motion: a quantitative clinical study. Orthop J Sports Med 2019;7(12). https://doi.org/10.1177/2325967119890382.

29. Duc SR, Zanetti M, Kramer J, et al. Magnetic resonance imaging of anterior cruciate ligament tears: evaluation of standard orthogonal and tailored paracoronal images. Acta Radiol 2005;46(7):729–33.

30. Katahira K, Yamashita Y, Takahashi M, et al. MR imaging of the anterior cruciate ligament: value of thin slice direct oblique coronal technique. Radiat Med 2001;19(1):1–7.

31. Ahn JH, Lee SH, Yoo JC, et al. Measurement of the graft angles for the anterior cruciate ligament reconstruction with transtibial technique using postoperative magnetic resonance imaging in comparative study. Knee Surg Sports Traumatol Arthrosc 2007;15(11):1293–300.

32. Fujimoto E, Sumen Y, Deie M, et al. Anterior cruciate ligament graft impingement against the posterior cruciate ligament: diagnosis using MRI plus three-dimensional reconstruction software. Magn Reson Imaging 2004;22(8):1125–9.

33. Pearle AD, Shannon FJ, Granchi C, et al. Comparison of 3-dimensional obliquity and anisometric characteristics of anterior cruciate ligament graft positions using surgical navigation. Am J Sports Med 2008;36(8):1534–41.

34. Steckel H, Vadala G, Davis D, et al. 2D and 3D 3-tesla magnetic resonance imaging of the double bundle structure in anterior cruciate ligament anatomy. Knee Surg Sports Traumatol Arthrosc 2006; 14(11):1151–8.

35. Ayerza MA, Muscolo DL, Costa-Paz M, et al. Comparison of sagittal obliquity of the reconstructed anterior cruciate ligament with native anterior cruciate ligament using magnetic resonance imaging. Arthroscopy 2003;19(3):257–61.

36. Hosseini A, Lodhia P, Van de Velde SK, et al. Tunnel position and graft orientation in failed anterior cruciate ligament reconstruction: a clinical and imaging analysis. Int Orthop 2012;36(4):845–52.

37. Forsythe B, Kopf S, Wong AK, et al. The location of femoral and tibial tunnels in anatomic double-bundle anterior cruciate ligament reconstruction analyzed by three-dimensional computed tomography models. J Bone Joint Surg Am 2010;92(6):1418–26.

38. Marchant BG, Noyes FR, Barber-Westin SD, et al. Prevalence of nonanatomical graft placement in a series of failed anterior cruciate ligament reconstructions. Am J Sports Med 2010;38(10):1987–96.

39. Howell SM. Principles for placing the tibial tunnel and avoiding roof impingement during reconstruction of a torn anterior cruciate ligament. Knee Surg Sports Traumatol Arthrosc 1998;6(Suppl 1):S49–55.

40. Morgan CD, Kalman VR, Grawl DM. Definitive landmarks for reproducible tibial tunnel placement in anterior cruciate ligament reconstruction. Arthroscopy 1995;11(3):275–88.

41. Steiner ME, Battaglia TC, Heming JF, et al. Independent drilling outperforms conventional transtibial drilling in anterior cruciate ligament reconstruction. Am J Sports Med 2009;37(10):1912–9.

42. Arnold MP, Kooloos J, van Kampen A. Single-incision technique misses the anatomical femoral anterior cruciate ligament insertion: a cadaver study. Knee Surg Sports Traumatol Arthrosc 2001;9(4):194–9.

43. Andriacchi TP, Briant PL, Bevill SL, et al. Rotational changes at the knee after ACL injury cause cartilage thinning. Clin Orthop Relat Res 2006;442:39–44.

44. Busam ML, Provencher MT, Bach BR Jr. Complications of anterior cruciate ligament reconstruction with bone-patellar tendon-bone constructs: care and prevention. Am J Sports Med 2008;36(2):379–94.

45. George MS, Dunn WR, Spindler KP. Current concepts review: revision anterior cruciate ligament reconstruction. Am J Sports Med 2006;34(12):2026–37.

46. Lubowitz JH. Anteromedial portal technique for the anterior cruciate ligament femoral socket: pitfalls and solutions. Arthroscopy 2009;25(1):95–101.

47. Marwan Y, Böttcher J, Laverdière C, et al. Three-dimensional magnetic resonance imaging for guiding tibial and femoral tunnel position in anterior cruciate ligament reconstruction: a cadaveric study. Orthop J Sports Med 2020;8(3). https://doi.org/10.1177/2325967120909913.

48. Claes S, Verdonk P, Forsyth R, et al. The "ligamentization" process in anterior cruciate ligament reconstruction: what happens to the human graft? A systematic review of the literature. Am J Sports Med 2011;39(11):2476–83.

49. Rougraff B, Shelbourne KD, Gerth PK, et al. Arthroscopic and histologic analysis of human patellar tendon autografts used for anterior cruciate ligament reconstruction. Am J Sports Med 1993;21(2):277–84.

50. Rougraff BT, Shelbourne KD. Early histologic appearance of human patellar tendon autografts used for anterior cruciate ligament reconstruction. Knee Surg Sports Traumatol Arthrosc 1999;7(1):9–14.

51. Sanchez M, Anitua E, Azofra J, et al. Ligamentization of tendon grafts treated with an endogenous preparation rich in growth factors: gross morphology and histology. Arthroscopy 2010;26(4):470–80.

52. Jansson KA, Harilainen A, Sandelin J, et al. Bone tunnel enlargement after anterior cruciate ligament reconstruction with the hamstring autograft and endobutton fixation technique. A clinical, radiographic and magnetic resonance imaging study with 2 years follow-up. Knee Surg Sports Traumatol Arthrosc 1999;7(5):290–5.

53. Zhang S, Liu S, Yang L, et al. Morphological Changes of the Femoral Tunnel and Their Correlation With Hamstring Tendon Autograft Maturation up to 2 Years After Anterior Cruciate Ligament Reconstruction Using Femoral Cortical Suspension. Am J Sports Med 2020;48(3):554–64.

54. Panos JA, Webster KE, Hewett TE. Anterior cruciate ligament grafts display differential maturation patterns on magnetic resonance imaging following reconstruction: a systematic review. Knee Surg Sports Traumatol Arthrosc 2020;28(7):2124–38.

55. Wright RW, Gill CS, Chen L, et al. Outcome of revision anterior cruciate ligament reconstruction: a systematic review. J Bone Joint Surg Am 2012;94(6):531–6.

56. Janarv PM, Nystrom A, Werner S, et al. Anterior cruciate ligament injuries in skeletally immature patients. J Pediatr Orthop 1996;16(5):673–7.

57. Souryal TO, Freeman TR. Intercondylar notch size and anterior cruciate ligament injuries in athletes. A prospective study. Am J Sports Med 1993;21(4):535–9.

58. McCarthy CJ, Harty JA. Follow-up study on transphyseal ACL reconstruction in Irish adolescents with no cases of leg length discrepancy or angular deformity. Ir J Med Sci 2020;189(4):1323–9.

59. Collins MS, Unruh KP, Bond JR, et al. Magnetic resonance imaging of surgically confirmed anterior cruciate ligament graft disruption. Skeletal Radiol 2008;37(3):233–43.

60. Saupe N, White LM, Chiavaras MM, et al. Anterior cruciate ligament reconstruction grafts: MR imaging features at long-term follow-up–correlation with functional and clinical evaluation. Radiology 2008; 249(2):581–90.

61. van Eck CF, Kropf EJ, Romanowski JR, et al. ACL graft re-rupture after double-bundle reconstruction: factors that influence the intra-articular pattern of injury. Knee Surg Sports Traumatol Arthrosc 2011; 19(3):340–6.

62. Teraoka T, Hashimoto Y, Takahashi S, et al. The relationship between graft intensity on MRI and tibial tunnel placement in anatomical double-bundle ACL reconstruction. Eur J Orthop Surg Traumatol 2019;29(8):1749–58.

63. Naraghi AM, Gupta S, Jacks LM, et al. Anterior cruciate ligament reconstruction: MR imaging signs of anterior knee laxity in the presence of an intact graft. Radiology 2012;263(3):802–10.

64. Viala P, Marchand P, Lecouvet F, et al. Imaging of the postoperative knee. Diagn Interv Imaging 2016; 97(7–8):823–37.

65. Van der Bracht H, Bellemans J, Victor J, et al. Can a tibial tunnel in ACL surgery be placed anatomically without impinging on the femoral notch? A risk factor analysis. Knee Surg Sports Traumatol Arthrosc 2014;22(2):291–7.

66. Facchetti L, Schwaiger BJ, Gersing AS, et al. Cyclops lesions detected by MRI are frequent findings after ACL surgical reconstruction but do not impact clinical outcome over 2 years. Eur Radiol 2017;27(8):3499–508.

67. Simpfendorfer C, Miniaci A, Subhas N, et al. Pseudocyclops: two cases of ACL graft partial tears mimicking cyclops lesions on MRI. Skeletal Radiol 2015;44(8):1169–73.

68. Zappia M, Capasso R, Berritto D, et al. Anterior cruciate ligament reconstruction: MR imaging findings. Musculoskelet Surg 2017;101(Suppl 1):23–35.

69. Pelfort X, Monllau JC, Puig L, et al. Iliotibial band friction syndrome after anterior cruciate ligament reconstruction using the transfix device: report of two cases and review of the literature. Knee Surg Sports Traumatol Arthrosc 2006;14(6):586–9.

70. Fauno P, Kaalund S. Tunnel widening after hamstring anterior cruciate ligament reconstruction is influenced by the type of graft fixation used: a prospective randomized study. Arthroscopy 2005; 21(11):1337–41.

71. Struewer J, Efe T, Frangen TM, et al. Prevalence and influence of tibial tunnel widening after isolated anterior cruciate ligament reconstruction using patella-bone-tendon-bone-graft: long-term follow-up. Orthop Rev (Pavia) 2012;4(2):e21.

72. Peyrache MD, Djian P, Christel P, et al. Tibial tunnel enlargement after anterior cruciate ligament reconstruction by autogenous bone-patellar tendon-bone graft. Knee Surg Sports Traumatol Arthrosc 1996; 4(1):2–8.

73. Ghazikhanian V, Beltran J, Nikac V, et al. Tibial tunnel and pretibial cysts following ACL graft reconstruction: MR imaging diagnosis. Skeletal Radiol 2012; 41(11):1375–9.

74. Deie M, Sumen Y, Ochi M, et al. Pretibial cyst formation after anterior cruciate ligament reconstruction using auto hamstring grafts: two case reports in a prospective study of 89 cases. Magn Reson Imaging 2000;18(8):973–7.

75. Peskun CJ, Whelan DB. Outcomes of operative and nonoperative treatment of multiligament knee injuries: an evidence-based review. Sports Med Arthrosc Rev 2011;19(2):167–73.

76. Ng JWG, Myint Y, Ali FM. Management of multiligament knee injuries. EFORT Open Rev 2020;5(3): 145–55.

77. Medina O, Arom GA, Yeranosian MG, et al. Vascular and nerve injury after knee dislocation: a systematic review. Clin Orthop Relat Res 2014;472(9):2621–9.

78. Samson D, Ng CY, Power D. An evidence-based algorithm for the management of common peroneal nerve injury associated with traumatic knee dislocation. EFORT Open Rev 2016;1(10):362–7.

79. Levy BA, Dajani KA, Whelan DB, et al. Decision making in the multiligament-injured knee: an evidence-based systematic review. Arthroscopy 2009;25(4):430–8.

80. Sims WF, Jacobson KE. The posteromedial corner of the knee: medial-sided injury patterns revisited. Am J Sports Med 2004;32(2):337–45.

81. Tibor LM, Marchant MH Jr, Taylor DC, et al. Management of medial-sided knee injuries, part 2: posteromedial corner. Am J Sports Med 2011;39(6):1332–40.

82. Laprade RF, Griffith CJ, Coobs BR, et al. Improving outcomes for posterolateral knee injuries. J Orthop Res 2014;32(4):485–91.

83. Alcalá-Galiano A, Baeva M, Ismael M, et al. Imaging of posterior cruciate ligament (PCL) reconstruction: normal postsurgical appearance and complications. Skeletal Radiol 2014;43(12):1659–68.

84. Narvy SJ, Pearl M, Vrla M, et al. Anatomy of the femoral footprint of the posterior cruciate ligament: a systematic review. Arthroscopy 2015;31(2): 345–54.

85. Parkar AP, Alcala-Galiano A. Rupture of the posterior cruciate ligament: preoperative and postoperative assessment. Semin Musculoskelet Radiol 2016; 20(1):43–51.

86. Lee YS, Ra HJ, Ahn JH, et al. Posterior cruciate ligament tibial insertion anatomy and implications for tibial tunnel placement. Arthroscopy 2011;27(2): 182–7.

87. Park HJ, Lee SY, Choi YJ, et al. The usefulness of the oblique coronal plane of three-dimensional isotropic T2-weighted fast spin-echo (VISTA) knee MRI in the evaluation of posterior cruciate ligament reconstruction with allograft: comparison with the oblique coronal plane of two-dimensional fast spin-echo T2-weighted sequences. Eur J Radiol 2019;114:105–10.

88. Park HJ, Lee SY, Chung EC, et al. The usefulness of the oblique coronal plane in knee MRI on the evaluation of the posterior cruciate ligament. Acta Radiol 2014;55(8):961–8.

89. Chiang LY, Lee CH, Tong KM, et al. Posterior cruciate ligament reconstruction implemented by the Ligament Advanced Reinforcement System over a minimum follow-up of 10 years. Knee 2020;27(1): 165–72.

90. Vaquero-Picado A, Rodriguez-Merchan EC. Isolated posterior cruciate ligament tears: an update of management. EFORT Open Rev 2017;2(4):89–96.

Postoperative MR Imaging of the Knee Meniscus

Mariam A. Malik, MD*, Jonathan C. Baker, MD

KEYWORDS

- Meniscus • Postoperative knee • Meniscus repair • Meniscectomy • MR arthrography

KEY POINTS

- Diagnostic imaging of the postoperative knee can be difficult to interpret, but understanding treatment techniques and expected postoperative findings can help to improve diagnostic accuracy.
- Conventional MR imaging is often performed in patients with recurrent knee pain after meniscectomy, whereas direct MR arthrography is preferred by many clinicians to evaluate the meniscus after repair.
- Recurrent tear can be diagnosed with confidence based on (1) fluid signal intensity or gadolinium imbibition within a meniscus remnant, (2) a displaced fragment, or (3) a tear at a different site from the original injury.

INTRODUCTION

Meniscus tears are common knee injuries resulting from trauma or degeneration, and often require operative treatment due to pain or mechanical symptoms. Although success rates for operative treatment of meniscal tears are high, some patients will develop new, recurrent, or persistent symptoms after meniscus surgery. Imaging techniques to evaluate symptomatic patients following meniscus surgery include conventional noncontrast MR imaging, direct MR arthrography (DMRA), indirect MR arthrography (IMRA), and computed tomography arthrography. This article focuses on MR imaging assessment. Criteria for the diagnosis of a native meniscus tear include the presence of a displaced flap, abnormal morphology, or abnormal intrameniscal signal intensity contacting an articular surface. The latter 2 features are often seen as expected findings in an intact postoperative meniscus, making evaluation of the postoperative meniscus on MR imaging a diagnostic challenge for the radiologist. This article aims to review the normal anatomy and clinical treatment of meniscus tears, to outline the advantages and disadvantages of various MR imaging techniques, and to highlight with surgically proven cases the normal and abnormal MR imaging appearance of the postoperative meniscus.

MENISCUS ANATOMY, STRUCTURE, AND FUNCTION

The menisci are C-shaped fibrocartilaginous structures whose primary functions include weight-bearing and redistribution of axial forces at the knee joint, providing stability to the knee joint, and protecting the hyaline articular cartilage. The menisci are composed of peripheral circumferential collagen fibers that provide hoop strength, interwoven with radially oriented collagen fibers. Meniscus-deficient knees are at increased risk of developing premature osteoarthritis, secondary to increased contact pressures on the hyaline articular cartilage.[1]

After the age of 10 years, only the outer 10% to 30% of the meniscus remains vascularized (the "red zone," so named for its ruddy appearance at arthroscopy), receiving blood supply from branches of the geniculate arteries.[1,2] Because of this blood supply in the peripheral zone of the meniscus, tears in the outer portion may heal after suture repair. In contrast, the inner portion of the

Musculoskeletal Section, Mallinckrodt Institute of Radiology, 510 South Kingshighway Boulevard, Campus Box 8131, Saint Louis, MO 63110, USA
* Corresponding author.
E-mail address: malikm@wustl.edu

Magn Reson Imaging Clin N Am 30 (2022) 723–731
https://doi.org/10.1016/j.mric.2022.02.005
1064-9689/22/© 2022 Elsevier Inc. All rights reserved.

mri.theclinics.com

menisci (the "white zone") in adults is avascular and aneural.[3] This inner portion receives nutrition from synovial fluid. White zone tears will not heal with suture repair, and surgical treatment involves resection of the injured tissue. Studies have shown that within the meniscus there is zonal variation of matrix, density, and phenotype of meniscus cells. The inner portion contains more proteoglycan content and chondrocytes than the peripheral zone, which contains more of the fibroblastic cell type.[3] When compared with articular cartilage, the meniscus fibrocartilage has a higher collagen content, and lower proteoglycan and water content.[4]

TREATMENT OF MENISCUS TEARS

Current approaches to treating meniscus tears include nonoperative management, meniscus repair, meniscus resection (meniscectomy), and meniscus allograft transplant. The foremost goals of surgery are to relieve pain and optimize or restore the function of the knee. Total meniscectomy was performed in the past until surgeons recognized the association between removal of the entire meniscus and the high rate of postmeniscectomy osteoarthritis (**Fig. 1**). Subsequent studies have revealed a direct correlation between the amount of meniscus tissue removed and the rate of subsequent osteoarthritis. For this reason, current surgical approaches aim for meniscus preservation. Although surgical treatment may not provide long-term benefits to patients with degenerated knees, arthroscopic surgery remains a common form of treatment for meniscal tear. There are nearly 1 million meniscus surgeries performed in the United States each year.[5]

The overall condition of the injured meniscus as well as the location and type of tear determine whether a torn meniscus can be repaired, or will require partial resection or transplant. Factors associated with improved healing include tear acuity, patient age less than 30 years, shorter tear length (<25 mm), tear of the lateral meniscus, and concurrent anterior cruciate ligament (ACL) reconstruction. The medial meniscus is more tightly fixed than the lateral meniscus, and the decreased mobility of the medial meniscus makes it more susceptible to injury and tear. Knees with persistent ACL instability have a higher rate of repair failure. Concurrent ACL reconstruction is thought to promote a healing environment and is associated with improved healing of the torn meniscus.[6] Other techniques that stimulate healing include mechanical trephination to increase bleeding, synovial abrasion, and the application of fibrin clot or platelet-rich plasma.[1,7]

Each type of surgical approach results in different expected postoperative changes, detailed later. Understanding the differences in operative techniques is helpful to identify the expected postoperative changes on imaging.

Meniscus Repair

Whenever possible, arthroscopic repair is preferred over meniscectomy to preserve as much meniscus function as possible, and to forestall the development of premature degenerative osteoarthritis. Stein and colleagues found that at an average of nearly 9-year follow-up, 81% of patients with prior meniscus repair showed no radiographic signs of arthritis. This was significantly better than the 40% of patients in the meniscectomy group that showed no radiographic signs of arthritis.[8] The current trend demonstrates an increasing number of meniscus repairs, particularly in the young adult and adolescent patient populations.[9] A variety of surgical procedures have been devised to repair the torn meniscus, using sutures, darts, or arrows to reapproximate the torn edges of the meniscus via arthroscopic techniques that involve inside-out, outside-in, or all-inside approaches.[1] When the appropriate technique is applied to repair the torn meniscus, modern inside-out and all-inside repairs have a 90% success rate.[6,9] Even posterior root tears, which are functionally equivalent to a total meniscectomy, can be treated by side-to-side repair, suture anchors, or the transtibial pull-out repair. Posterior root tears are particularly important to recognize and treat due to the high risk for osteoarthritis in the affected compartment, resulting from loss of hoop strength when the meniscus posterior root is detached from its anchor at the tibia.[1]

Meniscus Resection

Maximal preservation of the meniscus tissue is imperative to maintain function, particularly of the peripheral fibers that provide hoop strength. However, many meniscus tears involving the inner margin or white zone are not amenable to repair. In these cases, partial meniscectomy is performed. The aim of arthroscopic partial meniscectomy is to remove the unstable meniscus tissue using a biter or shaver and to recontour the meniscus remnant to a stable structure, while minimizing the amount of resected tissue.[1] Although rates of meniscus repair are increasing, rates of partial meniscectomy are not changing significantly, and the latter procedure is still more commonly performed than repair.[9] The large majority of partial meniscectomies involve the posterior horn.[6]

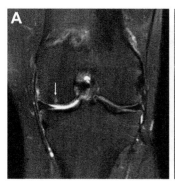
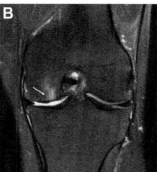

Fig. 1. 54-year-old man with 1-year history of medial left knee pain, swelling, and catching at initial presentation. (*A*) Coronal T2 fat-saturated image of the left knee at the time of initial presentation shows a small focus of subchondral edema and mild chondrosis along the medial femoral condyle (*white arrow*). (*B*) Coronal T2 fat-saturated image shows changes of interval partial meniscectomy, with progressive chondrosis and subchondral edema along the medial femoral condyle (*white arrow*).

Meniscus Replacement

Meniscus replacement using allograft transplantation is much less common than meniscus repair and partial meniscectomy. However, good outcomes are reported in more than 80% of patients.[3,10] Meniscus allografting can be considered for treatment of younger patients (<50 years) who have failed conservative measures. Allograft transplant is reserved for patients who have a stable knee joint with normal mechanical axis, normal articular cartilage or low-grade chondrosis, and either a large meniscus tear not amenable to repair or subtotal meniscectomy with persistent pain in the knee.[1,6] Allograft transplant has been shown to improve pain and activity level, and may hasten return to play for amateur and professional athletes.[1,11] Obesity is considered a contraindication to meniscus transplantation.[6] In allograft transplantation, the donor meniscus is harvested from a cadaveric knee. The meniscus remains attached to a tibial bone plug that includes the anterior and posterior root attachments. This is transferred en bloc to the recipient knee, where a matching slot has been carved in the tibia to accommodate the donor bone plug. Sutures are used to sew the grafted meniscus to the capsule of the recipient knee. Of note, synthetic grafts and augmentation are currently limited to investigational research trials in the United States, and use is not yet approved by the Food and Drug Administration. These will not be covered in the current review.

IMAGING FINDINGS OF MENISCUS TEAR

In native (nonoperated) knees, MR imaging has proven to be valuable for the diagnosis and characterization of meniscus injuries, with high sensitivity, specificity, and accuracy (approximately 85%–90%).[12,13] Three main MR imaging features are used to diagnose a native meniscus tear. The first is a displaced flap of meniscus tissue. The second criterion is abnormal morphology of the meniscus, consisting of truncation, blunting, or other surface irregularity that disturbs the normally well-defined "bowtie" appearance of the meniscus body and the sharp triangles formed by the anterior and posterior horns when seen in cross-section. The final criterion is the presence of increased intrameniscal signal intensity that unequivocally extends to an articular surface on short echo time (TE; proton density [PD] or T1-weighted) images, so-called surfacing signal.[12] When this abnormal signal intensity in a meniscus is identified on 2 consecutive images, or on one slice in 2 separate orthogonal planes such as sagittal and coronal images—the "two slice touch rule"—the positive predictive value for diagnosing tear is improved.[14] In the preoperative knee, these criteria allow for greater than 90% accuracy, and 85% to 95% specificity and sensitivity.[15]

MR IMAGING TECHNIQUES FOR ASSESSING THE POSTOPERATIVE MENISCUS
Conventional MR Imaging

Conventional MR imaging is often ordered by the treating physician to assess patients with knee pain after meniscus surgery. Conventional MR imaging relies on PD and fluid-sensitive, fat-suppressed sequences in multiple planes for the detection of recurrent meniscus tear. The advantages of conventional MR imaging include widespread availability, no need for an intravenous or intra-articular injection, the resulting lack of risks of joint infection and allergic reaction due to use of gadolinium-based contrast agents injected into the joint or intravenously, as well as the lower cost and shorter study acquisition time compared with DMRA and IMRA. Applegate and colleagues reported 66% accuracy in the diagnosis of recurrent meniscus tear by conventional MR imaging, compared with 88% by DMRA. Small partial meniscectomies (involving resection of <25% of the meniscus) are more common than larger partial meniscectomies or meniscus repair. Studies show that there is no significant benefit to MR arthrography in identifying recurrent tear when a <25% partial meniscectomy has been performed, with reported 89% accuracy in the diagnosis of recurrent tear on both conventional MR and MR arthrography. However, when the criteria for meniscus tear in the native knee is applied to a postoperative knee, which has undergone partial meniscectomy of greater than 25%, the diagnostic accuracy by conventional MR imaging falls to 65%, compared with 87% on MR arthrography.[16]

Direct MR Arthrography

DMRA refers to the intra-articular injection of dilute gadolinium contrast material into the knee joint before MR examination. The authors note that although the intra-articular administration of dilute gadolinium contrast is widely accepted and used, it is considered to be off-label use by the US Food and Drug Administration. Our preferred DMRA technique is to inject the knee joint capsule with 30 to 50 mL of a 1:200 dilution of gadolinium in sterile saline. The injection of dilute gadolinium into the joint distends the joint capsule, thereby separating and better outlining the intra-articular structures. The injectate also reduces the viscosity of the joint fluid, promoting the imbibition or uptake of contrast agent into a torn meniscus to highlight the tear. In addition, MR arthrography uses T1-weighted images to great advantage, with a higher signal-to-noise ratio and greater spatial resolution.[12] Some radiologists prefer DMRA to conventional MR imaging in the evaluation of meniscus repair for these reasons. Disadvantages include the potential risk of septic arthritis, allergic reaction, patient discomfort, cost, exposure to ionizing radiation if fluoroscopy is used to guide injection, and increased physician time to perform the injection.

Indirect MR Arthrography

With IMRA, gadolinium contrast agent is given intravenously. The patient then exercises the knee before the MR examination, with a 60–90 minute delay between injection and image acquisition. IMRA depends on the physiologic excretion of intravascular gadolinium by synovial cells into the joint. MR images show preferential contrast enhancement in areas of hyperemia, including sites of meniscus injury and tear.[17] Hyperemia can also be related to healed granulation tissue within a postoperative meniscus, which could lead to false-positive diagnosis.[18] IMRA is less commonly used but is a less invasive alternative

to DMRA. Physician time and fluoroscopy equipment are not required for indirect arthrography, as the technologist can administer the contrast independently.

INTERPRETING POSTOPERATIVE MR IMAGING OF THE MENISCUS

The variable MR imaging appearance of the postoperative meniscus may confound the accurate diagnosis of recurrent tear. Second-look arthroscopy is considered the gold standard for the diagnosis of recurrent meniscus tear, but MR imaging is usually performed first as a less invasive alternative. For the radiologist, comparison with prior imaging and operative reports can be immensely helpful to ascertain the original tear location and type, as well as to establish the type of procedure performed and the operative findings. In general, the MR imaging findings of a recurrent tear in the postoperative meniscus include any of the following: (1) displaced meniscus fragment, (2) abnormal signal extending to an articular surface at a different site from the original tear, or (3) fluid signal intensity on T2-weighted sequences or gadolinium uptake and T1 signal hyperintensity on DMRA T1-weighted, fat-suppressed sequences within the meniscus at the site of repair.[12] These features are discussed in detail in the following sections for the scenarios of partial meniscectomy, meniscus repair, and transplant.

Partial meniscectomy

A healed partial meniscectomy will display a truncated contour on postoperative MR imaging (**Figs. 2 and 3**). Diminutive morphology of the meniscus on MR imaging is a clue for partial resection. The margins should be smooth, including along the truncated edge. After a partial meniscectomy of more than 25%, the absence of a portion of the meniscus is more readily identifiable, and the remnant will appear blunted.

Irregular margins, abnormal morphology, and short TE signal abnormalities extending to the articular surface of the remnant meniscus can be seen in both healed and torn meniscal remnants. This decreases the specificity of these findings and may complicate the interpretation. Abnormal signal extending to the articular surface on short TE images is commonly seen, but a similar finding on T2-weighted images raises diagnostic accuracy for recurrent tear. Abnormally high T2 signal intensity within a fluid cleft of a torn meniscus is a specific but not sensitive characteristic of a recurrent tear.[12]

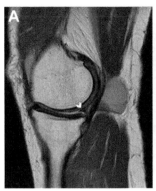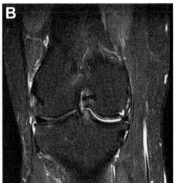

Fig. 2. 48-year-old woman with pain in the right knee after remote partial medial meniscectomy. (*A, B*) Sagittal PD and coronal T2 fat-saturated images show abnormal morphology and small size of the medial meniscus body and posterior horn, representing changes of prior partial meniscectomy (*arrowhead*). The borders of the meniscus are smooth, and there is no evidence of intrasubstance signal extending to an articular surface.

If the surgical history is unknown and the meniscus appears blunted, a displaced meniscus fragment should be sought. Medially, common locations for displaced fragments are in the medial gutter adjacent to the body, or in the posterior notch near the posterior cruciate ligament. Laterally, displaced fragments are frequently observed in the lateral gutter adjacent to the body, or posteriorly in the popliteal hiatus. Secondary findings on MR imaging that indicate prior surgery may be helpful to determine the significance of meniscus findings. These include small foci of susceptibility artifact from microscopic metallic fragments, focal thickening of the patellar tendon, or linear, low signal scarring in the Hoffa fat pad at the site of arthroscopy portals.[6]

Meniscus repair

A healed meniscus repair will maintain the normal meniscus morphology and will typically display intrameniscal signal hyperintensity at the repair site on short TE sequences that is lower intensity than joint fluid. On DMRA, the healed repair will not demonstrate gadolinium uptake on fat-suppressed T1-weighted sequences, a key finding that enables distinction of a healed repair from an unhealed repair or recurrent tear, both of which imbibe gadolinium (**Figs. 4 and 5**).

After meniscus repair, increased signal intensity extending to the articular surface is a common finding on short TE images and is attributed to granulation or fibrovascular tissue. This is

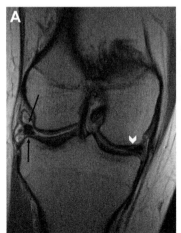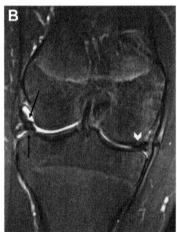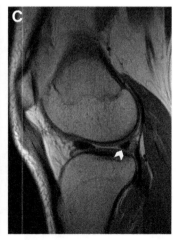

Fig. 3. 16-year-old girl with recurrent pain in the right knee after a cheerleading injury that occurred 6 weeks after partial meniscectomy and repair of the medial meniscus, and partial meniscectomy of the lateral meniscus. (*A*) Coronal PD image of the right knee shows a diminutive medial meniscus (*white arrowhead*) and abnormal morphology of the lateral meniscus (*black arrows*). The edges of both menisci are smooth. There is no abnormal intrasubstance signal. (*B*) Coronal T2 fat-saturated image shows abnormal morphology and size of the medial (*white arrowhead*) and lateral menisci (*black arrows*), with smooth borders that reflect prior partial meniscectomies. (*C*) Sagittal PD image of the lateral meniscus shows diminutive size of the posterior horn lateral meniscus reflecting prior partial meniscectomy, and intermediate T2 signal from prior meniscus repair (*arrowhead*).

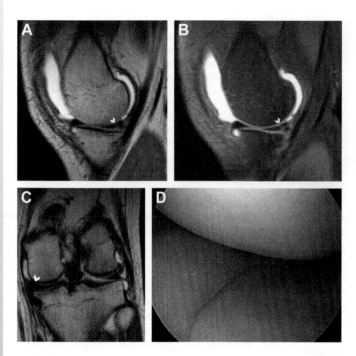

Fig. 4. 21-year-old woman with a history of prior medial meniscus repair and ACL reconstruction 4 months prior, who underwent direct MR arthrography and arthroscopy for evaluation of the cruciate graft and arthrofibrosis. (*A*) Sagittal PD image of the medial meniscus shows evidence of prior posterior horn meniscus repair (*arrowhead*). (*B*, *C*) Sagittal T1 fat-saturated and coronal T1 images from MR arthrogram show no contrast imbibition into the medial meniscus (*arrowhead*). (*D*) Arthroscopic image shows intact medial meniscus repair.

particularly pronounced in the first 12 weeks after surgery but can be seen in postoperative menisci even after more than 10 years.[3,19] The presence of a high T2 signal (equal to fluid, or greater than the signal of hyaline cartilage) increases sensitivity for identifying retear on nonarthrographic MR imaging, in the setting of meniscus repair.[20] Similar to the case of partial meniscectomy, the identification of either a displaced fragment or a signal abnormality in a new location within the repaired meniscus increases the diagnostic accuracy for retear, with up to 100% specificity (**Fig. 6**).[6,20]

Recurrent tear after repair can also be detected by the extension of gadolinium into the tear, based on the presence of a high T1 signal equal to that of

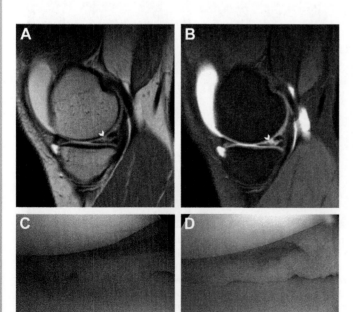

Fig. 5. 18-year-old girl with recurrent injury and medial right knee pain after prior partial meniscectomy 2 years prior. (*A*, *B*) Sagittal PD and T1 fat-saturated images demonstrate abnormal signals within the posterior horn medial meniscus, representing recurrent tear (*arrowhead*). (*C*, *D*) Arthroscopic images demonstrate recurrent tear before (*C*) and after (*D*) suture removal from prior repair.

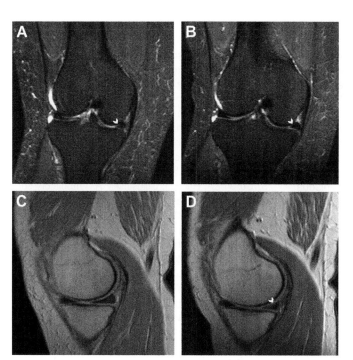

Fig. 6. 58-year-old woman with recurrent pain and occasional catching in the medial right knee after medial meniscus repair 3 years prior. (A, B) Coronal T2 fat-saturated images of the right knee demonstrate initial tear of the body of the medial meniscus (A) and healed meniscus repair 3 years later (B). (C, D) Sagittal PD images of the right knee medial meniscus at the time of initial injury (C) and 3 years later (D). New abnormally increased T2 signal along the superior articular surface of the posterior horn (arrowhead) was not present in the earlier study. This represents a new tear after interval meniscus repair of the posterior horn medial meniscus.

the injected contrast in the meniscus. Diagnostic accuracy is high when the abnormality reaching the surface is visualized on more than one image.[21] However, De Smet and colleagues noted that in 41% of recurrent tears, the intensity of the T1 signal reaching the articular surface is slightly lower than that of the intra-articular contrast agent. This finding is hypothesized to be related to visualization of slit-like tears limited by partial volume averaging, loose granulation tissue within the tear impeding contrast uptake, or insufficient stress being applied to the knee to force the contrast into the tear. The authors noted that reliance on the strict criterion of equal T1 signal intensity within the joint fluid and within the tear will cause the reader to overlook some recurrent tears.[21] In addition, other studies have recommended that T2 signal abnormality reaching the surface should be interpreted as a tear to increase diagnostic sensitivity.[6] Although many studies have suggested that MR arthrography has significantly improved specificity and sensitivity when compared with nonarthrographic MR imaging,[1,6,22,23] others including White and colleagues found no statistically significant differences among conventional MR imaging, DMRA, and IMRA for the diagnosis of recurrent meniscus tear.[24]

MENISCUS ALLOGRAFT TRANSPLANTATION

Postoperative MR imaging of a healed meniscus allograft will demonstrate identifiable meniscus tissue in the treated compartment, with incorporation of the bone plug to the recipient tibia. The transplanted meniscus may slightly overhang the edges of the tibial plateau due to slight size mismatch between the donor and recipient. Common findings after allograft transplant include shrinkage of the meniscus, the presence of suture, and diffusely increased signal throughout the grafted meniscus tissue. Graft extrusion, synovitis, and arthrofibrosis can also be seen postoperatively.[3] Diffusely increased signals within the graft and extrusion are frequently observed in studies that reported MR findings after meniscus transplantation.[1] However, these pathologic imaging findings do not correlate with clinical outcome.[1,25] MR imaging is primarily used to assess symptomatic patients for new tear, graft malposition, and the development of chondrosis. Meniscus allografts can fail by tearing within the graft, separating from the capsule, or at the implantation site (root avulsion, failed bone plug, or bridge).[1] We are aware of no evidence to prefer DMRA or IMRA over conventional MR imaging in this clinical scenario.

SUMMARY

The diagnosis of recurrent meniscus tear can be challenging after meniscus surgery, but familiarity with the commonly used surgical techniques and expected postoperative appearance will facilitate selection of the proper imaging modality and interpretation of the findings. After partial meniscectomy, the meniscus will display a truncated appearance with smooth borders. After meniscus repair, the morphology of the meniscus should be normal with variable high signal intensity at the repair site on short TE sequences. Recurrent tear will be diagnosed with confidence when there is fluid signal intensity or gadolinium imbibition in a meniscus remnant, when there is a displaced fragment, or when a tear occurs at a different site from the original injury. Conventional MR imaging performs well when less than 25% of the meniscus has been resected and for the assessment of allograft transplantation. We prefer to use DMRA in patients who have undergone meniscus repair.

CLINICS CARE POINTS

- T2 signal hyperintensity or contrast imbibition within the site of tear, abnormally increased T2 signal in a different region of the meniscus, or a displaced fragment are reliable findings to diagnose recurrent tear in the postoperative meniscus.

- After meniscus repair, high T2 signal in the site of prior tear can be seen for months to years after surgery, representing granulation tissue and healing. For these patients, direct MR arthrography can be helpful to differentiate between postoperative change and recurrent tear with the use of intra-articular gadolinium contrast.

- After meniscectomy, conventional MR imaging is acceptable to diagnose a new or recurrent meniscus tear using the same diagnostic criteria used for native meniscus tears, particularly when less than 25% of the meniscus has been removed. PD and T2-weighted sequences should be included in the protocol.

- If greater than 25% of the meniscus has been resected by partial meniscectomy, direct or indirect MR arthrography is more accurate for the diagnosis of recurrent tear.

DISCLOSURE

The authors have nothing to disclose.

REFERENCES

1. Baker JC, Friedman MV, Rubin DA. Imaging the postoperative knee meniscus: an evidence-based review. AJR Am J Roentgenol 2018;211(3):519–27.

2. Clark CR, Ogden JA. Development of the menisci of the human knee joint: morphological changes and their potential role in childhood meniscal injury. J Bone Joint Surg Am 1983;65(4):538–47.

3. Boutin RD, Fritz RC, Marder RA. Magnetic resonance imaging of the postoperative meniscus: resection, repair, and replacement. Magn Reson Imaging Clin N Am 2014;22:517–55.

4. Mow VC, Huiskes R. Basic orthopaedic biomechanics and mechano-biology. 3rd edition. Philadelphia: Lippincott Williams & Wilkins; 2005.

5. Cullen KA, Hall MJ, Golosinskiy A. Ambulatory surgery in the United States, 2006. Natl Health Stat Rep 2009;11:1–25.

6. Chapin R. Imaging of the postoperative meniscus. Radiol Clin North Am 2018;56(6):953–64.

7. Hutchison ID, Moran CJ, Potter HG, et al. Restoration of the meniscus: form and function. Am J Sports Med 2014;42:987–98.

8. Stein T, Mehling AP, Welsch F, et al. Long term outcome after arthroscopic meniscal repair versus arthroscopic partial meniscectomy for traumatic meniscal tears. Am J Sports Med 2010;38:1542–8.

9. Abrams GD, Frank RM, Gupta AK, et al. Trends in meniscus repair and meniscectomy in the United States, 2005-2011. Am J Sports Med 2013;41(10): 2333–9.

10. Lee AS, Kang RW, Kroin E, et al. Allograft meniscus transplantation. Sports Med Arthrosc Rev 2012;20: 106–14.

11. Zaffagnini S, Grassi A, Marcheggiani Muccioli GM, et al. Is sport activity possible after arthroscopic meniscal allograft transplantation? Midterm results in active patients. Am J Sports Med 2016;44: 625–32.

12. Recht MP, Kramer J. MR Imaging of the Postoperative Knee: A Pictorial Essay. Radiographics 2002; 22(4):765–74.

13. Resnick D, Kang HS. Disorders: specific joints. In: Internal derangements of joints: emphasis on MR imaging. Philadelphia, Pa: Saunders; 1997. p. 555–786.

14. Nguyen JC, De Smet AA, Graf BK, et al. MR Imaging-based diagnosis and Classification of Meniscal Tears. Radiographics 2014;34:981–99.

15. De Smet AA. How I diagnose meniscal tears on knee MRI. AJR Am J Roentgenol 2012;199:481–99.

16. Applegate GR, Flannigan BD, Tolin BS, et al. MR diagnosis of recurrent tears in the knee: value of intraarticular contrast material. AJR Am J Roentgenol 1993;161:821–5.

17. Vives MJ, Homesley D, Ciccotti MG, et al. Evaluation of recurring meniscal tears with gadolinium-enhanced magnetic resonance imaging. Am J Sports Med 2003;31:868–73.

18. Sanders TG. Imaging of the postoperative knee. Semin Musculoskelet Radiol 2011;15:383–407.

19. Fox MG. MR imaging of the meniscus: review, current trends, and clinical implications. Radiol Clin North Am 2007;45:1033–53.

20. Kijowski R, Rosas H, Williams A, et al. MRI characteristics of torn and untorn post-operative menisci. Skeletal Radiol 2017;46:1353–60.

21. De Smet AA, Horak DM, Davis KW, et al. Intensity of signal contacting meniscal surface in recurrent tears on MR arthrography compared with that of contrast material. AJR Am J Roentgenol 2006;187:W565–8.

22. Sciulli RL, Boutin RD, Brown RR, et al. Evaluation of the postoperative meniscus of the knee: a study comparing conventional arthrography, conventional MR imaging, MR arthrography with iodinated contrast material, and MR arthrography with gadolinium-based contrast material. Skeletal Radiol 1999;28:508–14.

23. Magee T. Accuracy of 3-Tesla MR and MR arthrography in diagnosis of meniscal retear in the postoperative knee. Skeletal Radiol 2014;43:1057–64.

24. White LM, Schweitzer ME, Weishaupt D, et al. Diagnosis of recurrent meniscal tears: prospective evaluation of conventional MR imaging, indirect MR arthrography, and direct MR arthrography. Radiology 2002;222:421–9.

25. Lee DH, Lee BS, Chung JW, et al. Changes in magnetic resonance imaging signal intensity of transplanted meniscus allografts are not associated with clinical outcomes. Arthroscopy 2011;27(9):1211–8.

Postoperative MRI of the Ankle and Foot

Hilary Umans, MD[a,b], Luis Cerezal, MD, PhD[c], James Linklater, OAM, FRANZCR[d], Jan Fritz, MD, PD, RMSK[e,*]

KEYWORDS

- MR imaging • Ankle • Foot • Surgery • Postoperative

KEY POINTS

- Successful MR imaging after foot and ankle instrumentation with metallic orthopedic implants depends on the appropriate use of basic and advanced metal artifact reduction techniques.
- Heavily T2-weighted pulse sequences are useful to assess tendon repairs and reconstruction.
- Anatomic repairs are often preferred over nonanatomic reconstruction in treating post-traumatic laxity and mechanical instability after lateral collateral ligament injuries.
- MR imaging is the imaging test of choice for morphologic grading of osteochondral lesions of the talus and assessing cartilage repair and restoration.
- The Magnetic Resonance Observation of Cartilage Repair Tissue scoring system is used for the semiquantitative assessment of neocartilage and correlation with surgical outcomes.

INTRODUCTION

There are myriad soft tissue and osseous procedures used in the surgical treatment of ankle and foot disorders, which threaten to make a review of the topic overwhelming for both the author and reader.[1–5] We have chosen a surgical approach to select the common types of procedures and discuss the normal and abnormal postoperative MR imaging appearances, highlighting potential complications. To this end, we focus on tendon repair, lateral ankle ligament repair and reconstruction, osteochondral lesions of the talar dome, total ankle arthroplasty, and select surgical complications.

Postoperative radiography is the first-line imaging test for assessing osseous procedures, anatomic alignment, and implant complications. Postoperative computed tomography (CT) scanning is most commonly used to evaluate the success of osseous bridging or lack thereof after arthrodesis. Larger metallic and prosthetic implants can cause various streak artifacts, which can be mitigated by metal artifact reduction techniques.[6,7]

Ultrasound examination permits the high-resolution evaluation of tendon or ligament repair. Advantages include dynamic imaging range of motion and stress maneuvers with real-time correlations of painful symptoms. Ultrasound examination is usually best used to examine superficial soft tissue structures. Ultrasound examination is typically unable to penetrate bone and joints and may not identify potentially clinically relevant regional abnormalities beyond the targeted anatomy.

As a multiplanar tomographic modality combining the highest soft tissue contrast and

[a] Lenox Hill Radiology & Imaging Associates, PC, 61 East 77th Street, New York, NY 10075, USA; [b] Department of Radiology, Albert Einstein College of Medicine, Bronx, NY, USA; [c] Department of Radiology, Diagnóstico Médico Cantabria, Castilla 6-Ground Floor, Santander, 39002, Spain; [d] Castlereagh Imaging & Illawarra Radiology Group, Level 1, 20-22 Mons Road, Westmead, Sydney, New South Wales 2145, Australia; [e] Department of Radiology, Division of Musculoskeletal Radiology, New York University Grossman School of Medicine, 660 1st Avenue, 3rd Floor, Room 313, New York, NY, USA
* Corresponding author.
E-mail address: jan.fritz@nyulangone.org
Twitter: DmcRadiologia (L.C.); JanFritzMSK (J.F.)

Magn Reson Imaging Clin N Am 30 (2022) 733–755
https://doi.org/10.1016/j.mric.2022.05.006
1064-9689/22/© 2022 Elsevier Inc. All rights reserved.

accuracy for evaluating marrow and soft tissue abnormalities, MR imaging permits the most comprehensive postoperative imaging evaluation despite the inherent challenges of mitigating hardware artifacts.

A 3.0 T MR image delivers higher signal-to-noise ratios and decreases the scan times of ankle and foot MR imaging examinations.[8–11] In addition to 2-dimensional MR imaging techniques, 3-dimensional isotropic MR imaging techniques offer the greatest spatial resolution and advanced postprocessing techniques to evaluate postoperative tendons, ligaments, and articular cartilage, including curved multiplanar reformation.[12–16] However, depending on the size and composition of metallic implants and prostheses, associated susceptibility artifacts can create challenges that may require advanced metal artifact reduction techniques.[17–20] Although it is possible to implement metal artifact reduction strategies at both 1.5 T and 3.0 T, metal artifact reduction may be easier to achieve at 1.5 T.[21] MR imaging at 1.2 T open configuration MR imaging systems with the magnetic field oriented vertically may exacerbate metallic artifacts, despite the lower field strength, and should be avoided in the postoperative setting. Lower field extremity and newer 0.55 T MR imaging systems with a horizontally oriented B0 magnetic field may offer the best solution to address exuberant metal artifacts.[22]

Postoperative MR Imaging with Metal Artifact Reduction

Metal artifact reduction MR imaging represents a group of techniques that reduce metallic orthopedic implant-related artifacts around orthopedic implants, such as plates, screws, rods, and total ankle arthroplasty systems, resulting in improved visualization of implant components, bone–implant interfaces, periprosthetic bone, and soft tissues.[23] Metal artifact reduction MR imaging can be grouped into basic and advanced techniques, which differ in the degree of achievable metal artifact reduction on MR images. The groups have different sequence software, licensing, and hardware requirements. Basic metal reduction MR imaging protocols often provide sufficient image quality for ankles with small implants, low-susceptibility titanium implants, and in the periphery of total ankle arthroplasty implants (Fig. 1). However, basic metal artifact reduction MR imaging protocols may be insufficient to evaluate total ankle arthroplasty components, bone–implant interfaces, and periprosthetic soft tissues in the immediate vicinity due to remaining metal artifacts. For such clinical scenarios, advanced metal artifact reduction MR imaging techniques are most valuable, including slice encoding for metal artifact correction (SEMAC) and multiacquisition variable-resonance image combination (MAVRIC).

Basic metal artifact reduction MR imaging techniques include fast and turbo spin echo pulse sequences, high receiver bandwidth, bandwidth-matched short tau inversion recovery (STIR) fat suppression, and the thinnest slice thickness, such as 3 mm in the foot and ankle with minimal or no interslice gaps (see Fig. 1) (Table 1).

Fast and turbo spin echo pulse sequences produce markedly fewer metal artifacts than gradient echo pulse sequences because the radiofrequency-induced spin refocusing of fast and turbo spin echo pulse sequences results in minimal pileup of metal artifacts, which is in contrast to the gradient inversion-induced spin refocusing of gradient echo pulse sequences.[24]

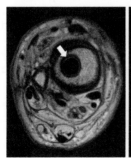 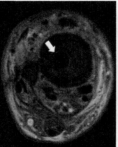 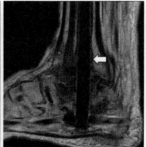 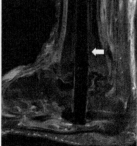

| Axial PD High-Bandwidth Turbo Spin Echo | Axial STIR High-Bandwidth Turbo Spin Echo | Sagittal PD High-Bandwidth Turbo Spin Echo | Sagittal STIR High-Bandwidth Turbo Spin Echo |

Fig. 1. Metal artifact reduction MR imaging after tibiotalocalcaneal fusion procedure demonstrates near circumferential osteolysis (*arrows*) around the retrograde intramedullary nail. Owing to the low magnetic susceptibility of the metallic implant, basic metal artifact reduction MR imaging techniques using high receiver bandwidth turbo spin echo pulse sequences with proton density (PD) weighting and STIR fat suppression is sufficient for near artifact-free MR imaging at 1.5 T field strength.

Table 1
Postoperative foot and ankle MR imaging protocol using basic metal artifact reduction techniques

Parameters	Coronal PD	Coronal STIR	Sagittal PD	Sagittal STIR	Axial PD	Axial STIR
Type	TSE	TSE	TSE	TSE	TSE	TSE
Repetition time (ms)/ Echo time (ms)	3800/26	3700/4.6	3800/26	3800/5.2	3800/31	4540/4.6
Receiver bandwidth (Hertz/pixel)	579	592	579	601	587	592
Number of Slices	34	24	32	22	41	30
Field-of-view (mm^2)	170 × 118	190 × 137	170 × 170	190 × 190	170 × 118	180 × 118
Matrix	320 × 240	256 × 204	320 × 240	256 × 204	320 × 240	256 × 204
Slice thickness/gap (mm)	3/0	4/0	3/0	4/0	3/0	4/0
Number of excitations/ concatenations	2/2	2/2	2/2	2/2	3/2	2/2
Turbo factor	19	16	19	19	19	16
Acquisition time (min:s)	4:43	4:35	4:43	4:43	5:06	5:02

Abbreviations: PD, proton density-weighted; TSE, turbo spin echo.

Contrary to previous assumptions, the isolated increase of the echo train length of fast and turbo spin echo pulse sequences does not reduce metal artifacts but may result in substantial blurring at higher turbo factors.[25]

Using high receiver or readout bandwidths of approximately 500 Hz per pixel will result in less in-plane signal displacement and metal artifacts, because the assignment of more frequencies per pixel effectively results in frequency displacement across fewer pixels.[23,26] Increasing the matrix size will result in greater spatial resolution, but may not decrease the degree of metallic artifacts.

The bandwidth of the second frequency-encoding gradient of the MR imaging system in the slice direction is usually not directly accessible for the user, but can be increased indirectly by decreasing the slice thickness. However, a thin slice thickness is practically limited by the associated signal-to-noise ratio loss. In our experience, a slice thickness of 3 mm is clinically viable for MR imaging of total ankle arthroplasty and other orthopedic implants.

STIR is the fat suppression technique of choice for MR imaging of orthopedic implants. STIR depends on T1 recovery constants of tissues, which are unaffected by metallic implants. STIR may require matching the excitation and readout bandwidths for homogeneous fat suppression.[27]

Dixon fat suppression may be advantageous for small implants that cause few artifacts to obviate STIR fat suppression and provide an avenue for postcontrast MR imaging without spectral fat suppression (**Fig. 2**). For postcontrast MR imaging cases with implants causing larger metallic artifacts and failure of T1 Dixon techniques, subtraction of matching non–fat-suppressed precontrast and postcontrast T1-weighted MR images is the method of choice[6] (**Fig. 3**).

Metal artifact reduction MR imaging at 1.5 T will result in fewer metal artifacts than at 3 T; however, with advanced metal artifact reduction techniques, similar diagnostic results may be achieved at 3 T, depending on the magnetic susceptibility of the TAA implant components.[18]

The view angle tilting technique can result in less apparent in-plane signal displacement and decrease metal artifacts. However, when using view angle tilting in isolation with 2-dimensional turbo spin echo pulse sequences at a high-receiver bandwidth of 500 to 600 Hz per pixel, the metal-reducing effect of view angle tilting is minimal, but can result in substantial blurring.[19]

SEMAC turbo spin echo and MAVRIC fast spin echo pulse sequences are advanced multispatial and multispectral metal artifact reduction MR imaging techniques that result in substantial metal artifact reduction in the through-plane z-direction.[28,29] Additional phase and frequency encoding steps are used to sample through-plane displaced signals, then used to form final composite MR images with minimal residual implant-induced metallic artifacts.

Modern SEMAC and MAVRIC pulse sequence types typically include elements of basic metal artifact reduction MR imaging techniques. Higher numbers of phase and frequency encoding steps result in more metal artifact reduction at the expense of longer acquisition times.[25] Compressed sensing-based undersampling can

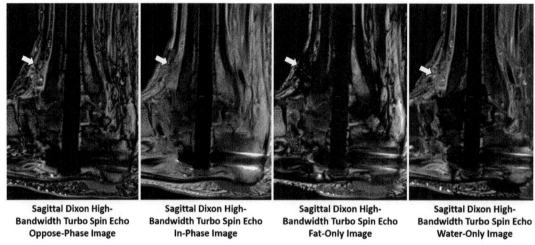

| Sagittal Dixon High-Bandwidth Turbo Spin Echo Oppose-Phase Image | Sagittal Dixon High-Bandwidth Turbo Spin Echo In-Phase Image | Sagittal Dixon High-Bandwidth Turbo Spin Echo Fat-Only Image | Sagittal Dixon High-Bandwidth Turbo Spin Echo Water-Only Image |

Fig. 2. Metal artifact reduction MR imaging after tibiotalocalcaneal fusion procedure demonstrates a focal extensor tendon discontinuity (*arrows*). Owing to the low magnetic susceptibility of the retrograde nail and fixation bolts, a T1-weighted high-bandwidth Dixon turbo spin echo pulse sequence can be used for contrast-enhanced metal artifact reduction MR imaging. The water-only image resembles a conventional fat-suppressed T1-weighted postcontrast MR image, demonstrating focal contrast enhancement at the area of the tendon discontinuity (*arrow*).

reduce acquisition times of SEMAC TSE by 60% to 70%.[20,30,31] **Table 1, Tables 2** and **3** summarize basic and advanced metal artifact reduction MR imaging protocols for postoperative foot and ankle MR imaging in patients with metallic orthopedic osteosynthesis and total arthroplasty implants.

MR Imaging of Tendon Repairs and Reconstruction

MR imaging after foot and ankle tendon surgery is used to assess postoperative pain, seeking to distinguish postoperative tendinitis and peritendinitis, hypertrophic scarring, failure of the

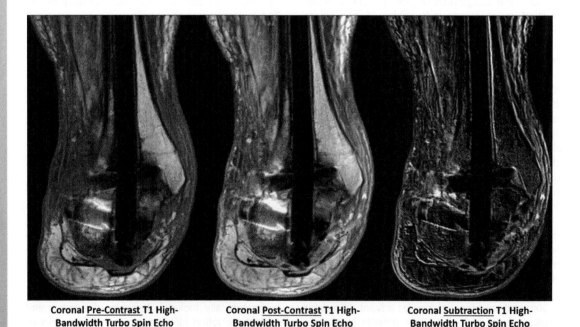

| Coronal Pre-Contrast T1 High-Bandwidth Turbo Spin Echo | Coronal Post-Contrast T1 High-Bandwidth Turbo Spin Echo | Coronal Subtraction T1 High-Bandwidth Turbo Spin Echo |

Fig. 3. Contrast-enhanced metal artifact reduction MR imaging after tibiotalocalcaneal fusion using T1-weighted high-bandwidth turbo spin echo pulse sequences. The subtraction MR image resulting from subtraction of precontrast from postcontrast MR images has a similar appearance to conventional fat-suppressed T1-weighted turbo spin echo MR images, providing a strategy to obviate spectral fat suppression.

Table 2
Postoperative foot and ankle MR imaging protocol using conventional SEMAC metal artifact reduction

Parameters	Coronal PD	Coronal STIR	Sagittal PD	Sagittal STIR	Axial PD	Axial STIR
Type	SEMAC	SEMAC	SEMAC	SEMAC	SEMAC	SEMAC
Repetition time/echo time (ms)	3530/28	3720/23	3530/28	2970/23	4150/28	2960/23
Receiver bandwidth (Hertz/pixel)	601	601	601	601	504	501
Number of slices	32	24	32	22	41	30
Field of view (mm²)	170 × 170	190 × 137	170 × 170	190 × 190	170 × 118	180 × 118
Matrix	320 × 240	256 × 204	320 × 240	256 × 204	320 × 240	256 × 204
Slice thickness/gap (mm)	3/0	4/0	3/0	4/0	3/0	4/0
Number of excitations/concatenations	1/1	1/1	1/1	1/1	1/1	1/1
Turbo factor/acceleration factor	11/3	11/3	11/3	11/3	11/3	11/3
View-angle tilting	100%	100%	100%	100%	100%	100%
SEMAC steps	11	11	11	11	11	11
Acquisition time (min:s)	8:30	7:35	8:30	6:04	9:07	8:05

Abbreviations: PD, proton density-weighted; TSE, turbo spin echo.

reconstruction, dehiscences, postoperative infection and post-traumatic neuroma formation.[32] MR imaging principles include using skin markers to localize symptoms, appropriate optimization of sequences to minimize metal artifact, and more heavily T2-weighted pulse sequences to aid the postoperative tendon (**Fig. 4**) and enthesis (**Fig. 5**) characterization.[33]

Occasionally, intravenous contrast can be helpful to evaluate the extent of tendinitis (**Fig. 6**) and peritendinitis and characterize suspected infection (**Fig. 7**). Distinguishing between normal postoperative imaging appearances and symptomatic postoperative tendinitis can present a diagnostic challenge. Correlation with surgical details and prior imaging examinations is helpful.

Table 3
Postoperative foot and ankle MR imaging protocol using compressed sensing SEMAC metal artifact reduction

Parameters	Coronal PD	Coronal STIR	Sagittal PD	Sagittal STIR	Axial PD	Axial STIR
Type	CS-SEMAC	CS-SEMAC	CS-SEMAC	CS-SEMAC	CS-SEMAC	CS-SEMAC
Repetition time/echo time (ms)	4200/28	3800/7.5	3800/28	4000/28	3800/31	4800/7.5
Receiver bandwidth (Hertz/pixel)	601	601	601	601	601	601
Number of slices	34	24	32	22	41	30
Field of view (mm²)	170 × 118	190 × 137	170 × 170	190 × 190	170 × 118	180 × 118
Matrix	320 × 240	256 × 204	320 × 240	256 × 204	320 × 240	256 × 204
Slice thickness/gap (mm)	3/0	4/0	3/0	4/0	3/0	4/0
Number of excitations/concatenations	1/1	1/2	1/1	1/2	1/1	1/2
Turbo factor/acceleration factor	11/8	19/8	11/8	17/8	11/8	19/8
View-angle tilting	100%	100%	100%	100%	100%	100%
SEMAC steps	19	19	19	19	19	19
Acquisition time (min:s)	5:38	4:51	5:06	5:06	4:54	5:53

Abbreviations: CS, compressed sensing; PD, proton density-weighted; TSE, turbo spin echo.

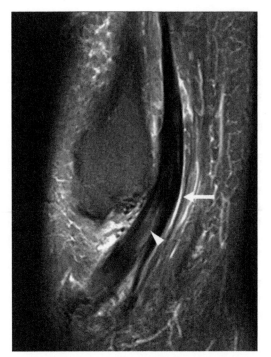

Fig. 4. Tendinosis and tenosynovitis following peroneus longus to brevis tenodesis. Sagittal fat-suppressed proton density-weighted MR image demonstrates the tenodesis construct, with focal tendon signal hyperintensity (*arrowhead*) and thickened peritendon space (*arrow*), indicating tendinosis and tenosynovitis.

Correlative ultrasound examinations may complement postoperative MR imaging to localize symptomatic abnormalities, more clearly identify intratendinous sutures, evaluate laxity with stress maneuvers, and assess tendon subluxation or friction syndromes with real-time dynamic imaging.[34]

MR Imaging of Ligament Repair and Reconstruction

Ankle sprains are common, accounting for 16% to 40% of sports injuries.[35] Eighty-five percent of sprains affect the anterior talofibular ligament (ATFL). Although most recover with conservative treatment, approximately 20% progress to chronic instability, which may necessitate ligament repair or reconstruction.[36] A greater percentage may experience chronic microinstability, which predisposes to degenerative joint disease. Ankle microinstability has been the focus of increased attention in the orthopedic literature and now influences the therapeutic approach of patients with chronic pain secondary to ankle sprains.[4]

The ATFL comprises 2 distinct bundles.[37] The superior fascicle of the ATFL is an intra-articular anatomic structure. The inferior fascicle has a common fibular insertion with the calcaneofibular ligament (CFL), and both are connected by arciform fibers, forming an isometric extra-articular anatomic and functional entity called the lateral fibulotalocalcaneal ligament complex.

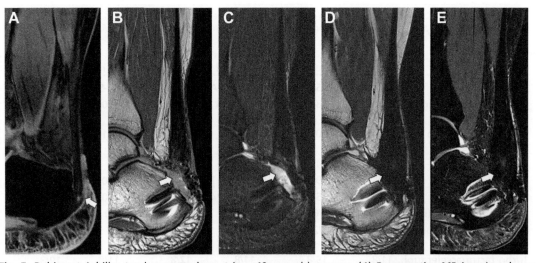

Fig. 5. Dehiscent Achilles tendon reattachment in a 40-year-old woman. (*A*) Preoperative MR imaging shows insertional tendinopathy characterized by subenthesial cyst formation and bony spur at the superficial margin (*arrow* in *A*). The patient underwent debridement of the distal Achilles tendon, calcaneoplasty, and Achilles tendon reattachment. Postoperative MR imaging demonstrates dehiscence of the Achilles tendon reattachment (*arrows* in *B* and *C*) with fluid collection at the point of dehiscence, containing foci of suture material. The patient underwent revision reattachment and subsequent mature reconstitution of the enthesis at 12 months (*arrows* in *D* and *E*) characterized by a low signal interface at the enthesis.

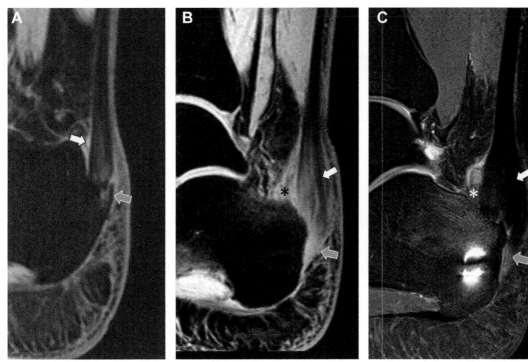

Fig. 6. A 50-year-old woman with postoperative Achilles tendinitis. (A) Preoperative MR imaging, including sagittal fat-suppressed T1-weighted gradient echo MR imaging, demonstrates tendon thickening and enhancement (*white arrow*) and bony spur at the superficial margin (*gray arrow*). The patient underwent Achilles tendon debridement and reattachment. Postoperative pain was slow to settle. Postoperative MR imaging obtained 6 months after surgery, including sagittal fat-suppressed T1-weighted gradient echo (B) and fat-suppressed T2-weighted (C) MR images, demonstrate marked thickening of the distal Achilles tendon (*white arrows*) with moderate tendon enhancement and T2 signal hyperintensity, reflecting postoperative tendinitis without dehiscence. Note the postoperative thickening of the retrocalcaneal bursa (*asterisks*).

Isolated injury of the superior fascicle of the ATFL is the most common lesion in ankle inversion sprains. This fascicle, similar to other intra-articular ligaments, has reduced healing capacity owing to synovial fluid inhibition of fibrin clot formation. Superior fascicle injury results in ankle microinstability, consisting of functional instability and minor degrees of mechanical instability of the ankle that are not detectable on clinical examination or imaging methods.[38] These patients are predisposed to recurrent ankle sprains and the subsequent development of other intra-articular pathology (soft tissue impingement, chondral and osteochondral lesions, and intra-articular bodies).[36]

Clinical distinction between post-traumatic laxity and mechanical instability and functional and subjective instability is required to determine the optimal management of individual cases. Functional and subjective instability may result from intra-articular abnormalities in the ankle, such as soft tissue impingement or articular

cartilage pathology, or alternatively, owing to extra-articular abnormalities such as peroneal tendinopathy, tendon tear, or tightness of the gastrocnemius soleus complex.

If there is adequate residual, viable ligament tissue, anatomic repair is preferred to restore the normal anatomy of the ATFL and, optionally, the CFL.[38] The original Broström procedure entailed open midsubstance suture repair of the torn native ATFL and CFL, although variations have used ligament anchors into the fibula with or without reinforcement with fibular periosteum[38,39] (Figs. 8–10). The Gould modification incorporated mobilization and reattachment of the extensor retinaculum to reinforce the primary lateral ligament repair, resulting in improved ankle and subtalar stability[35,38,39] (see Fig. 8; Fig. 11).

Indications for augmented ATFL repair using fiber tape include underlying ligamentous laxity, poor quality native ligament tissue for repair, and the presence of hindfoot varus. Arthroscopic ATFL repair has also been described, although

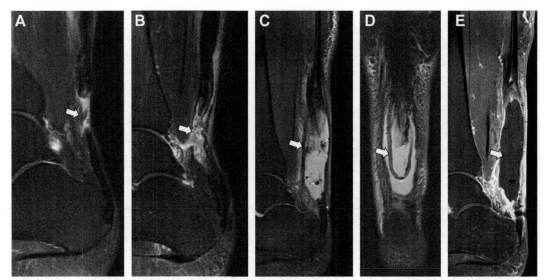

Fig. 7. A 60-year-old woman with Achilles tendon rupture treated with ligament augmentation reconstruction. (A) Preoperative sagittal fat-suppressed T2-weighted MR image demonstrates a subacute complete midsubstance Achilles tendon rupture (*arrow*), treated by primary surgical repair. (B) Postoperative sagittal fat-suppressed T2-weighted MR image demonstrates rerupture (*arrow*), which was subsequently treated with revision repair, augmented with a synthetic polyethylene terephthalate graft (ligament advanced reinforcement system [LARS]). The revision repair was complicated by infection and failed. (C) Postoperative sagittal fat-suppressed T2-weighted MR image demonstrates a retracted midsubstance Achilles tendon defect (*arrow*). (D) Postoperative coronal fat-suppressed T2-weighted MR image demonstrates the synthetic polyethylene terephthalate graft device (*arrow*) contiguous with the proximal tendon edge, whereas the distal component is lying within a mildly thick-walled fluid collection, which demonstrates moderate peripheral contrast enhancement on the sagittal fat-suppressed contrast-enhanced T1-weighted MR image (*arrow* in E). The failed graft was removed, and cultures confirmed bacterial infection. The postoperative course was complicated by wound breakdown requiring debridement and a vacuum-assisted closure dressing before finally healing.

because the approach precludes concomitant CFL repair, it is generally reserved for patients with minimal CFL laxity and no features of subtalar instability or hindfoot varus.[40]

Anatomic reconstruction may use tendon grafts or braided polyethylene to recreate the normal lateral ligament anatomy, varying on the types of autografts or allografts and surgical tunnels and fixation techniques.[2,41,42] Numerous nonanatomic reconstruction techniques use neighboring tendons, most commonly the peroneus brevis or extensor digitorum longus, to recreate the constraints of the torn lateral ligaments.

Although the Chrisman–Snook, Watson–Jones, and modified Evans procedures are the most widely described, they have been less commonly used in contemporary surgical practice[2,41,42] (Fig. 12). The modified Evans and Watson–Jones procedures sacrifice the peroneus brevis and limit subtalar motion. Advantages of the modified Evans procedure are that it is relatively easy, and proximal fixation accelerates rehabilitation and preserves the graft. The Watson–Jones procedure is advantageous in that it corrects anterior ankle

translation. The Chrisman–Snook procedure partially preserves the peroneus brevis, but is a demanding procedure with a higher risk of surgical complications. Outcomes are not as favorable as anatomic repairs, with a reported 7% to 10% postoperative rigidity or instability incidence. Approximately 4% fail owing to injury or rupture of the rerouted tendons[42] (Fig. 13). Nevertheless, surgical complications are relatively uncommon, with good to excellent outcomes reported in 80% to 95% of all types of procedures.[33]

Sammarco and colleagues[1] reported on 1516 lateral ligament procedure outcomes and found a 6.2% incidence of nerve injury, most commonly involving the superficial peroneal nerve, with symptoms presenting in the early postoperative period. Wound complications occurred in 2.7% of patients in the early postoperative period and are usually superficial, generally not requiring imaging characterization. Deep infections such as septic arthritis and osteomyelitis are exceedingly rare.

MR imaging may be used to evaluate poor clinical outcomes owing to persistent or recurrent

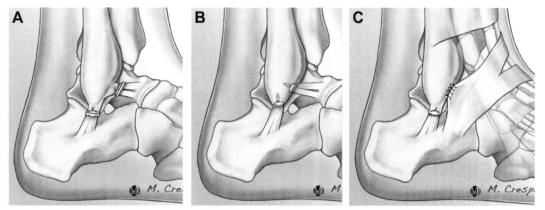

Fig. 8. Illustrations of anatomic repair techniques in chronic lateral ankle instability. (*A*) Broström anatomic repair consists of direct suture repair by overlapping the midsubstance of injured ATFL and CFL ligament ends. (*B*) Karlsson modification involves reattaching the ATFL and CFL ends through drill holes in their anatomic position in the distal fibula. (*C*) Gould or Broström modified technique (current technique of choice in chronic lateral ankle instability) implies suturing the ATFL and CFL and reinforcing the repair with reinsertion of the extensor retinaculum to the fibula.

instability, reinjury, or postsurgical pain (see **Fig. 13**). The goal of postoperative imaging is to identify the type of repair, assess the integrity of the surgical construct, and assess for complications. If there has been previous nonanatomic reconstruction, the torn remnants of the ATFL and CFL can be assessed for possible anatomic repair. If that is not an option, MR imaging can be used to assess the suitability for repositioning tenodesis.

Recurrent instability may result from inadequate reconstruction or reinjury. Postoperative stiffness

most commonly results from arthrofibrosis, but can be due to graft malpositioning or overtensioning.[43] Intra-articular causes of poor surgical outcomes include soft tissue impingement, syndesmotic widening, intra-articular ossicles, osteochondral lesion of the talus, degenerative cartilage loss, and osteophytes.[38]

MR Imaging of Osteochondral Lesions of the Talus

Ankle sprains are the most common sports injury, with concomitant osteochondral injury of the talus

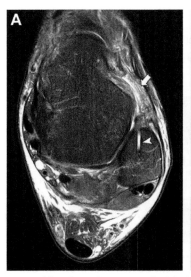
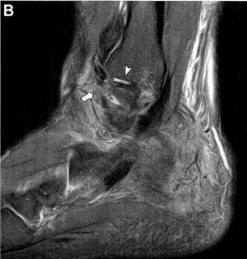

Fig. 9. A 26-year-old male patient treated with the modified Broström technique for chronic ankle instability after an acute ankle inversion sprain. Axial (*A*) and sagittal (*B*) fat-suppressed proton density-weighted MR images show a rupture of the repaired ligament (*arrow*) with associated edema in the adjacent soft tissues. Note the suture anchor into the anatomic origin of the ATFL to allow for the direct ligament to bone healing (*arrowhead*).

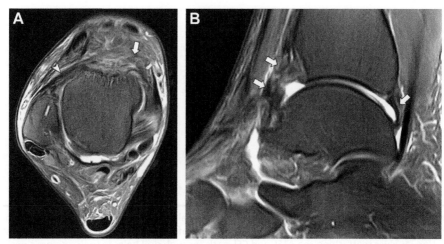

Fig. 10. A 24-year-old soccer player with postoperative pain and stiffness after modified Brömström technique repair, unresponsive to prolonged rehabilitation treatment. Axial (*A*) and sagittal (*B*) fat-suppressed proton density-weighted MR images show marked diffuse tibiotalar capsular thickening (*arrows*) and pericapsular inflammatory changes related to arthrofibrosis. The repaired ligament shows a normal appearance (*arrowhead* in *A*).

in 5% to 6.5% of all ankle sprains[38] (**Table 4**). Various surgical interventions exist to address osteochondral injury of the talus, including bone stimulation, tissue-based cartilage repair, and cell-based cartilage repair. The approach depends on the size and location of the lesion. Bone stimulation techniques include abrasion arthroplasty, subchondral drilling, and microfracture, which stimulate fibrocartilaginous repair tissue in the defect from bone marrow stem cells[44] (**Fig. 14**). Microfracture remains the most common cartilage repair surgery despite a lack of prospective clinical outcome studies. Favorable short-term outcomes have been reported with good lesion fill in individuals with low body mass index and short duration of preoperative symptoms. Although microfracture is commonly performed, fibrocartilage repair is thought to lack the structural, biochemical and biomechanical properties to support long-term joint function.[45,46]

Mosaicplasty, also known as autologous osteochondral autograft transplantation, is a tissue-based cartilage repair with harvested osteochondral plugs from non–weight-bearing joint surfaces to the defect[47] (**Fig. 15**). It is appropriate in defects measuring 1 to 4 cm^2, but relies on the availability of donor graft tissue and has the potential for donor site morbidity. This procedure restores autologous hyaline cartilage. Cadaveric allografts can fill larger defects, but carry the risk of immunologic rejection and disease transmission from the donor.

Cell-based cartilage repair has been performed using autologous chondrocyte implantation (ACI)

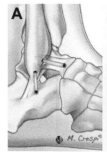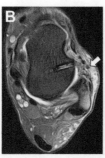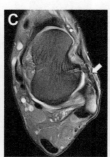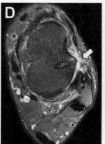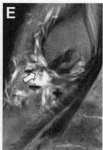

Fig. 11. Augmented ATFL repair using fiber tape. (*A*) Modified Bröstron repair technique with ligament augmentation with synthetic fiber tape. (*B–E*) Serial MR imaging of a patient treated with Broström-Gould procedure augmented with fiber tape. (*B*) Axial fat-suppressed proton density-weighted MR images at 3 months and (*C*) 12 months show a normal appearance of the repaired ATFL ligament (*arrows in B and C*). (*D, E*) Axial and sagittal fat-suppressed proton density-weighted MR images after acute ankle inversion sprain, 2 years after surgery, showing a complete tear of the ligament repair (*arrows in D and E*).

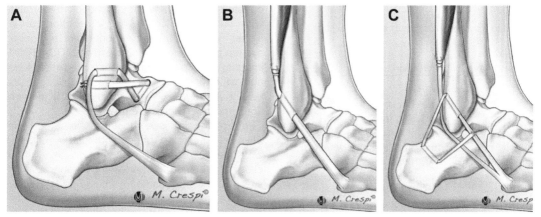

Fig. 12. Illustrations of the nonanatomic reconstruction for chronic lateral ankle instability. (A) Watson–Jones procedure: the peroneus brevis tendon is divided at the myotendinous junction and rerouted anteroposteriorly through the distal fibula to attach to the neck of the talus and back to the distal fibula. (B) Evans procedure: the peroneus brevis is divided at the myotendinous junction, passed retrograde through the fibular tunnel and sutured back to the myotendinous junction. (C) Chrisman–Snook procedure: the peroneus brevis tendon is divided longitudinally into 2 halves. One of the portions remains attached to the myotendinous junction. With the other slip, a tendinous loop is created through the lateral calcaneus, distal fibula, and again over the peroneus brevis tendon to reconstruct both the ATFL and the CFL.

through various techniques since the 1990s.[47,48] The first-generation procedure involved harvesting healthy chondrocytes from a non–weight-bearing surface, growth in culture for 3 to 5 weeks, and then implanting deep to a periosteal flap via arthrotomy.[49] The second-generation procedure used a collagen membrane in place of the periosteal flap.[46] A third-generation single-step procedure uses a biologic scaffold to culture the embedded chondrocytes trimmed to fit the defect, also known as matrix-associated ACI.[50] Matrix-associated ACI has the advantage of treating defects up to 12 cm[2] in high-demand individuals, producing reparative fibrocartilage with properties similar to hyaline cartilage.

MR Imaging Assessment of Cartilage Restoration

Morphologic MR imaging is routinely performed and may use the same MR imaging protocol recommended by the International Cartilage

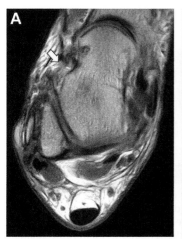
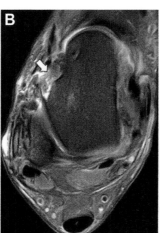
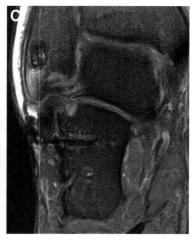

Fig. 13. A 38-year-old woman treated 5 years before for chronic ankle instability with the Chrisman–Snook procedure after an acute ankle sprain. (A–C) Axial T1 and axial and coronal fat-suppressed proton density-weighted MR images show the path of the graft through the fibula, talus, and calcaneus. A complete graft tear (arrows) is seen in A and B near the talar neck insertion.

Table 4	
MR imaging classification of osteochondral lesions of the talus	
Grade	**Description**
1	Normal
2	Partial thickness articular cartilage defect
3	Coapted full-thickness articular cartilage defect or exposed bone
4	Unstable but nondisplaced in situ chondral or osteochondral fragment
5	Displaced chondral or osteochondral fragment

Regeneration and Joint Preservation Society to evaluate native joint cartilage.[47] These include intermediate- and T2-weighted fast spin echo pulse sequences with and without fat suppression and T1-weighted gradient echo pulse sequences with spectral or water excitation fat suppression.

The Magnetic Resonance Observation of Cartilage Repair Tissue (MOCART) score analyzes a constellation of variables intended to correlate with surgical outcomes for osteochondral lesions[51,52] (**Fig. 16**). The components of the scoring system are outlined in **Table 5**. The MOCART MR imaging scoring system has been used in conjunction with various clinical scores to evaluate the healing and durability of various surgical interventions and predict treatment failure.

Ideally, repair tissue should be the same thickness and seem to be smooth and continuous with the surrounding native cartilage, without clefts at the interface between the reparative tissue and the surrounding cartilage. A low signal interface implies solid graft integration with adjacent native hyaline articular cartilage and the subchondral plate. The subchondral lamina should be intact, and there should be no subchondral marrow edema, granulation tissue, or cyst-like lesions. After microfracture, the reparative fibrocartilage can be thin and indistinct, but should eventually smoothly fill the defect 1 to 2 years after the procedure. The signal intensity of the reparative fibrocartilage is often hyperintense to native cartilage using T2 fast spin echo sequences, diminishing over time as the tissue matrix matures. Postoperative subchondral marrow edema should diminish over time. Persistent subchondral

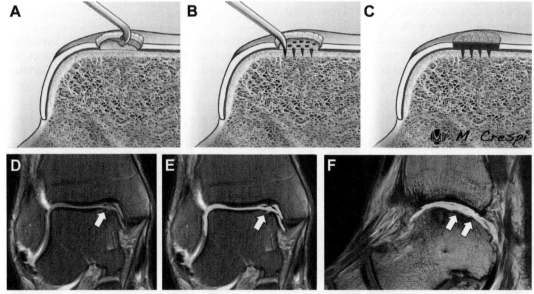

Fig. 14. Bone marrow stimulation microfracture technique. (*A–C*) Diagrams illustrating the bone marrow stimulation (microfracture) technique for cartilage repair. After curettage of the defect, removal of the calcified layer at the base of the defect is performed to facilitate clot adhesion (*A*). Bone marrow stimulation is achieved by perforating the subchondral bone at 3- to 4-mm intervals (*B*) to stimulate the formation of a fibrocartilaginous repair tissue (*C*). (*D–F*) A 42-year-old man with an osteochondral lesion of the medial talar dome treated with microfractures with good functional results. Coronal fat-suppressed proton density-weighted (*D*) and corresponding T2 mapping MR images (*E, F*) demonstrate a uniform defect filling with slight prolongation of T2 values, representing repair fibrocartilage (*arrows*).

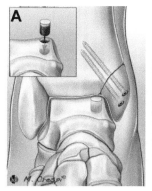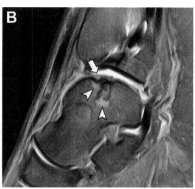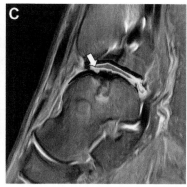

Fig. 15. Autologous osteochondral transplantation mosaicplasty technique. (*A*) Diagram illustrating the autologous osteochondral transplantation (mosaicplasty) technique to replace an osteochondral lesion of the talus. Depending on the location, it may require a tibial osteotomy for accessing the osteochondral lesion. (*B, C*) A 38-year-old man with an osteochondral lesion of the medial talar dome treated with mosaicplasty referred pain worse than before surgery. Sagittal fat-suppressed proton density-weighted (*B*) and corresponding T2 mapping (*C*) images, obtained with an 8-kg axial traction system, demonstrate an irregular surface and prolongation of T2 values in the graft (*arrows*). Note also subtle subchondral bone marrow edema surrounding the graft (*arrowheads*).

marrow edema and incomplete defect filling are morphologic imaging features of treatment failure. Overgrowth of the subchondral bone has been reported in up to 49% of cases, but does not indicate failure, as long as the defect has a smooth filling.[53–55]

Biochemical MR techniques are not routinely used in the postoperative assessment of cartilage repair, but complement morphologic imaging by evaluating cartilage structure and tissue repair maturation.

Several imaging techniques focus on assessing the glycosaminoglycan content in articular cartilage, including delayed gadolinium-enhanced MR imaging of cartilage. Compared with microfracture techniques, higher glycosaminoglycan concentrations have been shown after ACI. However, delayed gadolinium-enhanced MR imaging of cartilage poses the logistical challenge of delayed MR imaging after contrast administration and moderate exercise over varying time intervals appropriate for different joints.[53] In addition, most delayed gadolinium-enhanced MR imaging of cartilage techniques require the intravenous injection of a double dose of gadolinium.

Diffusion-weighted imaging exploits the mobility of water as it is influenced by the molecular structure of the biological tissue being imaged. In cartilage, proteoglycans, collagen fibers, and chondrocytes hinder diffusion. In a study by Apprich and colleagues,[53] there was no correlation between diffusion coefficient in follow-up imaging of repair cartilage after microfracture, whereas they demonstrated diminished diffusivity over time in those who had undergone ACI.

T2 mapping (multi-echo spin echo T2 imaging) (see **Figs. 14** and **15**) and T2* mapping (multi-echo gradient echo imaging) use T2 and T2*relaxation time measurements to evaluate the collagen content, orientation, and cartilage hydration. T2* techniques offer faster acquisition times and the potential for 3-dimensional acquisition. Quirbach and colleagues[54] showed no significant difference in T2 values between repair and healthy control cartilage, but demonstrated a significant difference in diffusion coefficient using diffusion-weighted imaging. By contrast, Pagliazzi and colleagues[55] found a statistically significant correlation between T2 map values and clinical outcomes in 20 patients with 5 and 7 years of clinical and MR imaging follow-up after ACI.

The MOCART score was devised to assess reparative cartilage in the knee[51,52] (see **Fig. 16**). Although it has been used, by extension, to assess cartilage repair in other joints, its usefulness without revision has been called into question.[56]

A combined morphologic and biologic imaging approach permits the assessment of both cartilage thickness and fill and reactive edema or cyst-like changes in the subchondral bone while providing information about the molecular structure of the repair tissue as it matures over time.[53–55]

General Postoperative Complications

Arthrofibrosis
Clinically presenting with pain, stiffness, limited range of motion, and tenderness on palpation, arthrofibrosis is a common complication of trauma and surgery. As a postoperative complication,

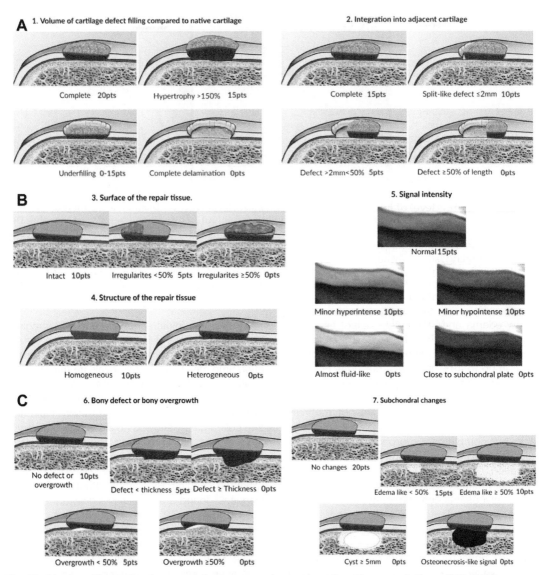

Fig. 16. Diagrams illustrating the magnetic resonance observation of cartilage repair tissue (MOCART) score system analyzing 7 variables of the surgical results of the osteochondral lesions, including volume and integrity (*A*), surface, structure, and signal (*B*), and bone and subchondral changes (*C*). The MOCART MR scoring system is combined with several clinical scores at follow-up of outcomes and complications of osteochondral lesions treatment procedures.

arthrofibrosis most commonly occurs after arthrotomy for open reduction and internal fracture fixation, talar dome osteochondral lesion grafting and resection of impingement spurs, but may also be seen after lateral ligament reconstruction and arthroscopy. It is also a common complication of metatarsophalangeal joint surgery after hallux valgus correction and lesser metatarsal Weil osteotomy.

Arthrofibrosis is thought to result from prolonged overexpression of cytokines leading to capsular and pericapsular fibrosis. Early diagnosis might permit successful conservative management. Arthroscopic debridement has reported inconclusive results for pain reduction and restored range of motion.

As compared with the normal ankle joint capsule which measures up to 1mm in thickness, arthrofibrosis is characterized by a minimum of 3mm of focal capsular thickening. There may or many not be superimposed infiltration of pericapsular fat, which is typically intermediate signal on proton density MR images within the first 6 months and becomes lower signal with chronicity.(57)[57]

Table 5
Magnetic resonance observation of cartilage repair tissue (MOCART) scoring system

MR Imaging Findings	Outcome Categories
Degree of defect fill	Complete (congruent with adjacent cartilage) Incomplete (below the level of adjacent cartilage)
Integration at border zone	Complete (no fissure at border zone) Incomplete (below the level of adjacent cartilage)
Surface of repair tissue	Intact (smooth) Damaged (irregular, fissure, fibrillation)
Structure of repair tissue	Homogeneous (no cleft) Inhomogeneous (cleft)
Signal intensity of repair tissue	Isointense to adjacent cartilage Moderately hyperintense to adjacent cartilage T2-weighted fast spin echo pulse seqeunces ± fat suppression or markedly hyperintense to adjacent cartilage 3D gradient echo pulse sequences with fat suppression
Subchondral lamina	Intact (smooth low signal-intensity line) Not intact (interrupted low signal-intensity line)
Subchondral bone	Intact (no marrow edema, granulation tissue, cysts) Disrupted (+ marrow edema, granulation tissue, cysts)
Adhesions	No/yes
Effusion	No/yes

Nerve Injury and Entrapment

Ankle arthroscopy for debridement of arthrofibrosis can be complicated by deep peroneal nerve injury. The superficial peroneal nerve lies anterior to the distal fibula and anterolateral recess of the ankle and is at greater risk with an anatomic repair of the lateral collateral ligaments. The sural nerve lies posterior to the peroneal compartment and is at greater risk with nonanatomic reconstructions of the lateral collateral ligaments that involve peroneal tenodesis (**Fig. 17**). The diagnosis is typically suspected clinically, with sensory deficits at the dorsolateral foot and toes, or painful paresthesia in the context of neuroma in continuity or scar entrapment of nerves and often a positive Tinel sign. This complication is often more readily evaluated by ultrasound examination than MR imaging, which requires skin markers to localize symptoms, high-resolution techniques, and often volumetric imaging sequences to provide an adequate neural assessment.

Vascular injury

Anterior tibial artery pseudoaneurysm is a rare complication of ankle arthroscopy, with a reported incidence of 0.0083%.[58] The relative risk depends on portal selection. The anterior central portal carries the greatest risk and is generally avoided. Anterior tibial artery pseudoaneurysm has been reported using both anteromedial and anterolateral portals.[5]

Anatomic variations of the anterior tibial artery and its branches pose a potential risk. Most pseudoaneurysms are diagnosed weeks after surgery based on clinical detection of an expansile, pulsatile mass.[59] Although ultrasound examination with color flow Doppler is typically diagnostic, MR imaging and MR angiography may be performed.

A pseudoaneurysm appears as an encapsulated mass with central heterogeneously dark T1 and T2 signal with a high signal rim and dark peripheral pseudocapsule (**Fig. 18**). Central contrast enhancement is nearly homogeneous, and arterial communication is evident, particularly on MR angiography. Pulsation artifact in the phase encoding direction across the mass supports the diagnosis.

Infection

Cellulitis commonly complicates ankle and foot surgery and does not require MR imaging. Deep soft tissue infection is rare after ankle arthroscopy, with an incidence of 2% in 101 cases reported in 2001 and 0.2% in a series of 905 cases reported in 2012.[60,61] In a 2019 review of 55 publications reviewing complications of ankle arthroscopy, there were no reported cases of osteomyelitis.[5]

Postoperative infection is not surprisingly more common after trauma than elective surgery, owing to contaminated tissues by way of penetrating injury. Seventy percent of open fractures are contaminated by *Staphylococcus aureus*, necessitating wound irrigation and antibiotic therapy. Although internal fixation can serve as a conduit and nidus for infection, animal studies have shown a higher risk of clinical infection in contaminated fractures treated without fixation.[62] In the context of peripheral joint arthroplasty, single organism infections by *Staphylococcus epidermidis* (31%) and *S aureus* (20%) are most common,[63] with mixed gram-positive and gram-negative infections reported in 8.3%.[64]

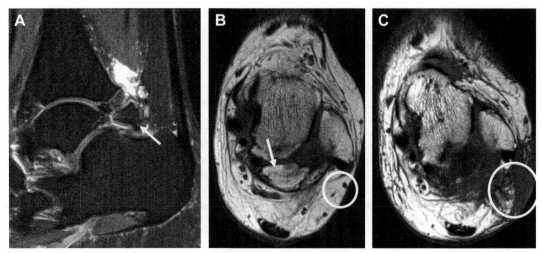

Fig. 17. A 50-year-old woman with posterior ankle impingement. (*A, B*) Preoperative sagittal T2-weighted fat-suppressed and axial T1-weighted MR images demonstrate a large os trigonum (*arrows*) with fluid signal coursing through the degenerated synchondrosis. The preoperative axial T1-weighted MR image shows preserved fat planes around the sural neurovascular bundle (*circle in B*). Nine months after excision of the os trigonum, the patient presented with pain along the sural nerve distribution. (*C*) Postoperative T1-weighted MR image shows perineural scarring (*circle*) and entrapment of the sural nerve along the healed surgical access.

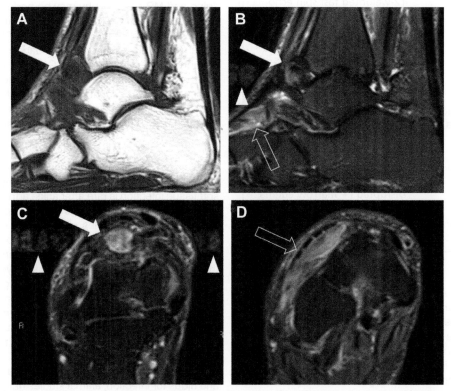

Fig. 18. A 69-year-old woman with pain and a pulsatile mass after arthroscopy via an anterolateral portal. Sagittal T1-weighted (*A*), sagittal (*B*), and oblique axial (*C*) T2-weighted fat-suppressed MR images show a pseudoaneurysm of the anterior tibial artery (*white arrows*) at the anterior ankle with heterogeneous dark T1 and T2 signal in the sagittal plane and pulsation artifact (*arrowheads*) in the phase encoding directions. (*D*) Oblique axial T2-weighted MR image at the midfoot level shows acute denervation edema of the extensor digitorum brevis muscle (*open arrow*) owing to compressive neuropathy of the superficial peroneal nerve by the pseudoaneurysm. (Courtesy of Vu Bui, MD)

Radiographs are the mainstay of postoperative surveillance of deep infection, but lack sensitivity and specificity for detecting osteomyelitis absent clear cortical destruction and contiguous localized osteopenia or frank bone loss. CT scans afford comparatively superior bone detail for detecting cortical erosion and destruction, sequestra, and periosteal new bone formation, and although it lacks soft tissue contrast, abscesses and sinus tracts can be delineated on CT scans after the intravenous administration of iodinated contrast.

Ultrasound examination permits targeted high-resolution imaging, which is useful for distinguishing soft tissue edema from fluid collections; differentiating between abscess, seroma; and hematoma, and guiding tissue sampling, arthrocentesis, and drainage of collections. MR imaging affords superior soft tissue contrast and detection of marrow signal alteration, permitting global assessment of superficial and deep soft tissue infection and osteomyelitis (Fig. 19).

The foot and ankle are notable for osteomyelitis occurring almost exclusively by contiguous spread from a cutaneous source, which has implications in assessing diabetic pedal osteomyelitis. However, in the context of a previous surgery, the soft tissue envelope has been breached, which may permit deep infection to occur in the setting of healed soft tissues. The MR imaging hallmark of osteomyelitis is a bright marrow signal on fat-suppressed fluid-sensitive MR images with accompanying confluent dark T1 marrow signal. Marrow edema-like signal on fluid-sensitive MR images without concomitant dark T1 marrow signal may indicate reactive, stress-related or traumatic edema but may eventually develop into osteomyelitis with typical MR imaging features.[65]

The ghost sign, particularly useful for distinguishing osteomyelitis in the context of Charcot arthropathy, is considered specific for osteomyelitis and describes profound dark signal marrow replacement on T1-weighted images, which results in the seeming disappearance of bone, which enhances and reappears with the intravenous administration of gadolinium.[66]

Sax and colleagues[65] recently reported a series of 60 patients with diabetic pedal ulceration in whom 57% progressed to osteomyelitis after MR imaging with bright T2 or STIR signal with normal T1 marrow signal. They found that a bone marrow to joint fluid ratio equal to or greater than 53% strongly predicted the development of osteomyelitis. Although the

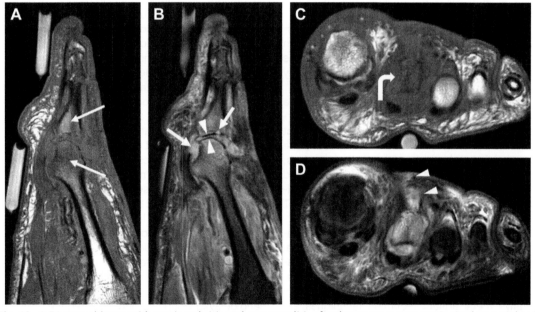

Fig. 19. A 74-year-old man with septic arthritis and osteomyelitis after hammertoe surgery. Sagittal T1-weighted (A) and T2-weighted fat-suppressed (B) MR images through the second metatarsophalangeal joint demonstrate full-thickness cartilage loss (arrowheads) with articular surface erosions on both sides of the joint (short arrows), and marrow signal alteration with darker T1 marrow replacement at the metatarsal head as compared with the proximal phalanx (long arrows). (C) Coronal T1-weighted MR image through the level of the second metatarsal head illustrates plantar articular erosion and marked marrow signal alteration, blurring the distinction between bone and joint fluid signal, resembling a ghost sign of osteomyelitis (bent arrow). (D) Coronal T2-weighted fat-suppressed MR image demonstrates fluid signal pointing dorsally along the surgical tract (arrowheads), resembling a sinus tract.

context is different, the implication that early osteomyelitis might be detectable before dark T1 marrow signal replacement is compelling in the postoperative setting where there is either a high risk or strong clinical suspicion of osteomyelitis.

Although marrow signal changes can be diagnostic for osteomyelitis without intravenous contrast, intravenous contrast enhancement increases the conspicuity of sinus tracts extending deep to the bone and can visualize devitalized soft tissue areas. Intravenous contrast may also increase diagnostic accuracy in the presence of metal artifacts.

Total Ankle Arthroplasty

First-generation total ankle arthroplasty systems required extensive bone resection and cement fixation. Because high complication rates accompany those implant systems, they are no longer used.[67] Second-generation total ankle arthroplasty systems were cementless and comprised 2 implant parts: a polyethylene bearing surface and the talar or tibial component.[67] Third-generation implants are cementless and include an independent, minimally constrained polyethylene component.[68] Fourth-generation implants are cementless, 2-component fixed-bearing devices that minimize bone resection and limit sagittal plane subluxation.[68]

The outcome literature is notable for inconsistent terminology and geographic differences in the registry of complications. In general, outcomes are compared between total ankle arthroplasty and ankle arthrodesis.[3,69]

Multislice and cone-beam CT scans evaluate implant integrity and assess bone–implant interfaces with the appropriate use of metal artifact reduction techniques. In addition, CT scans are excellent for evaluating periprosthetic bone loss, fracture detection and monitoring of healing, and concomitant arthrodesis procedures. Metal artifact reduction techniques include dual energy CT scan-based monoenergetic extrapolation and iterative metal artifact reduction techniques with inpainting–based recovery of missing data.[6] Dual energy CT scan-based monoenergetic extrapolation approximately 120 to 150 keV can successfully decrease bright streak artifacts, whereas iterative metal artifact reduction techniques are most useful to reduce dark streak artifacts. Although CT scans are commonly used, MR imaging may be more powerful for evaluating the bone–implant interfaces, periprosthetic bone, and synovium when appropriate metal artifact reduction techniques are used.

Depending on specific implant factors, including size, shape, and metal alloy, the combination of mono and extrapolation and iterative metal artifact reduction may be most powerful. Khodarahmi and colleagues[7] have shown that, for some ankle arthroplasty implants, the highest image quality can be obtained with iterative metal artifact reduction reconstruction of polychromatic data without applying dual energy-based monoenergetic extrapolation techniques.

MR imaging of total ankle arthroplasty requires protocol modification to mitigate implant-induced metal artifacts. Basic metal artifact reduction MR imaging strategies include a combination of fast spin echo sequences with increased receiver bandwidth and STIR imaging in place of frequency-selective fat suppression (see **Table 1**), similar to MR imaging of hip and knee arthroplasty implants.[17,18]

In the presence of abundant metal artifacts on MR imaging, advanced metal artifact reduction techniques, such as SEMAC, have been successfully used to achieve near metal artifact free MR imaging quality, significantly improving the visualization of bone and soft tissues near the implant interface (see **Table 2**).[20,70] Advanced metal artifact reduction techniques, including SEMAC, typically require longer acquisition times (see **Table 1**, **Table 2**). However, compressed sensing-based undersampling can substantially reduce the acquisition times by up to 70%[30,31] (see **Table 3**), thereby retaining the identical image quality.[20,70]

Radiologic complications after total ankle arthroplasty are common.[71,72] It has been reported that 62% will develop one or more imaging complications at a mean time of 74 weeks after arthroplasty.[73] Glazebrook and colleagues[73] categorized complications after total ankle arthroplasty into high-, intermediate-, and low-grade groups based on their impact on surgical outcome.

High-grade complications are associated with arthroplasty failure in more than 50% of patients, including aseptic loosening (**Fig. 20**), osteolysis, deep infection (**Fig. 21**)[74], and implant failure (as defined by revision). Intermediate-grade complications are associated with arthroplasty failure in more than 50% of patients, including implant subsidence, postoperative fracture, medial impingement by the implant, and technical error. Low-grade complications of intraoperative fracture and delayed wound healing rarely require revision.

The most common radiographic complication is periprosthetic bone resorption and osteolysis, reported in 34% of patients[75] (see **Fig. 20**). Aseptic loosening can result from failure of bony ingrowth in the early postoperative phase or may complicate an incorporated implant owing to mechanical overload or bone resorption months or years after arthroplasty. Osteolysis may be due

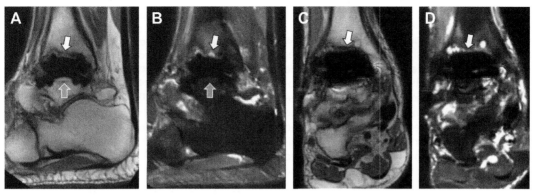

Fig. 20. A 62-year-old man presenting with pain during walking after tibiotalar resurfacing arthroplasty. Advanced metal artifact reduction MR imaging using sagittal proton density (A) and STIR (B) and coronal proton density (C) and STIR (D) compressed sensing SEMAC turbo spin echo pulse sequences shows bone resorption, cyst formation, and bone marrow edema pattern along the tibial bone-implant interface (white arrows), consistent with aseptic loosening. Normal MR imaging appearance of the talar bone implant interface (gray arrows).

to a foreign body reaction to particulate polyethylene debris, typically occurring years after implantation with contributions from component malalignment and incongruent polyethylene articulations of tibial and talar components. Categorized as an intermediate-grade complication, medial impingement owing to bony overgrowth is a common cause of pain after total ankle arthroplasty, reported as a cause in 63% of complications.[76]

de Cesar Netto and colleagues[20] assessed the clinical usefulness of near time equivalent high-bandwidth and compressed sensing SEMAC turbo spin echo metal artifact reduction MR imaging to identify causes of painful and dysfunctional total ankle arthroplasty implants with negative radiographs. Compressed sensing SEMAC MR imaging was superior to high-bandwidth MR imaging in showing the bone–implant interfaces, periprosthetic bone, tendons and joint capsule, bone marrow edema, interface osteolysis, tendinopathy, periprosthetic fractures, and synovitis. SEMAC MR imaging was found clinically useful because it either identified pain generators directly

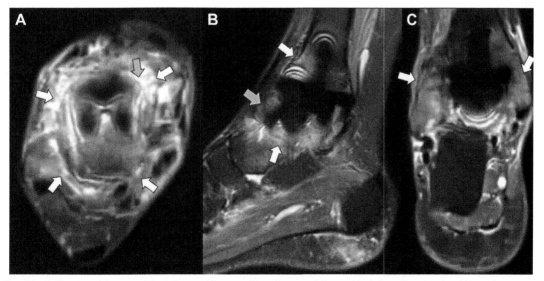

Fig. 21. A 68-year-old man with pain, swelling, and erythema of the ankle joint after total ankle replacement. Advanced metal artifact reduction MR imaging using axial (A), sagittal (B), and coronal (C) STIR compressed sensing SEMAC turbo spin echo pulse sequences shows the typical findings of a periprosthetic joint infection, including particulate synovitis (gray arrows in A and B), edematous, lamellated synovium (arrows in A), and periprosthetic bone marrow edema pattern (arrows in B and C).

or significantly reduced the number of differential diagnoses in symptomatic patients.

The anatomic tibiotalar relationship is a critical component for survivorship of total ankle replacement, which is evaluated with sagittal balance alignment measurements. Weight-bearing radiographs are typically used for sagittal balance assessments, but variations challenge reliable and repeatable measurements in rotational and angular alignments during radiograph acquisitions. de Cesar Netto and colleagues[70] evaluated the clinical usefulness of compressed sensing SEMAC MR imaging for standardized sagittal balance alignment measurements compared with weight-bearing radiographs. The authors found overall excellent agreements between radiographic and MR imaging measurements but higher reader agreements when MR imaging was used for images, which may be due to the better standardization of ankle positioning in boot-shaped MR imaging coils.

SUMMARY

Many soft tissue and osseous procedures and operations are used in the surgical treatment of ankle and foot disorders. Although radiography is the first-line imaging test for the routine postoperative surveillance and evaluation of pain and dysfunction, MR imaging is the most accurate imaging test for evaluating cases with negative radiographs and as a problem solving tool for the further characterization of unclear findings. Commonly used surgical techniques include tendon repair, lateral ankle ligament repair and reconstruction, osteochondral lesions of the talar dome, and total ankle arthroplasty. Familiarity with their normal and abnormal MR imaging appearances aids in accurate postoperative interpretation.

CLINICS CARE POINTS

- Postoperative MR imaging contributes useful information in the diagnostic workup of pain and dysfunction following repairs and reconstruction of tendons and ligaments, cartilage restoration procedures, ankle joint replacements, and arthrodesis.

- With basic and advanced metal artifact reduction, MR imaging is overall the most accurate test for assessing postoperative tendons, ligaments, synovium, vessels, and nerves and for evaluations of bone-implant interfaces in periprosthetic bone.

- After tendon repair and reconstruction, heavily T2-weighted MR imaging is useful to distinguish postoperative tendinitis and peritendinitis, hypertrophic scarring, failure of tendon reconstruction, repair dehiscence, postoperative infection, and post-traumatic neuroma formation.

- In lateral collateral ligament tears with post-traumatic laxity and mechanical instability, anatomic repairs include the Broström, Karlsson, and Gould techniques and modifications, whereas nonanatomic reconstruction techniques include Chrisman–Snook, Watson–Jones, and modified Evans procedures.

- MR imaging is accurate for morphologic classification of osteochondral lesions of the talus and evaluation of bone stimulation, such as microfracturing, tissue-based cartilage repair, and cell-based cartilage repair.

- The MOCART score analyzes a constellation of variables following cartilage repair and restoration procedures, intended to correlate with surgical outcomes for osteochondral lesions.

DISCLOSURE

H. Umans: Nothing to disclose. L. Cerezal: Nothing to disclose. J. Linklater: Nothing to disclose. J. Fritz received institutional research support from Siemens AG, BTG International Ltd., Zimmer Biomed, DePuy Synthes, QED, and SyntheticMR; is a scientific advisor for Siemens AG, SyntheticMR, GE Healthcare, QED, BTG, ImageBiopsy Lab, Boston Scientific, and Mirata Pharma; and has shared patents with Siemens Healthcare, Johns Hopkins University, and New York University.

REFERENCES

1. Sammarco VJ. Complications of lateral ankle ligament reconstruction. Clin Orthop Relat Res 2001; 391:123–32.
2. Shakked RJ, Karnovsky S, Drakos MC. Operative treatment of lateral ligament instability. Curr Rev Musculoskelet Med 2017;10(1):113–21.
3. Shih CL, Chen SJ, Huang PJ. Clinical outcomes of total ankle arthroplasty versus ankle arthrodesis for the treatment of end-stage ankle arthritis in the last decade: a systematic review and meta-analysis. J Foot Ankle Surg 2020;59(5):1032–9.
4. Vega J, Guelfi M. Arthroscopic assessment and treatment of medial collateral ligament complex. Foot Ankle Clin 2021;26(2):305–13.
5. Zekry M, Shahban SA, El Gamal T, et al. A literature review of the complications following anterior and

posterior ankle arthroscopy. Foot Ankle Surg 2019; 25(5):553–8.

6. Khodarahmi I, Fishman EK, Fritz J. Dedicated CT and MRI Techniques for the evaluation of the post-operative knee. Semin Musculoskelet Radiol 2018; 22(4):444–56.

7. Khodarahmi I, Haroun RR, Lee M, et al. Metal artifact reduction computed tomography of arthroplasty implants: effects of combined modeled iterative reconstruction and dual-energy virtual monoenergetic extrapolation at higher photon energies. Invest Radiol 2018;53(12):728–35.

8. Khodarahmi I, Fritz J. The value of 3 Tesla field strength for musculoskeletal magnetic resonance imaging. Invest Radiol 2021;56(11):749–63.

9. Fritz J, Fritz B, Zhang J, et al. Simultaneous multi-slice accelerated turbo spin echo magnetic resonance imaging: comparison and combination with in-plane parallel imaging acceleration for high-resolution magnetic resonance imaging of the knee. Invest Radiol 2017;52(9):529–37.

10. Fritz J, Guggenberger R, Del Grande F. Rapid musculoskeletal MRI in 2021: clinical application of advanced accelerated techniques. AJR Am J Roentgenol 2021;216(3):718–33.

11. Del Grande F, Guggenberger R, Fritz J. Rapid musculoskeletal MRI in 2021: value and optimized use of widely accessible techniques. AJR Am J Roentgenol 2021;216(3):704–17.

12. Fritz B, Bensler S, Thawait GK, et al. CAIPIRINHA-accelerated 10-min 3D TSE MRI of the ankle for the diagnosis of painful ankle conditions: performance evaluation in 70 patients. Eur Radiol 2019;29(2):609–19.

13. Fritz B, Fritz J, Sutter R. 3D MRI of the ankle: a concise state-of-the-art review. Semin Musculoskelet Radiol 2021;25(3):514–26.

14. Kalia V, Fritz B, Johnson R, et al. CAIPIRINHA accelerated SPACE enables 10-min isotropic 3D TSE MRI of the ankle for optimized visualization of curved and oblique ligaments and tendons. Eur Radiol 2017; 27(9):3652–61.

15. Fritz J, Fritz B, Thawait GG, et al. Three-dimensional CAIPIRINHA SPACE TSE for 5-minute high-resolution MRI of the knee. Invest Radiol 2016; 51(10):609–17.

16. Fritz J, Raithel E, Thawait GK, et al. Six-fold acceleration of high-spatial resolution 3D SPACE MRI of the knee through incoherent k-space undersampling and iterative reconstruction-first experience. Invest Radiol 2016;51(6):400–9.

17. Fritz J, Lurie B, Miller TT, et al. MR imaging of hip arthroplasty implants. Radiographics 2014;34(4):E106–32.

18. Fritz J, Lurie B, Potter HG. MR imaging of knee arthroplasty implants. Radiographics 2015;35(5): 1483–501.

19. Khodarahmi I, Isaac A, Fishman EK, et al. Metal about the hip and artifact reduction techniques: from basic concepts to advanced imaging. Semin Musculoskelet Radiol 2019;23(3):e68–81.

20. de Cesar Netto C, Fonseca LF, Fritz B, et al. Metal artifact reduction MRI of total ankle arthroplasty implants. Eur Radiol 2018;28(5):2216–27.

21. Khodarahmi I, Nittka M, Fritz J. Leaps in technology: advanced MR imaging after total hip arthroplasty. Semin Musculoskelet Radiol 2017;21(5):604–15.

22. Khodarahmi I, Brinkmann IM, Lin DJ, et al. New-Generation Low-Field Magnetic Resonance Imaging of Hip Arthroplasty Implants Using Slice Encoding for Metal Artifact Correction: First In Vitro Experience at 0.55 T and Comparison With 1.5 T. Invest Radiol 2022;2. doi:10.1097/RLI.0000000000000866. Epub ahead of print. PMID: 35239614.

23. Jungmann PM, Agten CA, Pfirrmann CW, et al. Advances in MRI around metal. J Magn Reson Imaging 2017;46(4):972–91.

24. Sofka CM. Postoperative magnetic resonance imaging of the foot and ankle. J Magn Reson Imaging 2013;37(3):556–65.

25. Kumar NM, de Cesar Netto C, Schon LC, et al. Metal artifact reduction magnetic resonance imaging around arthroplasty implants: the negative effect of long echo trains on the implant-related artifact. Invest Radiol 2017;52(5):310–6.

26. Olsen RV, Munk PL, Lee MJ, et al. Metal artifact reduction sequence: early clinical applications. Radiographics 2000;20(3):699–712.

27. Ulbrich EJ, Sutter R, Aguiar RF, et al. STIR sequence with increased receiver bandwidth of the inversion pulse for reduction of metallic artifacts. AJR Am J Roentgenol 2012;199(6):W735–42.

28. Sutter R, Ulbrich EJ, Jellus V, et al. Reduction of metal artifacts in patients with total hip arthroplasty with slice-encoding metal artifact correction and view-angle tilting MR imaging. Radiology 2012;265(1):204–14.

29. Hayter CL, Koff MF, Shah P, et al. MRI after arthroplasty: comparison of MAVRIC and conventional fast spin-echo techniques. AJR Am J Roentgenol 2011;197(3):W405–11.

30. Fritz J, Ahlawat S, Demehri S, et al. Compressed sensing SEMAC: 8-fold accelerated high resolution metal artifact reduction MRI of cobalt-chromium knee arthroplasty implants. Invest Radiol 2016; 51(10):666–76.

31. Fritz J, Fritz B, Thawait GK, et al. Advanced metal artifact reduction MRI of metal-on-metal hip resurfacing arthroplasty implants: compressed sensing acceleration enables the time-neutral use of SEMAC. Skeletal Radiol 2016;45(10):1345–56.

32. Kumar Y, Alian A, Ahlawat S, et al. Peroneal tendon pathology: pre- and post-operative high resolution US and MR imaging. Eur J Radiol 2017;92:132–44.

33. Jesse MK, Hunt KJ, Strickland C. Postoperative Imaging of the Ankle. AJR Am J Roentgenol 2018; 211(3):496–505.

34. Chianca V, Zappia M, Oliva F, et al. Post-operative MRI and US appearance of the Achilles tendons. J Ultrasound 2020;23(3):387–95.

35. Halabchi F, Hassabi M. Acute ankle sprain in athletes: clinical aspects and algorithmic approach. World J Orthop 2020;11(12):534–58.

36. Al-Mohrej OA, Al-Kenani NS. Chronic ankle instability: current perspectives. Avicenna J Med 2016; 6(4):103–8.

37. Vega J, Malagelada F, Manzanares Cespedes MC, et al. The lateral fibulotalocalcaneal ligament complex: an ankle stabilizing isometric structure. Knee Surg Sports Traumatol Arthrosc 2020;28(1):8–17.

38. Alparslan L, Chiodo CP. Lateral ankle instability: MR imaging of associated injuries and surgical treatment procedures. Semin Musculoskelet Radiol 2008;12(4):346–58.

39. Yang Y, Zhou X, Zhang M, et al. Lateral wall osteotomy combined with embedded biodegradable implants for displaced intra-articular calcaneal fractures. J Orthop Surg Res 2019;14(1):74.

40. Michels F, Pereira H, Calder J, et al. Searching for consensus in the approach to patients with chronic lateral ankle instability: ask the expert. Knee Surg Sports Traumatol Arthrosc 2018;26(7):2095–102.

41. Madoff SD, Kaye J, Newman JS. Postoperative foot and ankle MR imaging. Magn Reson Imaging Clin N Am 2017;25(1):195–209.

42. Bergin D, Morrison WB. Postoperative imaging of the ankle and foot. Radiol Clin North Am 2006; 44(3):391–406.

43. Zanetti M, Saupe N, Espinosa N. Postoperative MR imaging of the foot and ankle: tendon repair, ligament repair, and Morton's neuroma resection. Semin Musculoskelet Radiol 2010;14(3):357–64.

44. LiMarzi GM, Scherer KF, Richardson ML, et al. CT and MR imaging of the postoperative ankle and foot. Radiographics 2016;36(6):1828–48.

45. Bartlett W, Gooding CR, Carrington RW, et al. Autologous chondrocyte implantation at the knee using a bilayer collagen membrane with bone graft. A preliminary report. J Bone Joint Surg Br 2005;87(3):330–2.

46. Choi YS, Potter HG, Chun TJ. MR imaging of cartilage repair in the knee and ankle. Radiographics 2008;28(4):1043–59.

47. Niemeyer P, Porichis S, Steinwachs M, et al. Long-term outcomes after first-generation autologous chondrocyte implantation for cartilage defects of the knee. Am J Sports Med 2014;42(1):150–7.

48. Ahmad J, Jones K. Comparison of osteochondral autografts and allografts for treatment of recurrent or large talar osteochondral lesions. Foot Ankle Int 2016;37(1):40–50.

49. Giza E, Sullivan M, Ocel D, et al. Matrix-induced autologous chondrocyte implantation of talus articular defects. Foot Ankle Int 2010;31(9):747–53.

50. Iordache E, Robertson EL, Hirschmann A, et al. Typical MRI-pattern suggests peak maturation of the ACI graft 2 years after third-generation ACI: a systematic review. Knee Surg Sports Traumatol Arthrosc 2021;29(11):3664–77.

51. Migliorini F, Maffulli N, Eschweiler J, et al. Reliability of the MOCART score: a systematic review. J Orthop Trauma 2021;22(1):39.

52. Schreiner MM, Raudner M, Rohrich S, et al. Reliability of the MOCART (Magnetic Resonance Observation of Cartilage Repair Tissue) 2.0 knee score for different cartilage repair techniques-a retrospective observational study. Eur Radiol 2021;31(8):5734–45.

53. Apprich S, Trattnig S, Welsch GH, et al. Assessment of articular cartilage repair tissue after matrix-associated autologous chondrocyte transplantation or the microfracture technique in the ankle joint using diffusion-weighted imaging at 3 Tesla. Osteoarthritis Cartilage 2012;20(7):703–11.

54. Quirbach S, Trattnig S, Marlovits S, et al. Initial results of in vivo high-resolution morphological and biochemical cartilage imaging of patients after matrix-associated autologous chondrocyte transplantation (MACT) of the ankle. Skeletal Radiol 2009;38(8):751–60.

55. Pagliazzi G, Vannini F, Battaglia M, et al. Autologous chondrocyte implantation for talar osteochondral lesions: comparison between 5-year follow-up magnetic resonance imaging findings and 7-year follow-up clinical results. J Foot Ankle Surg 2018; 57(2):221–5.

56. Trattnig S, Welsch G, Domayer S, et al. MR imaging of postoperative talar dome lesions. Semin Musculoskelet Radiol 2012;16(3):177–84.

57. Linklater JM, Fessa CK. Imaging findings in arthrofibrosis of the ankle and foot. Semin Musculoskelet Radiol 2012;16(3):185–91.

58. Mariani PP, Mancini L, Giorgini TL. Pseudoaneurysm as a complication of ankle arthroscopy. Arthroscopy 2001;17(4):400–2.

59. Yamada T, Gloviczki P, Bower TC, et al. Variations of the arterial anatomy of the foot. Am J Surg 1993; 166(2):130–5. ; discussion 5.

60. Ferkel RD, Karzel RP, Del Pizzo W, et al. Arthroscopic treatment of anterolateral impingement of the ankle. Am J Sports Med 1991;19(5):440–6.

61. Zengerink M, van Dijk CN. Complications in ankle arthroscopy. Knee Surg Sports Traumatol Arthrosc 2012;20(8):1420–31.

62. Worlock P, Slack R, Harvey L, et al. The prevention of infection in open fractures: an experimental study of the effect of fracture stability. Injury 1994;25(1):31–8.

63. Della Valle CJ, Bogner E, Desai P, et al. Analysis of frozen sections of intraoperative specimens obtained at the time of reoperation after hip or knee resection arthroplasty for the treatment of infection. J Bone Joint Surg Am 1999;81(5):684–9.

64. Beiner JM, Grauer J, Kwon BK, et al. Postoperative wound infections of the spine. Neurosurg Focus 2003;15(3):E14.

65. Sax AJ, Halpern EJ, Zoga AC, et al. Predicting osteomyelitis in patients whose initial MRI demonstrated bone marrow edema without corresponding T1 signal marrow replacement. Skeletal Radiol 2020; 49(8):1239–47.

66. Donovan A, Schweitzer ME. Use of MR imaging in diagnosing diabetes-related pedal osteomyelitis. Radiographics 2010;30(3):723–36.

67. Rushing CJ, Zulauf E, Hyer CF, et al. Risk factors for early failure of fourth generation total ankle arthroplasty prostheses. J Foot Ankle Surg 2021;60(2): 312–7.

68. Cottom JM, DeVries JG, Hyer CF, et al. Current techniques in total ankle arthroplasty. Clin Podiatr Med Surg 2022;39(2):273–93.

69. Veljkovic AN, Daniels TR, Glazebrook MA, et al. Outcomes of total ankle replacement, arthroscopic ankle arthrodesis, and open ankle arthrodesis for isolated non-deformed end-stage ankle arthritis. J Bone Joint Surg Am 2019;101(17): 1523–9.

70. de Cesar Netto C, Schon LC, da Fonseca LF, et al. Metal artifact reduction MRI for total ankle replacement sagittal balance evaluation. Foot Ankle Surg 2019;25(6):739–47.

71. Mulcahy H, Chew FS. Current concepts in total ankle replacement for radiologists: complications. AJR Am J Roentgenol 2015;205(6):1244–50.

72. Bae JH, Lee JW, Kim SH, et al. Femoral matched tibia component rotation has little effect on the tibial torsion after total knee arthroplasty. Knee Surg Sports Traumatol Arthrosc 2022;30(2):698–704.

73. Glazebrook MA, Arsenault K, Dunbar M. Evidence-based classification of complications in total ankle arthroplasty. Foot Ankle Int 2009;30(10):945–9.

74. Fritz Jan, Meshram Prashant, Stern Steven E, Fritz Benjamin, Srikumaran Uma, McFarland Edward G. Diagnostic Performance of Advanced Metal Artifact Reduction MRI for Periprosthetic Shoulder Infection. J Bone Joint Surg Am 2022;Epub ahead of print. https://doi.org/10.2106/JBJS.21.00912.

75. Lee AY, Ha AS, Petscavage JM, et al. Total ankle arthroplasty: a radiographic outcome study. AJR Am J Roentgenol 2013;200(6):1310–6.

76. Spirt AA, Assal M, Hansen ST Jr. Complications and failure after total ankle arthroplasty. J Bone Joint Surg Am 2004;86(6):1172–8.

UNITED STATES POSTAL SERVICE®

Statement of Ownership, Management, and Circulation
(All Periodicals Publications Except Requester Publications)

1. Publication Title	2. Publication Number	3. Filing Date
MAGNETIC RESONANCE IMAGING CLINICS OF NORTH AMERICA	011 – 909	9/18/2022

4. Issue Frequency	5. Number of Issues Published Annually	6. Annual Subscription Price
FEB, MAY, AUG, NOV	4	$408.00

7. Complete Mailing Address of Known Office of Publication (Not printer) (Street, city, county, state, and ZIP+4®)

ELSEVIER INC.
230 Park Avenue, Suite 800
New York, NY 10169

Contact Person
Malathi Samayan

Telephone (Include area code)
91-44-4299-4507

8. Complete Mailing Address of Headquarters or General Business Office of Publisher (Not printer)

ELSEVIER INC.
230 Park Avenue, Suite 800
New York, NY 10169

9. Full Names and Complete Mailing Addresses of Publisher, Editor, and Managing Editor (Do not leave blank)

Publisher (Name and complete mailing address)

DOLORES MELONI, ELSEVIER INC.
1600 JOHN F KENNEDY BLVD. SUITE 1800
PHILADELPHIA, PA 19103-2899

Editor (Name and complete mailing address)

JOHN VASSALLO, ELSEVIER INC.
1600 JOHN F KENNEDY BLVD. SUITE 1800
PHILADELPHIA, PA 19103-2899

Managing Editor (Name and complete mailing address)

PATRICK MANLEY, ELSEVIER INC.
1600 JOHN F KENNEDY BLVD. SUITE 1800
PHILADELPHIA, PA 19103-2899

10. Owner (Do not leave blank. If the publication is owned by a corporation, give the name and address of the corporation immediately followed by the names and addresses of all stockholders owning or holding 1 percent or more of the total amount of stock. If not owned by a corporation, give the names and addresses of the individual owners. If owned by a partnership or other unincorporated firm, give its name and address as well as those of each individual owner. If the publication is published by a nonprofit organization, give its name and address.)

Full Name	Complete Mailing Address
WHOLLY OWNED SUBSIDIARY OF REED/ELSEVIER, US HOLDINGS	1600 JOHN F KENNEDY BLVD. SUITE 1800 PHILADELPHIA, PA 19103-2899

11. Known Bondholders, Mortgagees, and Other Security Holders Owning or Holding 1 Percent or More of Total Amount of Bonds, Mortgages, or Other Securities. If none, check box. ☐ None

Full Name	Complete Mailing Address
N/A	

12. Tax Status (For completion by nonprofit organizations authorized to mail at nonprofit rates) (Check one)
The purpose, function, and nonprofit status of this organization and the exempt status for federal income tax purposes:
☒ Has Not Changed During Preceding 12 Months
☐ Has Changed During Preceding 12 Months (Publisher must submit explanation of change with this statement)

PS Form 3526, July 2014 (Page 1 of 4 (see instructions page 4)) PSN: 7530-01-000-9931 PRIVACY NOTICE: See our privacy policy on www.usps.com.

13. Publication Title	14. Issue Date for Circulation Data Below
MAGNETIC RESONANCE IMAGING CLINICS OF NORTH AMERICA	MAY 2022

15. Extent and Nature of Circulation		Average No. Copies Each Issue During Preceding 12 Months	No. Copies of Single Issue Published Nearest to Filing Date
a. Total Number of Copies (Net press run)		363	322
b. Paid Circulation (By Mail and Outside the Mail)	(1) Mailed Outside-County Paid Subscriptions Stated on PS Form 3541 (Include paid distribution above nominal rate, advertiser's proof copies, and exchange copies)	280	250
	(2) Mailed In-County Paid Subscriptions Stated on PS Form 3541 (Include paid distribution above nominal rate, advertiser's proof copies, and exchange copies)	0	0
	(3) Paid Distribution Outside the Mails Including Sales Through Dealers and Carriers, Street Vendors, Counter Sales, and Other Paid Distribution Outside USPS®	66	59
	(4) Paid Distribution by Other Classes of Mail Through the USPS (e.g., First-Class Mail®)	0	0
c. Total Paid Distribution (Sum of 15b (1), (2), (3), and (4))	▶	346	309
d. Free or Nominal Rate Distribution (By Mail and Outside the Mail)	(1) Free or Nominal Rate Outside-County Copies included on PS Form 3541	17	13
	(2) Free or Nominal Rate In-County Copies Included on PS Form 3541	0	0
	(3) Free or Nominal Rate Copies Mailed at Other Classes Through the USPS (e.g., First-Class Mail)	0	0
	(4) Free or Nominal Rate Distribution Outside the Mail (Carriers or other means)	0	0
e. Total Free or Nominal Rate Distribution (Sum of 15d (1), (2), (3) and (4))	▶	17	13
f. Total Distribution (Sum of 15c and 15e)	▶	363	322
g. Copies not Distributed (See instructions to Publishers #4 (page #3))	▶	0	0
h. Total (Sum of 15f and g)	▶	363	322
i. Percent Paid (15c divided by 15f times 100)		95.31%	95.96%

* If you are claiming electronic copies, go to line 16 on page 3. If you are not claiming electronic copies, skip to line 17 on page 3.

PS Form 3526, July 2014 (Page 2 of 4)

16. Electronic Copy Circulation		Average No. Copies Each Issue During Preceding 12 Months	No. Copies of Single Issue Published Nearest to Filing Date
a. Paid Electronic Copies	▶		
b. Total Paid Print Copies (Line 15c) + Paid Electronic Copies (Line 16a)	▶		
c. Total Print Distribution (Line 15f) + Paid Electronic Copies (Line 16a)	▶		
d. Percent Paid (Both Print & Electronic Copies) (16b divided by 16c × 100)	▶		

☒ I certify that 50% of all my distributed copies (electronic and print) are paid above a nominal price.

17. Publication of Statement of Ownership

☒ If the publication is a general publication, publication of this statement is required. Will be printed in the NOVEMBER 2022 issue of this publication. ☐ Publication not required.

18. Signature and Title of Editor, Publisher, Business Manager, or Owner

Malathi Samayan

Malathi Samayan - Distribution Controller

Date 9/18/2022

I certify that all information furnished on this form is true and complete. I understand that anyone who furnishes false or misleading information on this form or who omits material or information requested on the form may be subject to criminal sanctions (including fines and imprisonment) and/or civil sanctions (including civil penalties).

PS Form 3526, July 2014 (Page 3 of 4) PRIVACY NOTICE: See our privacy policy on www.usps.com.

Moving?

Make sure your subscription moves with you!

To notify us of your new address, find your **Clinics Account Number** (located on your mailing label above your name), and contact customer service at:

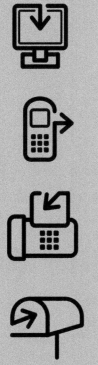

Email: journalscustomerservice-usa@elsevier.com

800-654-2452 (subscribers in the U.S. & Canada)
314-447-8871 (subscribers outside of the U.S. & Canada)

Fax number: 314-447-8029

Elsevier Health Sciences Division
Subscription Customer Service
3251 Riverport Lane
Maryland Heights, MO 63043

Printed and bound by CPI Group (UK) Ltd, Croydon, CR0 4YY

08/05/2025

01864700-0018